Snapshots of Hemodynamics

Nicolaas Westerhof • Nikolaos Stergiopulos
Mark I.M. Noble • Berend E. Westerhof

Snapshots of Hemodynamics

An Aid for Clinical Research and Graduate Education

Third Edition

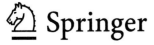 Springer

Nicolaas Westerhof
Department of Pulmonary Diseases
Amsterdam Cardiovascular Sciences
VU University Medical Center
Amsterdam
The Netherlands

Mark I.M. Noble
Cardiovascular Medicine
Department of Medicine and Therapeutics
University of Aberdeen
Aberdeen
United Kingdom

Nikolaos Stergiopulos
Laboratory of Hemodynamics
and Cardiovascular Technology
Ecole Polytechnique Fédérale
de Lausanne (EPFL)
Institute of Bioengineering
Lausanne
Switzerland

Berend E. Westerhof
Department of Pulmonary Diseases
Amsterdam Cardiovascular Sciences
VU University Medical Center
Amsterdam
The Netherlands

ISBN 978-3-319-91931-7   ISBN 978-3-319-91932-4   (eBook)
https://doi.org/10.1007/978-3-319-91932-4

Library of Congress Control Number: 2018952091

This Springer imprint is published by the registered company Springer Nature Switzerland AG.
The registered company address is: Gewerbestrasse 11, 6330 Cham, Switzerland

Preface

This book is written in a quick reference style to help clinical and basic researchers, as well as graduate students, in the understanding of hemodynamics. Hemodynamics makes it possible to characterize, in a quantitative way, and presently more and more with noninvasive techniques, the function of the heart and the arterial system, separately and in combination.

We have made the layout of this book such that it gives an overview of individual topics, in short chapters. Every chapter starts with a "Box" containing a figure and caption, describing the main aspects of the subject. It is often sufficient to study the contents of this Box alone to obtain the essential information on the subject, and it is then not necessary to read the whole chapter.

Each chapter is further written in such a way that one is able to grasp the basic and applied principles of the hemodynamic topic. The part called "Description" can be used to get more detailed information. The chapters end with a section "Physiological and Clinical Relevance" to place the information into perspective. If more details or broader perspectives are desired, one can go to the other, related, chapters to which the text refers or to the limited number of references given in each chapter.

More comprehensive information on the subjects discussed can be found in text-books on physiology and cardiology, as well as in special books on hemodynamics. A number of these books are listed in the section "Reference Books" (Appendix 5).

Amsterdam, The Netherlands   Nicolaas Westerhof
Lausanne, Switzerland   Nikolaos Stergiopulos
Aberdeen, United Kingdom   Mark I. M. Noble
Amsterdam, The Netherlands   Berend E. Westerhof

How to Use Snapshots of Hemodynamics

Chapter 2 Law of Poiseuille	Chapter number and title
The law of Poiseuille describes the relation between pressure drop, $\Delta P/l$, and blood flow, Q, in a stiff tube under steady flow conditions. This figure shows a tube with circular cross-section where the blood flows in a laminar fashion, i.e., each fluid layer stays at the same constant distance from the center. The flow depends strongly on the radius of the tube (fourth power), and also on the pressure drop over the tube length ($\Delta P/l$) and viscosity of blood (η). The velocity profile, $v(r)$, is parabolic (second formula). Resistance can be calculated as $R = \Delta P/Q = 8\eta \cdot l/\pi \cdot r_i^4$. The wall shear stress, τ, (third formula) acting on the intimal layer (endothelium) equals $\tau = 4\eta \cdot Q/(\pi \cdot r^3) = (\Delta P/l) \cdot (r_i/2)$.	The '**Box**' contains a figure and a short text that illustrates the main message of the chapter.
Description With laminar flow through a uniform tube the velocity profile over the cross-section is a parabola.	The '**Description**' section gives the essential background and discusses the different aspects of the subject.
Physiological and clinical relevance The more general form of Poiseuille's law given above, i.e., $Q = \Delta P/R$ allows the derivation of resistance, R, from measurements of mean pressure and mean flow.	The '**Physiological and clinical relevance**' section places the subject in a broader pathophysiological context and shows clinical applications.
References 1. Murgo JP, Westerhof N, Giolma JP, Altobelli SA. Aortic input impedance in normal man: relationship to pressure wave forms. Circulation. 1980;62:101–16.	A limited number of '**References**' is given. Major reference books are given in Appendix 5.

Contents

Part I
Basics of Hemodynamics

Chapter 1
Viscosity

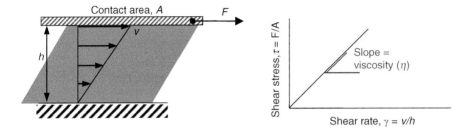

The definition of viscosity. A fluid is located between two parallel plates. The shear force, F, divided by the contact area, A, between the liquid and the plate gives the shear stress, $F/A = \tau$. The shear rate is the difference in velocity between the different fluid layers, and can here be calculated as the velocity of the top plate (the bottom plate does not move) divided by the distance between the plates, thus the shear rate is $\gamma = v/h$. The ratio of shear stress and shear rate is the viscosity, η, a material property (right figure). If a straight line is obtained, as for plasma, we call the fluid Newtonian. If we change the plate's velocity or change the distance between the plates, shear stress and shear rate will change.

1.1 Description

Consider the experiment shown in the Figure in the Box. The top plate is moved with constant velocity, v, by the action of a shear force F, while the bottom plate is kept in place (velocity is zero). The result is that the different layers of blood move with different velocities. The difference in velocity in the different blood layers causes a shearing action between them.

The rate of shear, γ, is the relative displacement of one fluid layer with respect to the next. In the example given in the Box, the velocity profile is linear, from zero at the bottom to velocity v at the top plate. Therefore, the slope of the velocity profile, and thus the rate of shear, is equal to v/h, h being the distance

© Springer International Publishing AG, part of Springer Nature 2019
N. Westerhof et al., *Snapshots of Hemodynamics*,
https://doi.org/10.1007/978-3-319-91932-4_1

Fig. 1.1 Velocity and
shear rate, for a general
profile, shear rate is highest
at the wall

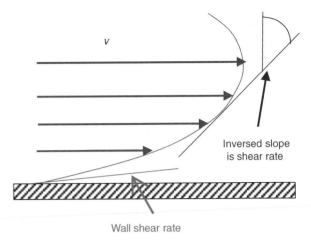

Wall shear rate

between the plates. The units of shear rate are 1/s. The force needed to obtain a certain velocity, is proportional to the contact area, A, between fluid and plates. It is therefore convenient, instead of force, to use the term shear stress, defined as the force per area $\tau = F/A$, with units Pa or N/m². The shear rate is highest where the difference in velocities is highest. In a tube the highest shear rate is at the wall, and inversely proportional to the slope of the velocity profile, as shown in Fig. 1.1.

We may think of the following experiment: we pull the top plate at different velocities v and we measure the shear force F to accomplish this. Then we plot the shear stress, τ, against the shear rate, γ. The resulting relation is given in the Figure in the Box and the slope is the viscosity:

$$\eta = shear\ stress\ /\ shear\ rate = \tau\ /\ \gamma$$

The units of viscosity are Pa·s = Ns/m², or Poise (dynes·s/cm²), with 1 Pa·s = 10 Poise. Viscosity is sometimes called dynamic viscosity in contrast to the kinematic viscosity, which is defined as viscosity divided by density ρ, thus η/ρ.

Fluids with a straight relationship between shear stress and shear rate are called Newtonian fluids, i.e., viscosity does not depend on shear stress or shear rate. This is not the case for blood (Fig. 1.2).

1.1.1 Viscosity of Blood

Blood consists of plasma and particles, with 99% of the particle volume taken by the red blood cells, RBC's, or erythrocytes. Thus, the red blood cells mainly determine the difference between plasma and blood viscosity (Fig. 1.2). The viscosity of blood therefore depends on the viscosity of the plasma, in combination with the hematocrit (volume % of red blood cells, Hct) and red cell deformability. Higher

Fig. 1.2 Viscosity of plasma and blood

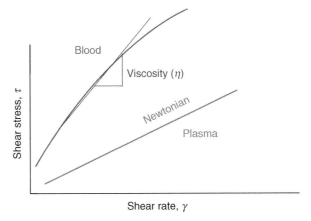

Fig. 1.3 Viscosity as a function of hematocrit

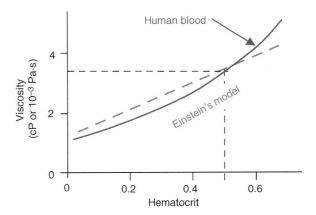

hematocrit and less deformable cells imply higher viscosity. The relation between hematocrit and viscosity is complex and many formulas exist. One of the simplest relations is the one derived by Einstein (Fig. 1.3):

$$\eta = \eta_{plasma} \cdot (1 + 2.5\text{Hct})$$

Einstein's relation for the viscosity of fluids containing particles applies only to very low particle concentrations. Nevertheless, it gives some indication. The viscosity of plasma is about 0.015 Poise (1.5 centipoise, cP) and the viscosity of whole blood at a physiological hematocrit of 40–45% is about 3.2 cP, or 3.2 10^{-3} Pa·s.

Blood viscosity depends not only on plasma viscosity and hematocrit, but also on the size, shape and flexibility of the red blood cells. For instance, the hematocrit of camel blood is about half of that of human blood, but the camel's red blood cells are more rigid, and the overall effect is a similar blood viscosity.

1.1.2   Anomalous Viscosity or Non-Newtonian Behavior of Blood

The viscosity of blood depends on its velocity. More exactly formulated, when shear rate increases, viscosity decreases (Fig. 1.4). At high shear rates the doughnut-shaped RBCs orient themselves in the direction of flow and viscosity is lower. For extremely low shear rates formation of RBC aggregates may occur, thereby increasing viscosity to very high values. It has even been suggested that a certain minimum shear stress is required before the blood will start to flow, the so-called yield stress. In large and medium size arteries shear rates are higher than 100 s^{-1}, and the viscosity is practically independent of velocity, and can be assumed constant. The physiological range of wall shear stress is 10–20 dynes/cm^2, or 1–2 Pa, i.e. about 0.0075–0.015 mmHg. Several equations exist that relate shear stress and shear rate of blood, e.g., Casson fluid, and Herschel-Bulkley fluid [1, 2].

Viscosity also depends on the size of a blood vessel (Fig. 1.5). In small blood vessels and at low velocities, blood viscosity apparently decreases with decreasing vessel size. This is known as the Fahraeus-Lindqvist effect, and it begins to play a role in vessels smaller than 1 mm in diameter. Therefore the non-Newtonian character of blood mainly plays a role in the microcirculation [3]. See also Chap. 6 on resistance in capillaries.

Red blood cells show axial accumulation, which is called plasma skimming, while the concentration of platelets appears highest at the wall.

Viscosity depends on temperature. A decrease of 1 °C in temperature yields a 2% increase in viscosity. Thus, in a cold foot blood viscosity is much higher than in the brain.

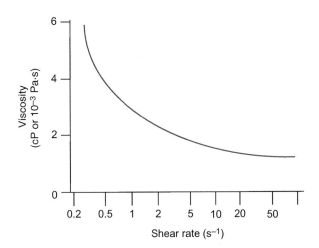

Fig. 1.4 Viscosity of blood as function of shear rate for hematocrit of 48

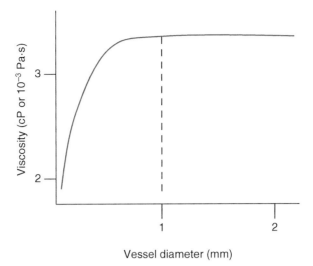

Fig. 1.5 Blood viscosity as function of vessel size

1.1.3 How to Measure Viscosity

Blood viscosity is measured using viscometers. Viscometers consist essentially of two rotating surfaces, as a model of the two plates shown in the Box Figure. Blood is usually prevented from air contact and temperature is controlled. When comparing data on viscosity one should always keep in mind that results are often device dependent.

1.2 Physiological and Clinical Relevance

The anomalous character of blood viscosity results from the red blood cells, and the effects are mainly found in the microcirculation at low shear rates and small vessel diameters. The effects are of little importance for the hemodynamics of large arteries. Thus, in large vessel hemodynamics, it may be assumed that viscosity is independent of vessel size and shear rate.

Determination of blood viscosity *in vivo* is virtually impossible. In principle, the mean pressure drop over a blood vessel and the mean flow through it, together with vessel size, can be used to derive viscosity on the basis of Poiseuille's law (Chap. 2). However, the vessel diameter in Poiseuille's law appears as the fourth power, so that a small error in the vessel diameter leads to a considerable error in the calculated viscosity. Also, the mean pressure difference over a uniform segment of conduit artery is typically a fraction of 1 mmHg. Moreover, hematocrit is not the same in all vessels due to plasma skimming effects, and side branches may receive blood with lower hematocrit. Finally, Poiseuille's law may only be applied when there are no effects of inlet length (see Chap. 2) and pressure and flow are not pulsatile.

The main purpose of the circulation is to supply the tissues with oxygen and substrates and to remove CO_2 and metabolites. Blood flow is also important for hormonal transport. Oxygen supply is the product of flow and oxygen content of the blood. The hematocrit determines the (maximum) oxygen carrying capacity of blood and its viscosity, and therefore the resistance to blood flow. These counteracting effects on oxygen transport result in an optimal hematocrit of about 45% in the human at sea level, with a small difference between males and females. It appears that in mammals, blood viscosity is similar, but the hematocrit is not because of the different size, shape and flexibility of the red blood cells as mentioned above.

Low hematocrit, as in anemia, decreases oxygen content and viscosity of blood. The former lowers oxygen supply and the latter increases blood flow thus increasing supply. Inversely, polycythemia increases oxygen content but lowers blood flow. At high altitude, where oxygen tension is lower and thus oxygen saturation in the blood is lower, a larger hematocrit is advantageous. In endurance sports higher hematocrit is more efficacious during increased oxygen demand. This is the reason why Erytropoetin (EPO) is sometimes used by the athletes.

References

1. Merrill EW. Rheology of blood. Physiol Rev. 1969;49:863–88.
2. Scott Blair GW, Spanner DC. An introduction to biorheology. Amsterdam: Elsevier Scientific Publishing; 1974.
3. Pries AR, Secomb TW, Gessner T, Sperandio MB, Gross JF, Gaehtgens P. Resistance to blood flow in microvessels in vivo. Circ Res. 1994;75:904–15.

Chapter 2
Law of Poiseuille

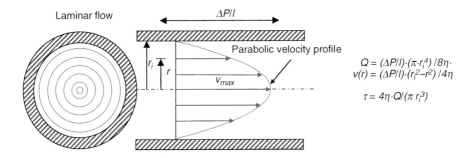

Laminar flow

$\Delta P/l$

Parabolic velocity profile

v_{max}

r_i r

$Q = (\Delta P/l)\cdot(\pi\cdot r_i^4)/8\eta\cdot$
$v(r) = (\Delta P/l)\cdot(r_i^2 - r^2)/4\eta$

$\tau = 4\eta\cdot Q/(\pi\, r_i^3)$

The law of Poiseuille describes the relation between pressure drop, $\Delta P/l$, and blood flow, Q, in a stiff tube under steady flow conditions. This figure shows a tube with circular cross-section where the blood flows in a laminar fashion, i.e., each fluid layer stays at the same constant distance from the center (left). The flow depends strongly on the radius of the tube (fourth power), the pressure drop over the tube length ($\Delta P/l$) and viscosity of blood (η). The velocity profile, $v(r)$, is parabolic (second formula). The wall shear stress, τ, (third formula) acting on the intimal layer (endothelium) equals $4\eta\, Q/(\pi\, r^3) = (\Delta P/l)\cdot(r_i/2)$. Resistance can be calculated as $R = \Delta P/Q = 8\, \eta l/\pi\, r_i^4$.

2.1 Description

With laminar and steady flow through a uniform tube with inner radius r_i, the velocity profile over the cross-section is a parabola. The formula that describes the velocity (v) as a function of the radius, r is:

$$v_r = \frac{\Delta P \cdot \left(r_i^2 - r^2\right)}{4 \cdot \eta \cdot l} = v_{max}\left(1 - r^2/r_i^2\right)$$

© Springer International Publishing AG, part of Springer Nature 2019
N. Westerhof et al., *Snapshots of Hemodynamics*,
https://doi.org/10.1007/978-3-319-91932-4_2

ΔP is the pressure drop over the tube of length (l), and η is blood viscosity. At the axis ($r = 0$), velocity is maximal, v_{max}, with $v_{max} = \Delta P r_i^2/4 \eta\ l$, while at the wall ($r = r_i$) the velocity is assumed to be zero. Mean velocity is:

$$v_{mean} = \frac{\Delta P \cdot r_i^2}{8 \cdot \eta \cdot l} = v_{max} / 2 = Q / \pi \cdot r_i^2$$

and v_{mean} is found at $r \approx 0.7\ r_i$.

Blood (volume) flow (Q) is mean velocity, v_{mean}, times the cross-sectional area of the tube, πr_i^2, giving:

$$Q = \frac{\Delta P \cdot \pi \cdot r_i^4}{8 \cdot \eta \cdot l}$$

This is Poiseuille's law relating the pressure difference, ΔP, and the steady flow, Q, through a uniform (constant radius) and stiff blood vessel. Hagen, in 1860, theoretically derived the law and therefore it is sometimes called the law of Hagen-Poiseuille. The law can be derived from very basic physics (Newton's law) or the Navier-Stokes equations that form the basis of all fluid dynamics (see Appendix 4).

The major assumptions for Poiseuille's law to hold are:

The tube is stiff, straight, and uniform
Blood is Newtonian, i.e., viscosity is constant
The flow is laminar and steady, not pulsatile, and the velocity at the wall is zero (no slip at the wall).

In curved vessels and distal to branching points the velocity profile is not parabolic and the blood flow profile needs some length of straight tube to develop, this length is called inlet length (Fig. 2.1). The inlet length, l_{inlet}, depends on the Reynolds number (Re, see Chap. 4) as:

$$l_{inlet} / D \approx 0.06\,\mathrm{Re}$$

with D vessel diameter. For the aorta mean blood flow is about 6 l/min, and the diameter 3 cm, so that the mean blood velocity is $\sim$ 15 cm/s. The Reynolds number is therefore $\sim$ 1350. This means that l_{inlet}/D is $\sim$ 80, and the inlet length $\sim$ 240 cm, which is much longer than the length of the entire aorta. In the common iliac artery, the Reynolds number is about 500 and diameter 0.6 cm giving an inlet length of $\sim$ 18 cm. In other, more peripheral arteries the inlet length is much shorter but their physical length is shorter as well. Clearly, a parabolic flow profile is not even approximated in the arterial system. Nevertheless, the law of Poiseuille can be used as a concept relating pressure drop to flow.

A less detailed and thus more general form of Poiseuille's law is $Q = \Delta P/R$ with resistance R being:

$$R = 8\eta \cdot l / \pi r_i^4$$

Fig. 2.1 Inlet length. Flow entering a side branch results in skewed velocity profile. It takes a certain inlet length, inlet length, before the velocity develops into a parabolic profile again

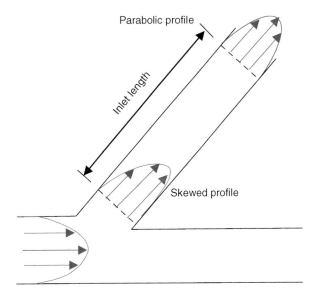

This law is an analogous to Ohm's law of electricity, where resistance equals voltage drop/current. In this analogy, the voltage difference is compared to pressure drop and current to volume flow. In hemodynamics, we also call it Ohm's law. Thus:

$$\Delta P / Q = R$$

This means that resistance can be calculated from (mean, time averaged) pressure and mean flow measurements.

Use of Ohm's law (Chap. 6) allows the calculation of resistance of a whole vessel bed. Application of Poiseuille's law to individual vessels of different lengths and diameters, to derive total resistance is virtually impossible, but Ohm's law is simple to use.

2.1.1   Calculation of Wall Shear Stress

The wall shear rate can be calculated from the slope of the velocity profile near the wall (angle θ in Fig. 2.2), which is the velocity gradient close to the wall (see Chap. 1). The derivative of the parabolic velocity profile gives the shear rate $\gamma = (\Delta P/l)\cdot r/2\eta$. Shear stress is shear rate times viscosity $\tau = (\Delta P/l)\cdot r/2$. The shear rate at the vessel axis, $r = 0$, is zero, and at the wall, $r = r_i$, it is $\tau = (\Delta P/l)\cdot r_i /2$, so the blood cells encounter a range of shear rates and shear stresses over the vessel's cross-section and is highest at the wall (Wall Shear Stress). Wall shear stress acts on the endothelium cells.

The shear stress at the wall can also be calculated from basic principles (Fig. 2.3). For an arterial segment of length l, the force resulting from the pressure difference

Fig. 2.2 The shear rate can be calculated from the 'rate of change of velocity' as indicated by angle Θ. Shear rate at the wall is largest. Relations between shear rate and flow or pressure gradient are given in the text

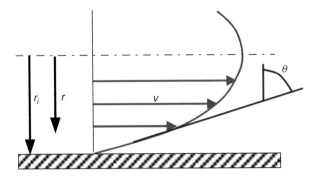

Fig. 2.3 Shear stress at the wall can also be calculated directly by the balance of pressure, $\Delta P = P_1 - P_2$, *and* frictional forces: $\tau = (\Delta P/l)\cdot(r_i/2)$

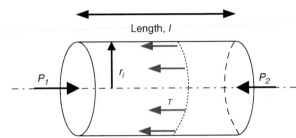

$(P_1 - P_2) = \Delta P$, times the cross-sectional area, πr_i^2, should equal the opposing force generated by friction. This frictional force on the wall equals the shear stress, τ times the lateral surface, $2\pi r_i \cdot l$. Equating these forces gives, $\Delta P \cdot \pi r_i^2 = \tau \cdot 2\pi r_i \cdot l$, and

$$\tau = \left(\Delta P / l\right)\cdot\left(r_i / 2\right)$$

Blood viscosity is not present in the formulas, thus with constant perfusion pressure a change in blood viscosity does not affect wall shear stress.

The wall shear stress may also be expressed as a function of volume flow assuming Poiseuille's law to hold:

$$\tau = 4\eta \cdot Q / \pi r_i^3$$

this is a more useful formula for estimating shear stress because flow and radius can be measured noninvasively using ultrasound or MRI, whereas a pressure gradient cannot.

2.1.2 *Example of the Use of Poiseuille's Law to Obtain Viscosity*

A relatively simple way to obtain viscosity is to use a reservoir that empties through a capillary (Fig. 2.4). Knowing the dimensions of the capillary and using Poiseuille's law viscosity can be calculated. Even simpler is the determination of viscosity

Fig. 2.4 A wide bore
reservoir maintaining
constant pressure, provides
the blood flow through a
capillary. The application
of Poiseuille's law, or
comparison with water,
gives absolute and relative
viscosity, respectively

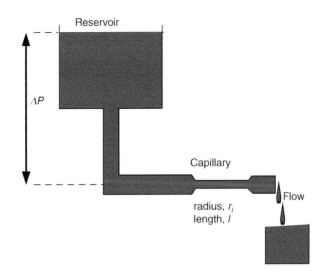

relative to that of water. In that case only a beaker and stopwatch are required. The
amounts of blood and water obtained for a chosen time are inversely proportional to
their viscosities. The practical design based on this principle is the Ostwald
viscometer.

2.1.3 Murray's Law

Murray's law (1926) was originally proposed by Hess in 1913 and assumes that the
energy required for blood flow plus the energy needed to maintain the vasculature is
assumed minimal [1]. The first term equals pressure times flow and, using
Poiseuille's law, this is $P{\cdot}Q = Q^2{\cdot}8{\cdot}\eta{\cdot}l/\pi r_i^4$. The second term is assumed proportional
to vessel volume and thus equals $b{\cdot}\pi\, r_i^2 l$, with b a proportionality constant. The total
energy, E_m, is:

$$E_m = Q^2 \cdot 8\eta \cdot l \, / \, \pi r_i^4 + b \cdot \pi r_i^2 l$$

The minimal value is found for $dE_m/dr = 0$ and this leads to:

$$Q = (\pi/4l)\cdot(b/\eta)^{0.5} \times r_i^3 = k \cdot r_i^3$$

For a bifurcation it holds that

$$Q_{mother} = Q_{daughter1} + Q_{daughter2}$$

and thus

$$k_m r^3_{\,mother} = k_{d,1} r^3_{\,daughter1} + k_{d,2} r^3_{\,daughter2}$$

with two equal daughters and lengths, and equal k's, it holds that:

$$r^3_{mother} = 2 \cdot r^3_{daughter}$$

and we find that

$$r_{daughter} = \left(\frac{1}{2}\right)^{1/3} r_{mother} \approx 0.79 r_{mother}$$

The area of both daughters together is thus $2 \cdot 0.79^2 \approx 1.25$ the area of the mother vessel. This area ratio is close to the area ratio predicted by Womersley on the basis of the oscillatory flow theory (Chap. 8), where minimal reflection of waves at a bifurcation (Chap. 12), is found when the area ratio is between 1.15 and 1.33 [2]. Thus, Murray's law suggests a minimal size of blood vessels and an optimum area of bifurcation [1]. It can be shown that the constant k relates to shear rate, as $k = \pi\gamma$ $/4 \approx 0.75\gamma$. The finding that wall shear differs considerably between mammalian vessels implies that Murray's law cannot simply be applied to the whole arterial system [3, 4].

2.2   Physiological and Clinical Relevance

The more general form of Poiseuille's law given above, namely Ohm's law, $Q = \Delta P/R$ allows us to derive resistance, R, from mean pressure and mean flow measurement (Chap. 6).

The wall shear stress, i.e., the shear force on the endothelial cells plays an important role in the short term, seconds to minutes, and the long term, weeks, months or years. Short-term effects are vasomotor tone and flow mediated dilatation (FMD). Long-term effects are vascular remodeling, endothelial damage, changes in barrier function, and atherosclerosis (Chap. 29).

Shear stress plays a role in the embryonic development of the cardiovascular system. On the one hand shear stress, through gene expression, affects (ab)normal cardiovascular growth [5], and on the other hand it activates blood-forming stem cells [6].

It is still not possible to directly measure wall shear stress or shear rate *in vivo*. Shear rate is therefore best estimated from the velocity profile. Velocity profiles can be measured with MRI and Ultrasound Doppler. From the velocity profile the velocity gradient, dv/dr, is then calculated. However, the calculations to obtain shear rate at the vessel wall require extrapolation, because very near the wall velocity cannot be measured. To calculate wall shear stress the blood viscosity near the wall has to be known as well, but viscosity close to the wall is not known because of plasma skimming (Chap. 1). Also, the change in vessel diameter over the heartbeat is almost impossible to account for.

Wall shear stresses are about 10–20 dynes/cm^2 (0.01 mmHg), which is about $10,000$ times less than the circumferential stress in the vessel wall, the hoop stress (Chap. 9). Despite this enormous difference in magnitude, both stresses are equally important in the functional wall behavior in physiological and pathological conditions (see Chaps. 29 and 30).

References

1. Weibel ER. Symmorphosis. Cambridge, MA: Harvard University Press; 2000.
2. Womersley JR. The mathematical analysis of the arterial circulation in a state of oscillatory motion. 1957, Wright Air Dev. Center, Tech Report WADC-TR-56-614.
3. Cheng C, Helderman F, Tempel D, Segers D, Hierck B, Poelmann R, et al. Large variations in absolute wall shear stress levels within one species and between species. Atherosclerosis. 2007;195:225–35.
4. Reneman RS, Hoeks AP. Wall shear stress as measured in vivo: consequences for the design of the arterial system. Med Biol Eng Comput. 2008;46:499–507.
5. Poelmann RE, Gittenberger-de Groot AC, Hierck BP. The development of the heart and microcirculation: role of shear stress. Med Biol Eng Comput. 2008;46:479–84.
6. Adamo L, Naveiras O, Wenzel PL, McKinney-Freeman S, Mack PJ, Gracia-Sancho J, et al. Biomechanical forces promote embryonic haematopoiesis. Nature. 2009;459:1131–5.

Chapter 3
Bernoulli's Equation

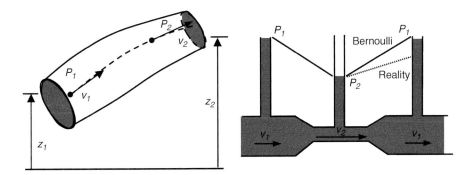

Bernoulli's equation relates blood pressure, P, and blood flow velocity, v. It expresses the conservation of energy in the flowing blood. If pressure losses due to friction or turbulence are neglected, Bernoulli's equation states that the sum of mechanical energy expressed in terms of pressure, P, kinetic energy based on blood velocity, $\frac{1}{2} \cdot \rho \cdot v^2$, and potential energy, $\rho\, g\, z$, stays constant. For a blood vessel in the supine human the term $\rho\, g\, z$ is usually neglected, and $P + \frac{1}{2}\, \rho \cdot v^2 =$ constant. Thus, when velocity is high, ($v_2 > v_1$, right hand figure), pressure is low. In reality pressure distal to the narrowing section does not recover completely as suggested by Bernoulli's equation. The law helps to understand the effect of valvular stenosis and coarctation. The pressure drop over a stenosed valve can be estimated by $\Delta P = 4v_s^2$ with ΔP in mmHg and v_s, the maximal velocity in the stenosis, given in m·s^{-1}.

© Springer International Publishing AG, part of Springer Nature 2019
N. Westerhof et al., *Snapshots of Hemodynamics*,
https://doi.org/10.1007/978-3-319-91932-4_3

3.1 Description

The Bernoulli equation can be viewed as an energy law. It relates blood pressure (P) to flow velocity (v). Bernoulli's law says that if we follow a blood particle along its path (dashed line in left Figure in the Box) the following sum remains constant:

$$P + \tfrac{1}{2} \cdot \rho \cdot v^2 + \rho \cdot g \cdot z = \text{constant}$$

where ρ is blood density, g acceleration of gravity, and z elevation with respect to a horizontal reference surface (i.e., ground level or heart level). One can derive Bernoulli's equation from Newton's law: Pressure forces + gravitational forces = mass times acceleration.

Strictly speaking, the Bernoulli equation is applicable only if there are no viscous losses and blood flow is steady.

3.2 Physiological and Clinical Relevance

Bernoulli's law tells us that when a fluid particle decelerates pressure increases. Conversely, when a fluid particle accelerates, such as when going through a (severe) stenosis, pressure drops.

Because of the direct relationship between pressure and velocity, the Bernoulli equation has found several interesting clinical applications, such as the Gorlin [1] equation for estimating the severity of an aortic or mitral valve stenosis.

Let us consider flow through a stenosed valve according to Fig. 3.1.

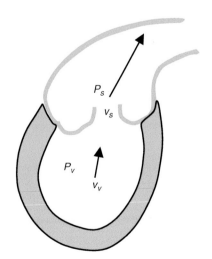

Fig. 3.1 Pressures, P_v and P_s, and velocities, v_v, and v_s, in ventricular lumen, v and valvular stenosis

3.2.1 Applying Bernoulli's Law

Consider the pressure and velocity over a valvular stenosis. When height differences are neglected

$$P_v + \tfrac{1}{2} \cdot \rho \cdot v_v^{\,2} = P_s + \tfrac{1}{2} \cdot \rho \cdot v_s^{\,2}$$

with subscripts v and s pertaining to ventricle and valve respectively.

$$P_v - P_s = \tfrac{1}{2} \cdot \rho \cdot \left(v_s^{\,2} - v_v^{\,2} \right)$$

The flow Q is the same at both locations, thus $A_v \cdot v_v = A_s \cdot v_s = Q$, where A_v and A_s are the cross-sectional areas of ventricle and valve, respectively. Substituting this into the Bernoulli's equation we obtain:

$$\Delta P = P_v - P_s = \tfrac{1}{2} \cdot \rho \cdot Q^2 \cdot \left(1/A_s^{\,2} - 1/A_v^{\,2} \right)$$

Since the cross-sectional area of the stenosed valve A_s is much smaller than the cross-sectional area of the ventricle ($A_s \ll A_v$), the equation can be simplified to:

$$\Delta P = \tfrac{1}{2} \cdot \rho \cdot Q^2 / A_s^{\,2} = \tfrac{1}{2} \cdot \rho \cdot v_s^{\,2}$$

When blood velocity in the stenosis, v_s is expressed in m/s, the pressure drop (ΔP, in mmHg) is approximately $4 \cdot v_s^2$.

This relation has been used to estimate effective area, A_s, of a valvular stenosis by measuring flow and pressure gradient (e.g., using a pressure wire).

$$A_s = Q \sqrt{\frac{\rho}{2\Delta P}}$$

When the pressure is in mmHg and flow in ml/s, this gives an effective area: A_s (in cm²) = $0.02 \cdot Q / \sqrt{\Delta P}$. If pressure recovery downstream of the vena contracta is included then: $A_s = 0.0225 \cdot Q / \sqrt{\Delta P} = Q/(44\sqrt{\Delta P})$, [2].

3.2.2 Calculation of Aortic Valvular Area

Doppler velocimetry applied to both the valvular annulus and the aorta allows for the direct calculation of relative valve area (Fig. 3.2). Since volume flow is the same, the product of velocity and area (Q) is also the same at both locations. Thus

$$A_{valve} = A_{aorta} v_{aorta} / v_{valve}$$

Fig. 3.2 Relative aortic
valve area can be derived
from Doppler velocity
measurements, in aorta and
valve, and aortic area

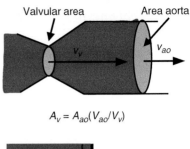

$$A_v = A_{ao}(V_{ao}/V_v)$$

Fig. 3.3 Vena contracta
effect is the result of the
inability of the fluid to turn
a sharp corner. The
contraction coefficient
A_{jet}/A_{valve} depends on the
anatomical shape

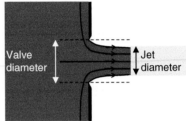

3.2.3   Jets and Vena Contracta

Jets and vena contracta (Fig. 3.3) are formed when blood flow emerges from an
opening such as a valve and play a role in valvular stenosis and regurgitation. The
contraction coefficient, i.e., the area ratio of the jet and the valve (dashed) depends
on the shape of the valve. The coanda effect is the phenomenon that a jet along the,
atrial or ventricular, wall appears smaller than a free jet. Estimation of valvular
area from the jet area is therefore not straightforward. Computational flow dynamics, i.e., the numerical solution of the Navier-Stokes equations, allows the calculation flow velocity in complex geometries and makes it possible to learn more about
jets.

3.2.4   Kinetic Energy

Bernoulli's equation pertains to conservation of energy. The term $\frac{1}{2}{\cdot}\rho{\cdot}v^2$ is the
kinetic energy. At peak systole (P = 120 mmHg), the blood flowing in the lower
abdominal aorta with a peak velocity $v \approx 0.5$ m/s hits the wall of the apex of the iliac
bifurcation. If it would come to a rest there, velocity is negligible ($v = 0$). On the
basis of the Bernoulli equation this implies a pressure rise in systole of $\frac{1}{2}{\cdot}\rho{\cdot}v^2 = 1/2{\cdot}$
$1060{\cdot}(0.5)^2 = 130$ N/m$^2 \approx 0.13$ kPa or about 1 mmHg.

O'Rourke [3] introduced the terms lateral pressure and impact pressure (Fig. 3.4).
To calculate power or energy the impact pressure should be used. For the calculation
of impedance (Chap. 24) a linear system is required and lateral pressure is preferred,
but it does change in a stenosis (Fig. 3.4). In unstenosed vessels the differences

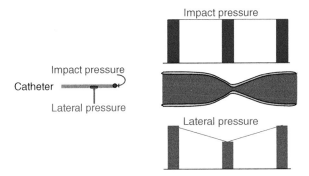

Fig. 3.4 A catheter with a lateral sensor (green) measures pressure without the contribution of blood velocity. The end-sensor measures impact pressure, pressure plus $\frac{1}{2}\rho \cdot v^2$. When the catheter is moved through a stenosis the lateral pressure is lower in the stenosis while impact pressure, $P + \frac{1}{2}\rho \cdot v^2$ is constant

between lateral and impact pressure are not large. Therefore, the lateral measurement is generally accepted as standard method.

3.2.5   The Hydrostatic Pressure

Most measurements are performed in the supine position. However, most activity takes place in the standing position. Pressures in the arterial and venous systems in the supine and the (motionless) standing position differ considerably. In the supine subject the mean pressures in major arteries are all about 100 mmHg and in the major veins about 5 mmHg, respectively. In the standing position the hydrostatic pressure plays a role, with a height of 133 cm blood corresponding to a pressure of about 100 mmHg. Arterial pressure in the main head arteries is then about 50 mmHg and in the veins about −45 mmHg. Pressure in the arteries of the feet are about 190 mmHg and venous pressure about 95 mmHg [4]. Effectively, the arterio-venous pressure gradients are not much affected. Thus, the driving forces for the flow are not much different in the two positions, but the transmural pressures over the vessel wall are very different and this mainly has an effect on the venous and capillary systems since arteries are much stiffer than veins and capillaries. The result is venous pooling of blood which reduces cardiac filling and therefore has a, temporary, effect on the pump function of the heart. The capillary transmural pressure increase gives rise to edema formation. The high filling of the veins can in part be compensated by muscle contraction, the skeletal muscle pump.

When a person is lying in a reclined position the central venous pressure can be estimated in the veins of the neck and hand. The height difference between the point of collapse of superficial hand veins and the heart, is a measure of venous filling pressure. If the height difference is z in cm, the venous pressure can be estimated as $z/1.33$ mmHg, or with $z = 10$ cm the pressure it is 7.5 mmHg.

References

1. Gorlin R, Gorlin SG. Hydraulic formula for calculations of the area of the stenotic mitral valve value, orthocardiac values and central circulating shunts. Am Heart J. 1951;41:1–29.
2. Wilkinson JL. Haemodynamic calculations in the catheter laboratory. Heart. 2001;85:113–20.
3. O'Rourke MF. Impact pressure, lateral pressure, and impedance in the proximal aorta and pulmonary artery. J Appl Physiol. 1968;25:533–41.
4. Burton AC. Physiology and biophysics of the circulation. 2nd ed. Chicago: Year Book Medical Publ; 1972.

Chapter 4
Turbulence

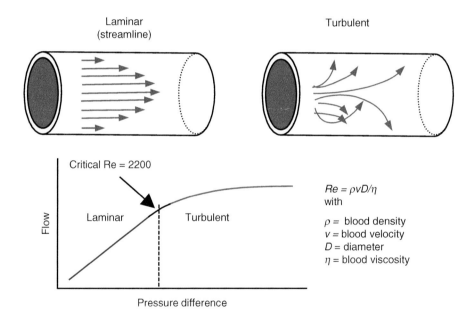

Laminar and turbulent flow. In laminar flow particles remain in a single layer (left), while in turbulent flow blood particles move erratically between layers (right). Turbulent flow is less efficient than laminar flow, i.e., a relatively larger pressure difference is required for the same amount of flow. Laminar flow may be steady or unsteady (pulsatile). The Reynolds number, $Re = \rho\,v\,D/\eta$, is a dimensionless number (no units) characterizing the flow. In a straight vessel, when the Reynolds number exceeds the critical value of 2200 flow becomes turbulent. Below the critical Reynolds number flow is laminar. In general, flow in the arterial system is laminar.

© Springer International Publishing AG, part of Springer Nature 2019
N. Westerhof et al., *Snapshots of Hemodynamics*,
https://doi.org/10.1007/978-3-319-91932-4_4

In the aorta for large cardiac outputs, as during exercise, flow can be turbulent. Flow distal to stenoses and stenotic valves is turbulent. Flows in vascular access grafts in hemodialysis patients can also be very high leading to turbulence.

4.1 Description

When flow in a straight cylindrical tube is relatively low, fluid particles move smoothly in concentric layers (Box Figure, left). This type of flow is called laminar flow. The relation between the pressure gradient and flow is linear and described by Poiseuille's laws. As flow increases, the smooth parallel fluid motion becomes wavy, leading to vortices propagated downstream, with more increase in flow the number of vortices increases and finally fluid motion becomes irregular [1]. This irregular and seemingly random fluid particle motion is called turbulence. Turbulent flow is energetically more costly than laminar flow, because part of the mechanical energy used to maintain flow (i.e., pressure gradient) is lost in the erratic motion between the fluid particles. The resistance to flow is thus higher and increases with flow, which is reflected by the change in slope in the relation between pressure drop and flow (Box Figure, right).

To judge whether a fluid flow is laminar or turbulent, the Reynolds number, Re, is often used. Re is defined as

$$Re = \rho \cdot v \cdot D / \eta,$$

with ρ the fluid density, v the mean fluid velocity, D the tube inner diameter and η fluid viscosity. The Reynolds number is dimensionless (has no units) and reflects the ratio of inertia and viscous effects. For low Reynolds numbers the viscous effects are dominant and laminar flow prevails. Thus, it is not only the fluid velocity that determines whether or not the flow is laminar, but tube size, viscosity and blood density also play a role.

There exists a transitional zone around the critical Reynolds number of 2200 where flow is neither strictly laminar nor strictly turbulent. Also, when flow is slowly increased turbulence may start at Reynolds numbers somewhat higher than 2200 and, inversely, when flow is decreased from a turbulent condition it may remain turbulent for Reynolds numbers smaller than 2200. In some hemodynamic texts the radius is used instead of the diameter; and the critical Reynolds number is then 1100.

4.2 Physiological and Clinical Relevance

At normal resting conditions arterial flows are laminar. For instance, in the human aorta at rest with a Cardiac Output, CO, of 6 l/min (100 ml/s) the Reynolds number can be calculated as follows. Mean velocity $v = CO/\pi r_i^2$, and with $r_i = 1.5$ cm,

$v = 6000/(60 \cdot \pi \cdot 1.5^2) \approx 15$ cm/s. Assuming blood density to be 1.06 g/cm^3 and blood viscosity to be 3.5 cP the Reynolds number equals Re $= v \cdot D \cdot \rho / \eta = 1.06 \cdot 15 \cdot 2 \cdot 1.5/0.035 \approx 1350$. This Reynolds number is below the critical number of 2200 and thus flow is laminar. With heavy exercise, where flow can increase by a factor of 5, the Reynolds number increases to values above 2200 and turbulence occurs.

The criterion for transition to turbulence, i.e., Re > 2200 applies to steady flow in straight uniform tubes. Because arterial flow is highly pulsatile and blood vessels are not uniform, this criterion does not strictly apply. For pulsatile flow laminar flow persists longer and transition to turbulence takes place at higher Reynolds numbers.

Turbulence is delayed when the fluid is accelerating whereas transition to turbulence occurs faster in decelerating flows. Loss of pressure due to turbulence is an effective means to decelerate flow fast. An example is turbulence distal to a stenosis. Fluid particles, which have been accelerated through the converging part of the stenosis decelerate fast in the distal expanding part of the vessel, the flow separates and turbulence develops. Turbulence in severe stenoses can be initiated for Reynolds numbers as low as 50.

Turbulence may affect endothelial function and plays an important role in certain pathologies. For example, it has been suggested that turbulence distal to a stenosis contributes to the phenomenon of post-stenotic dilatation (Chap. 5). Aortic dilatation in valvular stenosis is also known to exist. Turbulence occurring at the venous anastomoses of vascular access grafts used in hemodialysis patients is correlated with the local development of intima hyperplasia, which ultimately leads to a stenosis and graft failure.

Reference

1. Munson BR, Young DF, Okiishi TH. Fundamentals of fluid mechanics. New York: Wiley; 1994.

Chapter 5
Arterial Stenosis

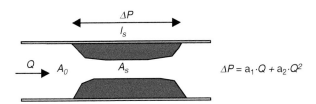

Aortic coarctation and arterial stenosis is a localized narrowing of the arterial lumen, typically as a result of atherosclerosis. A stenosis is quantified by the ratio A_s/A_0, called the area ratio, often expressed as % area occlusion, given as $(1 - A_s/A_0) \cdot 100$. The relation between pressure drop across the stenosis, ΔP, and flow, Q, is quadratic, which means that stenotic resistance increases with flow. The linear term in the pressure drop-flow equation accounts for the viscous losses within the stenosis, whereas the quadratic term accounts for losses due to turbulence. In severe stenoses (area occlusion more than 85%), turbulent losses dominate and the pressure drop is proportional to flow squared. Severe stenoses add significant resistance to flow and can be potentially harmful by preventing adequate blood supply to distal beds.

5.1 Description

Stenosis, from the Greek word for 'narrowing', is a medical term used to describe a localized constriction in an artery. Stenoses are usually caused by the development of atheromatous plaques in the sub intimal layer of the arterial wall, which subsequently protrude into the lumen of the artery, thus causing a narrowing and limiting the free passage of blood.

A coarctation or arterial stenosis consists of a converging section, a narrow section, with the minimal luminal section defining the degree of stenosis, and a diverging

© Springer International Publishing AG, part of Springer Nature 2019
N. Westerhof et al., *Snapshots of Hemodynamics*,
https://doi.org/10.1007/978-3-319-91932-4_5

Fig. 5.1 A coarctation consists of a converging section, a narrow section and a diverging section, each with their particular pressure-flow relations

Narrow section. If it is long and constant in diameter Poiseuille's law applies.

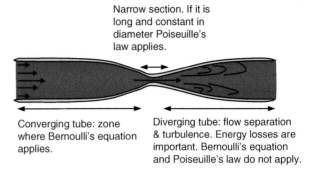

Converging tube: zone where Bernoulli's equation applies.

Diverging tube: flow separation & turbulence. Energy losses are important. Bernoulli's equation and Poiseuille's law do not apply.

section (Fig. 5.1). In the converging section, Bernoulli's equation holds (see Chap. 3). In the narrow section Poiseuille's law is assumed to apply, provided that this narrow section is long enough with approximately constant diameter. In the diverging section flow separates and is often turbulent with significant viscous losses, which means that in this region neither Bernoulli's nor Poiseuille's law applies.

The severity of a stenosis can be expressed as % area $(1 - A_s/A_o)\cdot 100$ or percentage of the normal diameter as $(1 - D_s/D_o)\cdot 100$, with subscripts s and o denoting stenotic and unstenosed vessel segments, respectively (Figure in the Box). Pressure losses over a coarctation can be treated through semi-empirical relations. Such a relationship was developed by Young & Tsai [1] who performed a series of experiments of steady and pulsatile flows in models of concentric and eccentric stenoses. Young and Tsai found that the pressure across a stenosis, ΔP, can be related to flow, Q, by the following relation:

$$\Delta P = \frac{8\pi \cdot \eta \cdot l_s}{A_s^2} \cdot Q + \frac{K_t \cdot \rho}{2A_0^2} \cdot \left[A_0 / A_s - 1\right]^2 \cdot Q^2 = a_1 Q + a_2 Q^2$$

where A_0 is the unobstructed cross-sectional lumen area and A_s the minimal free cross-sectional lumen area (see Box Figure). The first term of the stenosis equation accounts for the viscous losses (Poiseuille's law) as blood flows through the narrow coarctation lumen. The second term accounts for the pressure losses distal to the stenosis and it is derived from the mechanics of flow in a tube with an abrupt expansion. The K_t is an empirical coefficient approximately equal to 1.5, but strongly depending on the shape of the stenosis, smoother return to distal area corresponds with a smaller K_t. The equation is derived for steady flow, but for oscillatory pressure-flow relations a qualitatively similar equation holds [2].

5.1.1   Post Stenotic Dilatation

The arterial diameter distal of a stenoses is often increased, a phenomenon called post stenotic dilatation. The mechanism causing the dilatation is still not clear. It may be due to abnormal shear stress and turbulent flow downstream of the stenosis,

leading to extracellular matrix remodeling in the vessel wall. It has also been suggested that vessel wall vibrations distal to the stenosis cause the dilatation [3]
Another possible mechanism of post-stenotic dilatation is the effect of increased
shear stress within the stenosis upon platelets which become activated and release
the serotonin from their dense granules. Serotonin acts upon endothelial $5HT_1$
receptors to release nitric oxide which relaxes the vascular smooth muscle to produce dilatation.

5.2 Physiological and Clinical Relevance

The best way to characterize a stenosis is by constructing the relation between flow
through and pressure across the stenosis (See Fig. 5.2).

The empirical formula for the pressure drop across a stenosis shows that both
flow and area appear as quadratic terms. This is an important aspect of the hemodynamics of a coarctation. To illustrate the significance of the quadratic terms, let us
assume that the stenosis length, l_s, is very small so that the first term in the equation
above, $a_1 \cdot Q$, is negligible. The pressure drop is then proportional to the flow squared.
Suppose that a patient with a mild coarctation in the femoral artery has, at rest, a
pressure gradient over the narrowed section of 10 mmHg. When the patient starts
walking, and the peripheral bed dilates to allow for more perfusion flow through the
microcirculation, the gradient in pressure increases. When flow needs to increase by
a factor three the pressure gradient should be $10 \cdot 3^2 = 90$ mmHg. This is clearly
impossible and vasodilation, the decrease in peripheral resistance of the leg, does
not help to increase flow sufficiently.

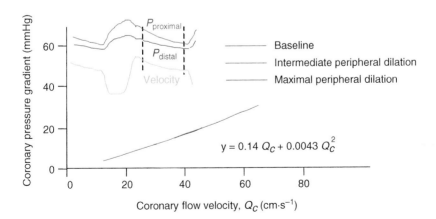

Fig. 5.2 Pressure drop over a coronary stenosis, as a function of blood flow velocity during diastole to minimize the effect of cardiac muscle contraction on the vasculature. The range of velocities
is obtained by vasodilation of the distal vessels. The quadratic expression can be applied. (Adapted
from Ref. [4], used by permission)

The pressure drop is inversely related to the square of the cross-sectional area in the stenosis. For an 80% area stenosis, the factor $(A_0/A_s - 1)^2$ equals $(1/0.2 - 1)^2 = 16$, whereas for a 90% stenosis this factor increases to 81. Thus a 90% stenosis is 81/16 or about 5 times more severe in terms of pressure drop than an 80% stenosis for a similar flow, i.e., it increases from 10 to 50 mmHg. This strongly nonlinear effect implies that complaints from ischemia will arise 'suddenly' when the narrowing becomes more severe, typically for a stenosis of >70%. Measurement from angiography is often not accurate enough to distinguish the small differences in area reduction.

From Bernoulli's equation it follows that at high velocity in a stenosis the pressure is low (Chap. 3). This implies that, as is the case during vasodilation, when flow and thus velocity is increases, the transmural pressure in the narrow section may decrease to low values. For compliant stenoses, (compliant wall) the decrease in transmural pressure may lead to extra narrowing, thereby worsening the situation.

5.2.1 Flow Reserve

Angiographic data often do not give accurate information about the functional hemodynamic aspects of a stenosis or coarctation. This has led several investigators to propose methods to obtain a quantitative description in terms of pressure-flow relations. One approach is the determination of flow reserve. The, absolute, flow reserve is defined as the ratio of flow during maximal (pharmacologic) dilatation and flow during control (Q_{max}/Q_{contr}). In Fig. 5.3, pressure distal to a stenosis, P_d, is plotted as a function of flow, while proximal (aortic) pressure is assumed to be constant. It is apparent that when the periphery is strongly dilated, i.e., the peripheral resistance decreases from R_{contr} to R_{min} the flow increases. However, in the presence of a severe stenosis (lower curve in Fig. 5.3), the flow increase is limited and distal pressure greatly decreases. In control conditions, at rest, flow may be hardly affected by the presence of the stenosis, since peripheral (physiological) dilation may compensate for the stenosis 'resistance', i.e., Q_{contr} depends on stenosis severity and on microvascular resistance. At maximal vasodilation a severe stenosis limits maximal flow Q_{max} considerably, but the peripheral resistance remains playing a role. Thus, in presence of a stenosis, flows are not determined by the stenosis alone, but by both the stenosis and the microvascular resistance. In other words, the flow reserve (Q_{max}/Q_{contr}) is not determined by the severity of a stenosis alone.

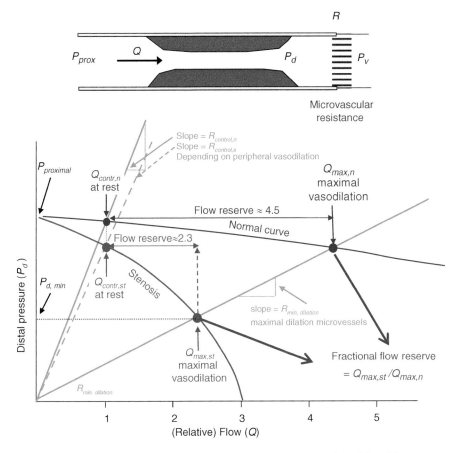

Fig. 5.3 In this figure pressure (distal of a stenosis) is plotted as a function of flow. Flow reserve is defined as the ratio of flow during maximal vasodilation and flow during control. Without stenosis the $Q_{max,n}/Q_{contr,n}$ is much larger than with a stenosis present, $Q_{max,st}/Q_{contr,s}$. With the stenosis the microcirculation may dilate to result in similar flow at rest (indicated by green). When the peripheral bed is maximally vasodilated, peripheral resistance decreases from R_{contr} to $R_{min,dilation}$ and flow increases, but distal pressure decreases. The decrease in distal pressure limits the maximal flow under vasodilation, thereby reducing the flow reserve. Thus, the flow reserve depends on the stenosis severity and microvascular resistance both in control and after maximal dilation. The Fractional Flow Reserve, FFR, is the ratio of the maximal flow with the stenosis present and maximal flow in the unaffected bed, $Q_{max,st}/Q_{max,n}$. The FFR depends on the stenosis severity and also on how much the distal bed can dilate. The FFR is close to the ratio of the distal pressure during dilation and the proximal pressure, $P_{distal,min}/P_{prox}$, if the maximally dilated bed distal to the stenosis is "normal". The, nonlinear, relation between pressure drop over the stenosis and flow through it, $(P_{prox} - P_{dmin})/Q$, depends on the stenosis severity only

5.2.2 *Fractional Flow Reserve*

Another estimate of stenosis severity is the Fractional Flow Reserve, FFR, which is the ratio of the maximal (pharmacologically induced) flow, $Q_{max,st}$ in the bed perfused by the stenosed artery and the maximal flow in a normal, not stenosed bed, $Q_{max,n}$. The FFR is thus

$$FFR = Q_{max,st} / Q_{max,n} = [(P_d - P_v) / R_{st,min}] / [(P_{prox} - P_v) / R_{contr,min}]$$
$$\cong P_d / P_{prox} \cong P_d / P_{aorta}$$

with P_d being the distal pressure during maximal dilation, and P_{prox} the proximal (aorta) pressure, and P_v venous or intercept pressure (Chap. 6). For coronary stenoses the proximal pressure equals aortic pressure. Under the assumption that the microvascular bed of the stenosed area has the same resistance as the bed of the normal area, $R_{st} = R_n$, and assuming that P_v is small with respect to P_d it holds that the FFR is close to the ratio P_d/P_{aorta} [5].

Although a normal periphery and the periphery distal to a stenosis may not have similar resistance, the FFR appears a workable parameter. The cut-off value of the FFR is 0.74, i.e. for values higher than 0.74 the stenosis is not considered functionally important. For segmented stenoses, i.e., stenoses severity changes over the vessel's length, and for multiple stenoses P_d should be measured distal of the last lesion.

Spaan et al. [6] have reviewed the principles and limitations of flow reserve.

References

1. Young DF, Tsai FY. Flow characteristics in models of arterial stenoses: I steady flow. J Biomech. 1973;6:395–410.
2. Newman DL, Westerhof N, Sipkema P. Modelling of aortic stenosis. J Biomech. 1979;12:229–35.
3. Roach MR, Stockley D. The effects of the geometry of a stenosis on poststenotic flow in models and poststenotic vibration of canine carotid arteries in vivo. J Biomech. 1980;13:623–34.
4. Marques KM, Spruijt HJ, Boer C, Westerhof N, Visser CA, Visser FC. The diastolic flow-pressure gradient relation in coronary stenoses in humans. J Am Coll Cardiol. 2002;39:1630–6.
5. Pijls NHJ, De Bruyne B. Coronary pressure. Dordrecht & Boston: Kluwer Academic Publishers; 1997.
6. Spaan JAE, Piek JJ, Hoffman JIE, Siebes M. Physiological basis of clinically used coronary hemodynamic indices. Circulation. 2006;113:446–55.

Chapter 6
Resistance

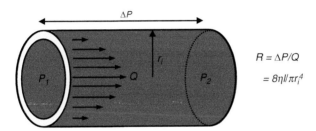

$$R = \Delta P/Q$$
$$= 8\eta l / \pi r_i^4$$

Resistance to blood flow is an important property of blood vessels. Resistance can be determined by the ratio of mean pressure difference over and mean flow through a blood vessel ($R = \Delta P/Q$, Ohm's law). For a single uniform vessel Poiseuille's law can predict its resistance, but in practice resistance is obtainable using Ohm's law. In other words, resistance although depending on the vascular geometry and blood viscosity, can be calculated directly from measurements of mean pressure difference, ΔP, and mean blood flow, Q. Detailed knowledge of the vascular geometry is not required. Ohm's law not only pertains to single blood vessels but may also be applied to combinations of vessels, whole organ beds, and the whole systemic or pulmonary circulation. Rules for addition of resistances are discussed below. Resistance should always be calculated from a mean pressure difference as indicated by ΔP. In the systemic circulation venous pressure is usually much lower than aortic pressure and ΔP is close to aortic pressure. However, this is not the case in the pulmonary circulation. The resistance in the systemic, and pulmonary circulation are mainly determined by the resistance of small arteries and arterioles, often called resistance arteries. This means that the mean pressure in all large, conduit arteries, is almost the same. The arterioles act as resistances to regulate flow to the local tissue.

© Springer International Publishing AG, part of Springer Nature 2019
N. Westerhof et al., *Snapshots of Hemodynamics*,
https://doi.org/10.1007/978-3-319-91932-4_6

6.1   Description

Poiseuille's law (Chap. 2) shows that resistance depends on the length and diameter of the vessel, and the viscosity of blood. However, even for a single blood vessel, it is difficult to derive the relation between pressure and flow on the basis of Poiseuille's law. The diameter of the vessel needs to be accurately known because of the fourth power law. Furthermore, the vessel should be uniform, and, especially for small vessels, the anomalous viscous properties of blood makes it impossible to use a single value for viscosity. Accurate calculation of resistance on the basis of Poiseuille's law is therefore virtually impossible. However, resistance can be calculated from the ratio of the *mean* pressure gradient and *mean* flow constituting a practical experimental approach. Thus, although Poiseuille's law makes it possible to arrive at several important conclusions regarding vascular function, in practice we use resistance as calculated using Ohm's law: the ratio of the mean pressure difference over the vessel or system and mean flow through it, $\Delta P/Q$ (Fig. 6.1).

To understand where resistance is located in the arterial tree we need to know some rules about resistances.

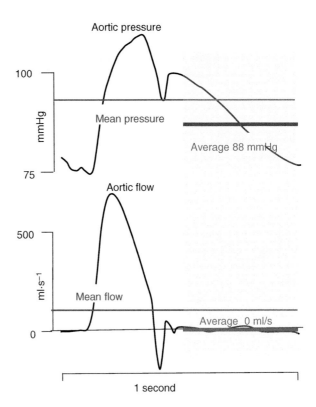

Fig. 6.1 Ohm's law quantifies the total arterial resistance by the ratio of <u>mean</u> pressure difference and <u>mean</u> flow. The instantaneous ratio of pressure and flow or the ratio of diastolic pressure and flow averaged over diastole only gives nonsensical results: divided by zero

6.1.1 Addition of Resistances

Two resistances in series result in a total resistance equal to the sum of the resistances. This rule can be derived as follows. The total pressure drop over two resistances in series is the sum of the individual pressure drops, i.e., $\Delta P_{total} = \Delta P_I + \Delta P_{II}$ and flow is the same through both. Thus $\Delta P_{total} = Q \cdot R_I + Q \cdot R_{II} = Q \cdot (R_I + R_{II}) = Q \cdot R_{total}$. Thus, $R_{total} = R_I + R_{II}$, i.e., the total resistance is the sum and thus larger than each individual resistance.

Two resistances in parallel add up in a so-called 'inverse' fashion (Fig. 6.2). When in parallel, the pressure drop, ΔP, over both daughter vessels is the same, and the two flows add up to total flow, Q_{total}, thus

$$Q_m = Q_{total} = Q_{d,1} + Q_{d,2} = \Delta P / R_1 + \Delta P / R_2 = \Delta P / \left(1 / R_1 + 1 / R_2\right) = \Delta P / R_{sum}$$

and we find

$$1 / R_{sum} = 1 / R_1 + 1 / R_2$$

For the two daughters and mother together, the resistance is then:

$$R_{total} = R_{mother} + R_{sum}$$

An easier calculation is through conductance (G), which is the inverse of resistance, $G = 1/R$. Ohm's law written in terms of conductance is $Q = \Delta P \cdot G$. Parallel conductances can be added directly: $G_{total} = G_1 + G_2$.

Thus, two equal resistances in parallel add to a total resistance of half the resistance of each. Ten equal arterioles in parallel result in an overall resistance equal to 1/10 of a single arteriole.

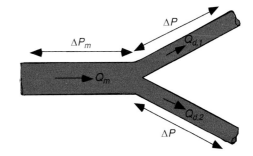

Fig. 6.2 A blood vessel, mother, divides into two smaller, daughter vessels. We determine the resistance of this network by proper addition of the two distal vessels in parallel and then add the resistance of the mother vessel. Note that we work from the distal end

6.1.2 *Physical Reason Why the Systemic Resistance Is Mainly Located in the Arterioles*

We first compare the resistance of the aorta with the resistance of an arteriole using Poiseuille's law. Comparing an aortic with radius of 15 mm and an (arbitrary) length of 50 cm with an arteriole with a radius of 7.5 micrometer and a length of 1 mm we can estimate the resistance ratio of the two. The radius ratio is 2000 and the length ratio is ~500, thus the resistance ratio is $(2000)^4/500$, i.e., $\sim3\cdot10^{10}$. Thus, the resistance of a single arteriole is $3\cdot10^{10}$ larger than of a 50 cm long aorta.

However, there is only one aorta and about $3\cdot10^8$ arterioles, and since these arterioles all sprout (indirectly) from the single aorta we can consider them as in parallel. Thus, the total arteriolar resistance is about $3\cdot10^{10}/3\cdot10^8 \approx 100$ times as large as the resistance of the aorta.

Therefore, the pressure drop over the aorta is about 1% of the total pressure drop over the systemic arterial system, which is about 100 mmHg. Indeed, the mean pressure in the dorsalis pedis artery is, in the supine human, only a few mmHg lower than mean pressure the ascending aorta.

6.1.3 *Resistance of Capillaries and Veins*

Capillaries have diameters that are of the same order as the smallest arterioles but their number is larger (4–5 capillaries per arteriole) and therefore their resistance is about 4–5 times smaller. The glycocalyx, the carbohydrate structures on the luminal surface of the microvascular endothelial cells, not only protects against edema, but also reduces the effective capillary diameter and thus increases capillary resistance [1]. At present an unresolved controversy is the mechanism of the low resistance of capillaries when the red cells (RBCs) have a diameter larger than the capillary. The red blood cells deform to squeeze through even though the pressure gradient is very small. An important role is thus played by the deformability of the RBCs [2], reduced RBC deformability as in Sickle Cell Anemia increases the resistance to capillary flow. The interaction of the capillary endothelial glycocalyx with the RBCs has been likened to skiing on compressible porous media which would reduce resistance to flow [3]. A possibly different mechanism is that the red blood cell endothelium interface consists of a layer of water that is not liquid [4]. Still capillaries contribute little to total systemic resistance.

In the systemic vascular system venules and veins have larger diameters than their accompanying arteries and often appear as two veins to one artery. Therefore, total venous resistance in the systemic circulation is about 1/20 of total resistance. It is still not entirely clear whether resistance and its regulation should be based on diameters or anatomical location [5].

However, in the pulmonary vascular system the veins appear to contribute to overall resistance (Chap. 28) [6].

6.1.4 Calculation of Vascular Resistance

The total resistance of the systemic circulation can be calculated as follows. When mean aortic pressure is taken to be about 105 mmHg and central venous pressure is about 5 mmHg the pressure difference is 100 mmHg. With a Cardiac Output of 6 l/min, thus 100 ml/s, the total resistance is $100/100 = 1$ mmHg·s·ml^{-1}. The units are mmHg·s·ml^{-1} and called peripheral resistance units, PRU. Often physical resistance units are used in the clinic and resistance is then expressed in dyn·s·cm^{-5} or Pa·s·m^{-3}. As can be seen from Appendix 7 the following holds: $7.5 \cdot 10^{-9}$ mmHg·s·ml^{-1} = 10^{-5} dyn·s·cm^{-5} = 1 Pa·s·m^{-3} or a resistance of 1 mmHg·s·ml^{-1} = $1.3 \cdot 10^{3}$ dyn·s·cm^{-5} = $1.3 \cdot 10^{8}$ Pa·s·m^{-3}.

For the systemic circulation subtraction of venous pressure is often omitted without introducing large errors. However, in the pulmonary circulation with mean pulmonary artery pressure of about 20 mmHg and a pulmonary venous pressure of 5 mmHg, use of the pressure difference is mandatory, and pulmonary resistance is $(20 - 5)/100 = 0.15$ PRU, which is about 15% of the resistance of the systemic circulation.

6.1.5 The Zero Flow Intercept Pressure, Starling Resistor and the Waterfall Model

Pressure-flow relations often show and intercept with the pressure axis: the zero-flow pressure intercept. This intercept depends on vasoactive state: with vasodilation the intercept is lower. It has been suggested that the intercept depends on microvascular compliance [7]. Sipkema et al. [8], using a thin-walled latex microtube, showed that the intercept pressure relates to the plateau of its pressure-volume relation. Thus, implicating vessel compliance as the explanation. Others have suggested that the rheological properties of blood play a role [9], but changing the perfusion fluid from blood to a crystalloid medium did not change the intercept pressure [10]. Sagawa et al. showed that the intercept pressure depends on smooth muscle tone [11]. Surface tension between blood and vessel wall [12] and the role of the glycocalyx have been suggested to play a role.

The calculation of resistance assumes the vascular system to be linear and resistance to be pressure independent. In reality the vessels are compliant implying that with increased pressure vessel diameters are larger (nonlinear pressure-flow relation) and resistance smaller. Linehan et al. developed a model to quantify the effect of hematocrit, Hct, and vessel distensibility, $\alpha = \Delta D/D_o \Delta P$, on pressure-flow relations [13].

$$P_a = \left\{ \left[\left(1 + \alpha P_v \right)^5 + 5\alpha \cdot Q \cdot R_o \left(Hct \right) \right]^{1/5} - 1 \right\} / \alpha$$

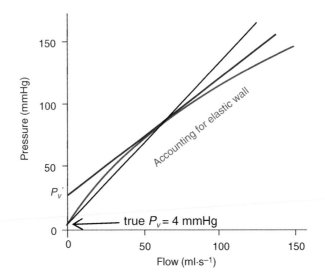

Fig. 6.3 A pressure-flow relation (red) fitted by the equation discussed in the text using human parameters, $\alpha = 0.025$ mmHg^{-1}, (wall thickness radius ratio of 0.1; Young modulus 400 kPa), $R_o(\text{Hct}) = 2$ mmHg·s·ml^{-1} and venous pressure $P_v = 4$ mmHg. It may be seen that a piecewise approximation with a straight line (blue) gives an apparent intercept, P_v' higher than true venous pressure, P_v. The apparent intercept depends on Hematocrit (not shown here). A linear approximation using $(P_a - P_v)/Q$ (black line) deviates from the flow-dependent true resistance

with P_a arterial and P_v venous pressure. At a known Hct the parameters α, $R_o(\text{Hct})$, the reference resistance, can be determined from a pressure-flow relation [13]. Figure 6.3 shows an example of a pressure-flow relation of the systemic arterial tree, as predicted by the above formula. The local slope is flow dependent and overestimates the 'zero-flow pressure intercept'.

The intercept pressure has led to the so-called Waterfall (Fig. 6.4) as arterial model. The 'Starling resistor', a compliant tube with adjustable external pressure (Fig. 6.5), was used as vascular model in heart studies. The Starling resistor is actually more a mechanical pressure control system than a resistor.

6.2   Physiological and Clinical Relevance

The small arteries and arterioles (Peripheral Resistance) mainly determine total systemic resistance. Resistance can be regulated by the arterioles, because they are muscular arteries and it follows from Poiseuille's law that rather small changes in diameter (and cross-sectional area) result in large resistance changes. A 10% change in diameter corresponds to a change in resistance by 1.1^4, or about 50%.

The resistance of the aorta and conduit arteries is so low that the mean pressure hardly decreases from heart to the small peripheral arteries, the pressure drop being

Fig. 6.4 The Waterfall model. The slope, 'resistance', and Arterial minus Waterfall pressure, $P_a - P_w$ determine flow. Venous pressures less than waterfall pressure P_w do not affect flow

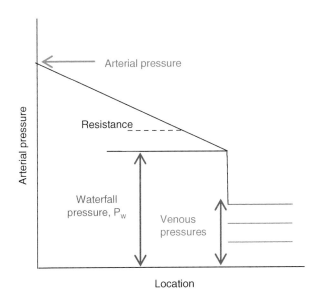

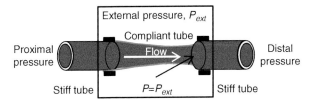

Fig. 6.5 The Starling resistor. The external pressure in the chamber, by partially decreasing the diameter of the compliant tube, results a tube pressure equal to external pressure. The term resistor is not correct. The Starling Resistor was used to study cardiac output as a function of ventricular filling under constant pressure load (Chaps. 14 and 15)

only a few mmHg. This means that in the supine human, *mean* blood pressure is practically the same in all conduit arteries, and therefore *mean* blood pressure may be determined in any conduit artery. This also implies that conduit arteries can be seen as a supply reservoir with (the local) peripheral resistances adjusting themselves such that the demand of flow to the (local) tissue is met.

When perfusion flow is high, e.g., during exercise, the large artery resistance could cause a sizable pressure drop. However, with increased flow the conduit arteries dilate through 'Flow Mediated Dilation', FMD, to decrease their resistance. An FMD of 7% gives a resistance decrease of more than 30%.

Vascular smooth muscle tone is regulated by the nervous and hormonal systems and through autoregulation (see also Chap. 19). Autoregulation is based on metabolic, myogenic, and endothelial mechanisms, as response to NO. With increased pressure arteriolar resistance increases thereby keeping capillary pressure constant to maintain tissue fluid equilibrium, the Starling equilibrium (see Appendix 4). The lateral area or exchange area is the area involved in the exchange of oxygen, substrates and metabolites between tissue and blood. This area is largest in the capillaries and can be calculated as $2\pi rl$, with l capillary length. The total exchange area of all capillaries together is about 6000 m^2.

The total cross-sectional area is the largest in capillaries, and velocity of blood is lowest allowing ample time for exchange with the tissues [14]. It is incorrect to apply Poiseuille's law using total cross-sectional area. The cross-sectional area (radius) of individual vessels should be used to calculate resistance and then resistances must be added in series and in parallel according to the anatomy.

6.2.1   Low Resistance of an Arterio-Venous Fistula

Several arterio-venous fistulas may exist, such as an open ductus arteriosus, and the fistula between the radial artery and vein made for dialysis. As an example, the latter an arterio-venous shunt causes a low resistance in parallel with the resistance of the lower arm. However, the shunt does not always cause ischemia in the hand for the following reason (steal syndrome). The mean blood pressure in the aorta is 100 mmHg and is in the radial artery normally about 3 mmHg lower, and thus 97 mmHg. The venous pressure is about 5 mmHg and in the vena cava pressure is 2 mmHg. The low resistance of the conduit arteries and veins will, with a large shunt flow, decrease arterial pressure by about 10 mmHg and increase the venous pressure by the same amount. The perfusion pressure for the hand is then $87 - 15 = 72$ mmHg, which is high enough to avoid ischemia. The fistula will, however, lower the total systemic peripheral resistance and increase Cardiac Output thereby affecting cardiac function.

Qualitatively stated: the conduit arterial system and venous system can be viewed as pressure reservoirs with resistance arteries as a resistor. Another way of stating this is that conduit arteries and veins are pressure sources, i.e., pressure is hardly affected by flow. The venous reservoir is much larger than the arterial reservoir and plays a major role in ventricular filling.

References

1. Vink H, Duling BR. Identification of distinct luminal domains for macromolecules, erythrocytes and leukocytes within mammalian capillaries. Circ Res. 1996;71:581–9.
2. Driessen GK, Haest CW, Heidtmann H, Kamp D, Schmid-Schönbein H. Effect of reduced red cell "deformability" on flow velocity in capillaries of rat mesentery. Pflugers Arch. 1980;388:75–8.
3. Feng J, Weinbaum S. Lubrication theory in highly compressible porous media: the mechanics of skiing, from RBCs to humans. J Fluid Mech. 2000;422:281–317.
4. Zheng J-M, Chin WC, Khijniak E, Khijniak E Jr, Pollack GH. Surfaces and interfacial water: evidence that hydrophilic surfaces have long-range impact. Adv Colloid Interface Sci. 2006;127:19–27.

5. Christensen KL, Mulvany MJ. Location of resistance arteries. J Vasc Res. 2001;38:1–12. Review.
6. Hakim TS, Kelly S. Occlusion pressures vs. micropipette pressures in the pulmonary circulation. J Appl Physiol. 1989;67:1277–85.
7. Spaan JA. Coronary diastolic pressure-flow relation and zero flow pressure explained on the basis of intramyocardial compliance. Circ Res. 1985;56:293–309.
8. Sipkema P, Westerhof N. Mechanics of a thin walled collapsible microtube. Ann Biomed Eng. 1989;17:203–17.
9. Schmid-Schönbein H. Critical closing pressure or yield shear stress as the cause of disturbed peripheral circulation? Acta Chir Scand Suppl. 1976;465:10–9.
10. Sagawa K, Eisner A. Static pressure-flow relation in the total systemic vascular bed of the dog and its modification by the baroreceptor reflex. Circ Res. 1975;36:406–13.
11. Van Dijk LC, Krams R, Sipkema P, Westerhof N. Changes in coronary pressure-flow relation after transition from blood to Tyrode perfusion. Am J Phys. 1988;255:H476–82.
12. Sherman IA. Interfacial tension effects in the microvasculature. Microvasc Res. 1981;22:296–307.
13. Linehan JH, Haworth ST, Nelin LD, Krenz GS, Dawson CA. A simple distensible vessel model for interpreting pulmonary vascular pressure-flow curves. J Appl Physiol. 1992;73:987–94.
14. Berne RM, Levy MN, Koeppen BM, Stanton BA. Physiology. 5th ed. St. Louis & Baltimore: Mosby-Elsevier; 2003.

Chapter 7
Inertance

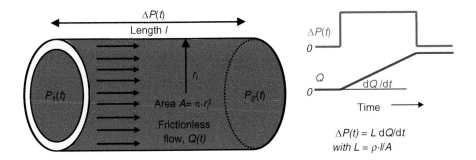

$$\Delta P(t) = L\, dQ/dt$$
$$\text{with } L = \rho \cdot l / A$$

Inertance relates the pressure drop with the acceleration of flow. This figure shows that when blood is subjected to an increase in pressure difference flow will change (right side). Assuming no friction, the relation between the pressure drop, $\Delta P(t) = P_1(t) - P_2(t)$, and the rate of change of blood flow dQ/dt, depends on the density of the blood, ρ, the cross-sectional area, $A = \pi r_i^2$, and the length, l, of the blood vessel. We call this combined effect the inertance, $L = \rho\, l/A$. Inertance pertains to oscillatory pressure and flow and plays a dominating role in large blood vessels, where the viscous resistance is small and pulsatility is considerable. Inertance and Poiseuille resistance together form the basis of the Oscillatory Flow Theory. The inertance and vessel compliance in combination determine the wave speed and the characteristic impedance of a blood vessel.

7.1 Description

Blood is accelerated and decelerated with every heartbeat, and the mass of the blood plays a role. The mass is density times volume, and the volume depends on the geometry of the blood vessel or heart. Blood density is a material property and is

© Springer International Publishing AG, part of Springer Nature 2019
N. Westerhof et al., *Snapshots of Hemodynamics*,
https://doi.org/10.1007/978-3-319-91932-4_7

about 1.06 g/cm^3. In hemodynamics, we calculate the effective mass and call it inertance. Inertance connects the oscillatory pressure drop with the rate of change of blood flow.

We can derive inertance by using Newton's law relating force, F, mass, m, and the rate of change of change of velocity, dv/dt, which is the acceleration, a:

$$F = m \cdot a = m \cdot \mathrm{d}v / \mathrm{d}t$$

For a blood vessel, the net force $F(t) = (P_1(t) - P_2(t)) \cdot A = \Delta P(t) \cdot A$, A being the luminal cross-sectional area. The mass in the segment equals blood density, ρ, times the volume (length times area): $\rho \cdot (l \cdot A)$. The acceleration is the rate of change of velocity with time, i.e., dv/dt. In terms of volume flow this is $(1/A) \cdot \mathrm{d}Q/\mathrm{d}t$. With Newton's equation this gives:

$$\Delta P(t) \cdot A = \rho \cdot l \cdot A \cdot (1/A) \cdot \mathrm{d}Q / \mathrm{d}t = \rho \cdot l \cdot \mathrm{d}Q / \mathrm{d}t$$

and

$$\Delta P = \rho \cdot l / A \cdot (\mathrm{d}Q / \mathrm{d}t) = L \cdot \mathrm{d}Q / \mathrm{d}t$$

where $L = \rho \cdot l/A$ is called inertance. We recall that resistance is inversely proportional to r^4 (Chap. 2) while inertance is inversely related to r^2. Thus, in large vessels the inertance plays a larger role than resistance while in small arteries and arterioles it is the resistance that plays the larger role.

The inertance in combination with the compliance of a vessel segment determines the characteristic impedance and the wave speed (see Chap. 12 and Appendix 3).

7.1.1   Addition of Series and Parallel Inertances

The principal rules for addition of inertance of vessels in parallel and in series are as for resistances (see Chap. 6).

7.2   Physiological and Clinical Relevance

The inertance is determined by the cross-sectional area and length of the blood vessel, and by blood density. Blood density varies little, even in pathologic conditions. Inertance is therefore primarily a geometrically determined parameter.

An example where the effect of the inertance can be seen is when left ventricular and aortic pressures are measured simultaneously (Fig. 7.1). During the ejection period aortic flow is first accelerating (early ejection) and then decelerating. When

Fig. 7.1 Inertance plays a role in accelerating and decelerating the blood. In early systole, when left ventricular pressure is higher than aortic pressure the blood accelerates, i.e., flow increases. In late systole, aortic pressure is higher than ventricular pressure the blood still flows forward but decreases (deceleration). The lower part of the figure shows the similarity in ΔP_{lv-ao} and dQ/dt, their ratio being inertance. (Adapted from Ref. [1], by permission)

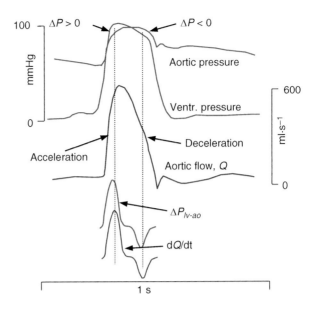

Fig. 7.2 Blood flow may be reversed, or negative, during part of the cardiac cycle. This results from inertia and reflections. With vasodilation the reflections decrease and flow reversal disappears (example from femoral artery). (Adapted from Ref. [2], by permission)

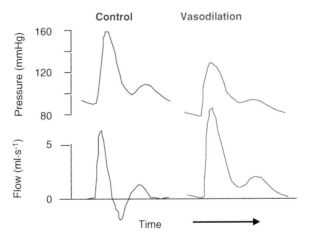

the blood is accelerating the left ventricular pressure is higher than aortic pressure. When the blood is decelerating the pressure difference reverses, as in the later phase of ejection. It may be seen that the pressure difference and the time derivative of flow are almost proportional in systole, suggesting constant inertance.

Inertance in combination with reflections (see Chaps. 12 and 22) can result in flow reversal, i.e., negative flow during part of the cardiac cycle (Fig. 7.2). The mean flow is, of course, always in the direction of the periphery. The negative flow is physiologic as well. The momentarily negative flow shows that Ohm's law cannot be applied to instantaneous values of pressure and flow, but only to their mean values (Chap. 6).

Fig. 7.3 During left
ventricular diastolic filling
inertia plays a role. Flow is
still forward, but
decelerates, while the
pressure difference
between atrium and
ventricle reverses.
(Adapted from [3], by
permission)

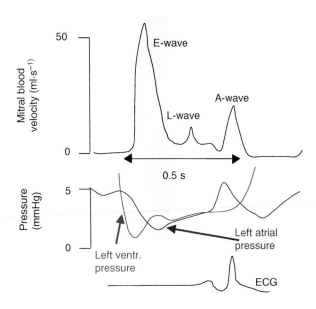

Another example (see Fig. 7.3) is the diastolic filling of the ventricle through the
mitral valve. As a result of the inertance, flow persists, but decelerates, when left
ventricular pressure is higher than left atrial pressure.

References

1. Noble MIM. The contribution of blood momentum to left ventricular ejection in the dog. Circ
   Res. 1968;23:663–70.
2. O'Rourke MF, Taylor MG. Vascular impedance of the femoral bed. Circ Res. 1966;18:126–39.
3. Solomon SB, Nikolic SD, Glantz SA, Yellin EL. Left ventricular diastolic function of remod-
   eled myocardium in dogs with pacing induced heart failure. Am J Phys. 1998;274:H945–54.

Chapter 8
Oscillatory Flow Theory

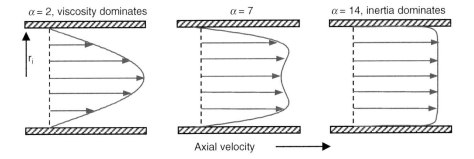

Oscillatory flow velocity profiles in a stiff tube during laminar sinusoidal flow resulting from a sinusoidal pressure gradient. The velocity profiles vary over the sinusoidal cycle and only the profile at the moment of maximal forward flow is depicted here. The velocity profile depends on the Womersley parameter, $\alpha^2 = r_i^2 \omega \rho / \eta$, where r_i is the internal radius, ω the circular frequency ($2\pi \cdot f$, f frequency), ρ blood density, and η blood viscosity. Womersley's parameter α expresses the relative importance of inertial effects over viscous (frictional) effects. For low values of the Womersley parameter ($\alpha < 3$, low frequency, small radius), viscous effects dominate and the profile becomes parabolic, as in Poiseuille flow (left figure). For a medium range of α values the velocity profile becomes flatter and the maximum velocity does not occur at the tube's center (middle figure). For large values of α, $\alpha > 10$, i.e., high frequency and/or large vessels the profile becomes flat, because inertial effects dominate. The theory is based on sinusoidal oscillations of pressure and flow. This implies that application of the theory to hemodynamics requires Fourier analysis (Appendix 1). From work on comprehensive models we conclude that the contribution of oscillatory flow theory only gives a small correction over and above the use of a resistance with a inertance in series (Appendix 3). However, in the calculation of wall shear and in the calculations and measurements of local flow profiles, the theory is of great importance.

© Springer International Publishing AG, part of Springer Nature 2019
N. Westerhof et al., *Snapshots of Hemodynamics*,
https://doi.org/10.1007/978-3-319-91932-4_8

8.1   Description

The pressure-flow relation for steady flow, where only frictional losses are playing a role (resistance, law of Poiseuille, Ohm's law), and the relation between oscillatory or pulsatile pressure and flow when only blood mass (inertance) is taken into consideration, are simplifications of reality.

The relation between oscillatory, sinusoidal, pressure drop and flow through a blood vessel can be derived from the Navier-Stokes equations. The assumptions are to a large extent similar to the derivation of Poiseuille's law: uniform and straight blood vessel, rigid wall, Newtonian viscosity, etc. The result is that flow is still laminar but pulsatile, i.e., not constant in time, and the flow profile is no longer parabolic. The theory is based on sinusoidal pressure-flow relations, and therefore called oscillatory flow theory.

The flow profile depends on the, circular, frequency of oscillation, ω, with $\omega = 2\pi f$, with f the frequency; the tube radius, r_i, the viscosity, η, and density, ρ, of the blood. These variables were taken together in a single dimensionless (no unit-less) parameter called Womersley's alpha parameter [1]:

$$\alpha^2 = r_i^2 \omega \cdot \rho / \eta$$

If the local pressure gradient, $\Delta P/l$, is of a sinusoidal shape with amplitude $\Delta P/l$ and circular frequency ω, then the corresponding velocity profile is given by the formula [1]:

$$v(r, t) = \text{Real}\left[\left((\Delta P / l) / i\omega\rho \right) \cdot \left\{ 1 - J_0 \left(\alpha \cdot y \cdot i^{3/2} \right) / J_0 \left(\alpha \cdot i^{3/2} \right) \right\} e^{i\omega t} \right]$$

where y is the relative radial position, $y = r/r_i$, and $i = \sqrt{-1}$. Flow is given as:

$$Q(t) = \text{Real}\left[\left(\pi r_i^2 \Delta P / i\omega\rho l \right) \cdot \left\{ 1 - 2J_1 \left(\alpha \cdot i^{3/2} \right) / \left(\alpha \cdot i^{3/2} \cdot J_0 \left(\alpha \cdot i^{3/2} \right) \right) \right\} e^{i\omega t} \right]$$

J_0 and J_1 are Bessel functions of order 0 and 1, respectively. The Real means that only the real part of the mathematically complex formula is taken.

Since the heart does not generate a single sine wave but a sum of sine waves (see Appendix 1) the flow profile *in vivo* is found by addition of the velocity profiles of the various Fourier harmonics, and is very complex. The relation between pressure drop and flow as given above is the so-called longitudinal impedance of a vessel segment (see Appendix 3). Experiments have shown that the theory is accurate.

For large α, i.e., $\alpha > 10$, i.e. large vessels or high frequencies inertia dominates the viscous effects with the result that phase velocity (wave speed), characteristic impedance and local wave reflection have simple relations with vessel properties and are frequency-independent (Chap. 12).

8.2   Physiological and Clinical Relevance

Womersley's oscillatory flow theory [1] reduces to Poiseuille's law for very low α. This means that in the periphery with small blood vessels (small r, thus small α) and little oscillation, there is no need for the oscillatory flow theory and we can describe the pressure-flow relations with Poiseuille's law. For the very large conduit arteries, where $\alpha > 10$, friction does not play a significant role and the pressure-flow relation can be described with inertance alone. For α values in between, the combination of resistance and inertance approximates the oscillatory pressure-flow relations (see Appendix 3). In studies on large arteries the assumption of large α appears reasonable and Pulse Wave Velocity, characteristic impedance etc. are then reduced to frequency independent parameters.

The oscillatory flow theory was intended to derive flow from a pressure difference at two locations in an artery [2]. However, a pressure difference over a few centimeters is extremely small and leads to large errors in the flow estimates, and the method proved too inaccurate to use.

Models of the entire arterial system have indicated that, even in intermediate size arteries, the oscillatory effects on the velocity profiles are not large in terms of the overall relations between pressure and flow. The main factors contributing to the pressure and flow wave shapes in the arterial tree are due to branching, non-uniformity and bending of the blood vessels etc. Thus, for global hemodynamics, i.e., wave travel, input impedance, Windkessel models etc., the longitudinal impedance of a segment of artery (Appendix 3) can be described, in a sufficiently accurate way, by an inertance only in the aorta and major arteries, by an inertance in series with a resistance in medium sized conduit vessels, and a resistance in peripheral arteries.

The oscillatory flow theory is, however, of importance when local phenomena are studied. For instance, detailed flow profiles and calculation of shear stress at the vascular wall require the use of the oscillatory flow theory.

There is another dimensionless number of importance in unsteady, oscillating flow problems: the Strouhal number, St. The Strouhal number can be written as $St = \omega D/v$, where D is diameter, ω circular frequency and v velocity. This unit-less number represents a measure of the ratio of inertial forces due to oscillatory flow and the inertial forces due to convective acceleration (acceleration due to the change of position of fluid particles in a fluid flow). It can be shown that the Strouhal number relates in combination with the Reynolds number (Re, Chap. 4) to the square of Womersley's parameter α:

$$St \cdot Re = \left(\omega D / v\right)\left(\rho v D / \eta\right) = D^2 \omega \rho / \eta = 4\alpha^2$$

The Strouhal number has been used in experimental studies of arterial flows in the past, such as vortex shedding phenomena distal of a cardiac (mitral) valve. It is widely accepted, however, that the most relevant parameter expressing the relative significance of inertial effects due to oscillatory flow is the Womersley parameter α.

Ultrasound Doppler velocity and other new flow measurement techniques (MRI) made the derivation of blood flow from the measurement of two pressures in the aorta a few centimeters apart using the oscillatory flow theory [2] obsolete.

References

1. Womersley JR. The mathematical analysis of the arterial circulation in a state of oscillatory motion. 1957, Wright Air Dev. Center, Tech Report WADC-TR-56-614.
2. Womersley JR. Method for the calculation of velocity, rate of flow and viscous drag in arteries when the pressure gradient is known. J Physiol. 1955;127:553–63.

Chapter 9
Law of Laplace

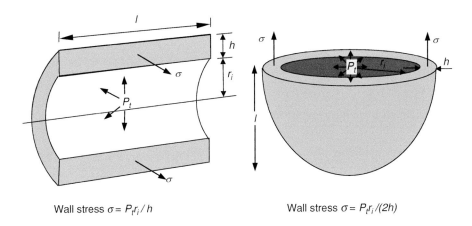

Wall stress $\sigma = P_t r_i / h$ Wall stress $\sigma = P_t r_i /(2h)$

The law of Laplace relates transmural pressure, P_t, with wall stress, σ. In a (cylindrical) blood vessel and in a (spherical) heart model there is a simple relation between pressure and circumferential wall stress. The law gives the average stress over the wall, thus how the stress varies over the wall cannot be derived. The law holds only for simple geometries, cardiac stress estimates are discussed in the text. Often transmural pressure can be approximated by pressure in the organ.

9.1 Description

The original law of Laplace pertains to soap bubbles with negligible wall thickness and radius r, and gives the relation between transmural pressure, i.e., pressure difference between inside and outside, P_t, and wall tension, T_s. Thus, for a thin-walled sphere as $T_s = P_t \cdot r$. The law can be used, for example, to calculate tension in alveoli,

© Springer International Publishing AG, part of Springer Nature 2019
N. Westerhof et al., *Snapshots of Hemodynamics*,
https://doi.org/10.1007/978-3-319-91932-4_9

where outside pressure (intra-thoracic pressure) is often neglected. This tension is directly related to surface tension and has the dimension N/m. The form of the law of Laplace most often used in hemodynamics gives the relation between transmural pressure within the lumen of a hollow organ minus external pressure, and the stress in the wall. We here use the Cauchy stress formulation, which is defined as the ratio of the normal (perpendicular) force acting on a surface divided by the area of the surface, stress, at its deformed configuration. Stress, σ, has the dimension N/m^2 (See Figure in the Box).

For a circular cylinder, as model of a blood vessel, the transmural pressure acts to push the two halves apart with a force equal to pressure times the area (left Figure in the Box). Thus the force is $2 \cdot P_t \cdot l \cdot r_i$. The two halves are kept together by wall stress, σ, acting in the wall only. This force is $2\sigma \cdot h \cdot l$. These forces are in equilibrium and: $2\,P_t \cdot l \cdot r_i = 2\sigma \cdot h \cdot l$, which gives circumferential stress $\sigma = P_t \cdot r_i/h$. This form of the law of Laplace is more correctly called Lamé's equation. For a sphere, a similar derivation holds and the result is $\sigma = P_t \cdot r_i/2\,h$.

We see that transmural pressure and wall stress are related by the ratio of radius over wall thickness.

9.1.1 Applicability of the Law of Laplace

The law of Laplace applies to cylindrical or spherical geometries, irrespective of whether the material is linear or nonlinear or if the wall is thin or thick. A limitation of Laplace's law is that it yields the average wall stress and thus it cannot give any information on the stress distribution across the wall. For cylindrical geometries, and assuming linearly elastic (Hookean) material the distribution of circumferential stress or hoop stress across the wall can be approximated by:

$$\sigma\left(r\right) = P_t \cdot r_i^2 \cdot \left(1 + r_o^2 \,/\, r^2\right) / \left(r_o^2 - r_i^2\right)$$

where r_i and r_o is the internal and external radius, respectively, and r is the position within the wall for which local stress is calculated.

There is a large body of literature, especially for the thick-walled left heart, where (local) wall stress or muscle fiber stress is related with transmural pressure for different complex geometries (for information see [1]).

Hefner [2] extended the Law of Laplace for the left ventricle by showing that the equatorial wall force (F) is $P_{lv} \cdot A_e$, where A_e = equatorial cavity cross-sectional area and P_{lv} ventricular pressure, assuming external (thorax) pressure negligible so that $P_t = P_{lv}$. The wall stress, σ, is given by F/A_w with A_w the equatorial cross-sectional area of the muscle ring. Thus $\sigma = P_{lv} \cdot A_e/A_w$.

Mirsky and Rankin [3] suggested an often used estimation of mid-wall stress. For an ellipsoidal heart shape the mid-wall stress is:

$$\sigma \,/\, P_t = \sigma \,/\, P_{lv}\left(D \,/\, 2h\right) \cdot \left(1 - h \,/\, D - D^2 \,/\, 2l^2\right)$$

with D and l the mid-wall diameter 2r, and mid-wall long axis, l, of the ventricle (see Figure in Box).

Arts et al. [4] derived a simple and practical relation between fiber stress, σ_f, and ventricular pressure, P_{lv}, which reads:

$$\sigma_f / P_{lv} \approx (1/3)\ln(1+V_w/V_{lv})$$

or in linearized form:

$$P_{lv} / \sigma_f \approx 1+3V_{lv}/V_w$$

where V_{lv} and V_w are ventricular lumen volume and ventricular wall volume, respectively.

Torrent-Guasp [5], performed anatomical studies in the heart and concluded that the heart muscle is arranged in such a way that contraction results in a figure eight wringing motion; the helical heart. Torsion or twisting of the ventricle during contraction implies more homogeneity of muscle shorting in the wall, but limiting the law of Laplace in cardiac mechanics [6]. Many relations between wall force or stress and ventricular pressure have been reported, but since measurement of wall force is still not possible [1, 3] it is difficult to decide which relation is best.

The Law of Laplace can be applied to diastole and systole, and during cardiac contraction, where the force is generated in the wall and the pressure the result of the contracting muscle.

9.1.2 Relation to the Youngs Modulus

Assuming that the arterial wall is relatively thin ($h \ll r_i$) and incompressible, one can use Laplace's Law to derive the following expression for the incremental elastic modulus (Chaps. 10 and 11):

$$E_{inc} = (r_i^2/h) \cdot \Delta P_t / \Delta r_i$$

where the Δr_i and the ΔP_t, are the change in internal radius and transmural pressure as occur during the cardiac cycle.

If the wall cannot be considered thin, as is often the case in muscular arteries, the Youngs modulus is best derived from the measurement of pressure and radius using the following expression [7]

$$E_{inc} = 3r_i^2 \cdot r_o \cdot (\Delta P_t / 2\Delta r_o)/(r_o^2 - r_i^2)$$

9.2 Physiological and Clinical Relevance

The law of Laplace, although basic and pertaining to simple geometries only, helps in understanding cardiac and vascular function. The law is therefore of great conceptual importance. For instance, the ratio r/h is a main determinant of the wall stress. Arterial pressures are higher than pressure in the veins and have relatively thicker walls (smaller r/h) than veins resulting in comparable wall stresses. The radius of curvature of the left ventricle is smaller at the apex than at the base, and so is the wall thickness. In other words, the ratio r/h at the ventricular apex and base is about the same resulting in similar wall stress at these locations. During ejection the ventricular volume decreases and the wall thickness increases, and with a high pressure at end-systole the wall stress may be lower [8].

In hypertension the cardiac muscle cells increase in thickness by building more contractile proteins in parallel, leading to concentric hypertrophy. The thicker wall, but similar lumen, i.e., decreased r/h, causes the systolic wall stress to return to presumably normal levels despite the higher pressure in systole (Fig. 9.1). When the heart dilates, often without much change in wall thickness, i.e., eccentric hypertrophy, the volume increase leads to an decrease in the ratio of wall thickness and wall stress increases. The higher muscle stress leads to higher oxygen consumption (Chap. 17), often too large for oxygen supply, thereby adding to the deleterious effect of the dilatation.

In trained athletes, depending on the type of exercise, cardiac dilatation may occur, enabling them to increase stroke volume, and, together with a greater Heart Rate reserve, Cardiac Output. The wall stress is normalized by an increase in wall thickness.

How stresses in the cells are sensed is still largely unknown.

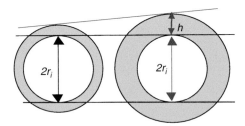

Fig. 9.1 In concentric hypertrophy, when compensated, ventricular pressure and wall thickness both are increased in approximately the same proportion, thus r_i/h is the same, and wall stress remains similar

References

1. Huisman RM, Sipkema P, Westerhof N, Elzinga G. Comparison of models used to calculate left ventricular wall force. Med Biol Eng Comput. 1980;18:133–44.
2. Hefner LL, Sheffield LT, Cobbs GC, Klip W. Relation between mural force and pressure in the left ventricle of the dog. Circ Res. 1962;11:654–63.
3. Mirsky I, Rankin JS. The effects of geometry, elasticity, and external pressures on the diastolic pressure-volume and stiffness-stress relations. How important is the pericardium? Circ Res. 1979;44:601–11. Review.
4. Arts T, Bovendeerd HHM, Prinzen FW, Reneman RS. Relation between left ventricular cavity pressure and volume and systolic fiber stress and strain in the wall. Biophys J. 1991;59:93–102.
5. Torrent-Guasp F, Kocica MJ, Corno AF, Komeda M, Carreras-Costa F, Flotats A, et al. Towards new understanding of the heart structure and function. Eur J Cardiothorac Surg. 2005;27:191–201. Review.
6. Arts T, Reneman RS, Veenstra PC. A model of the mechanics of the left ventricle. Ann Biomed Eng. 1979;7:299–318.
7. Love AEH. A treatise on mathematical elasticity. 3rd ed. London & New York: Cambridge University Press; 1952.
8. Chirinos JA, Segers P, Gupta AK, Swillens A, Rietzschel ER, De Buyzere ML, et al. Time-varying myocardial stress and systolic pressure-stress relationship: role in myocardial-arterial coupling in hypertension. Circulation. 2009;119:2798–807.

Chapter 10
Elasticity

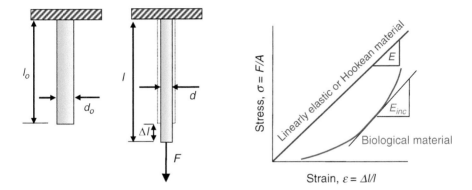

The Youngs modulus of elasticity is a material constant. A strip of material subjected to a force will lengthen. Force, F, per cross-sectional area, $A = \frac{1}{4}\pi d_0^2$, is stress, $\sigma = F/A$, and the relative length change, $\varepsilon = \Delta l/l_0$, is the strain. Stress-strain relations of elastic materials are given at the right. If the stress-strain relationship is linear, the material obeys Hooke's law and the slope of the relation is called the Youngs modulus of elasticity, E. The stress-strain relation of biological tissues is not linear, and the local slope gives the incremental elastic modulus, E_{inc}, which is strain (or stress) dependent. The Youngs modulus of elasticity is actually stiffness modulus.

10.1 Description

When a force, F, is applied to a (round) specimen with cross-sectional area $A = \frac{1}{4}\pi d^2$, and length l_0, the length will be increased by Δl (Left Figure in Box). With a specimen of larger cross-sectional area the same force will result in a smaller length

© Springer International Publishing AG, part of Springer Nature 2019
N. Westerhof et al., *Snapshots of Hemodynamics*,
https://doi.org/10.1007/978-3-319-91932-4_10

change. Also, when the starting length of the specimen, l_0, is longer the same force will result in a larger length change. To be able to give a unique characterization of the material, independent of the sample size, we normalize force by the area and the LaGrangian stress is obtained, $\sigma = F/A$. Similarly we normalize the length change to the starting length, l_o, and obtain strain, $\varepsilon = \Delta l/l_o$.

The relation between stress and strain is given in the right part of the Figure in the Box. When the relation is straight we say that the law of Hooke applies, and the material is called Hookean or linearly elastic. The slope of the graph is called the Youngs modulus of elasticity $E = \sigma/\varepsilon$. The Youngs modulus is a material property and is a measure of the stiffness, not the elasticity, of the material. The units of the Youngs modulus are force per area, thus the same units as for stress and pressure, i.e., $N/m^2 = Pa$, or mmHg.

When lengthened the specimen also gets thinner. The strain in the transverse direction, ε_t, is $\varepsilon_t = \Delta d/d_o = (d - d_0)/d_0$. The ratio of the transverse strain and the longitudinal strain, $\varepsilon_t/\varepsilon$, is called the Poisson ratio. When with stretch the specimen's volume is remaining constant, as appears to be the case for most biological tissues, the Poisson ratio is close to 0.5.

Biological materials almost always exhibit a nonlinear, i.e., curved, stress-strain relationship with convexity towards the strain axis (Right panel, Figure in the Box). The curved relation implies that the material cannot be characterized by a single Youngs modulus. The solution is to introduce an incremental modulus, E_{inc}, defined as the local slope of the stress-strain relation. For biological tissue the incremental elastic modulus increases with strain, i.e., the biological material becomes stiffer with increasing stress and strain.

There are no clear conventions about the choice of the horizontal and vertical axes for stress and strain. This often leads to confusion when the slope of the relation is determined. It should be remembered that biological relations are convex towards the strain axis, i.e., the strain is limited. This limitation is mainly the contribution of collagen fibers and protects against overstretch and damage (see below and Fig. 10.1).

10.1.1   Viscoelasticity

Viscoelasticity (see Figs. 10.2 and 10.3) means that a material is not only elastic but also has viscous ('fluid-like') properties. Viscoelasticity can be made visible and quantified in different ways. If one wants to stretch (increase strain) a viscoelastic material rapidly to a new length, initially a larger force is needed for the same amount of stretch as for a purely elastic material. With time the viscous contribution to the stress decreases. This is called stress relaxation. Inversely, with a sudden increase in stress the strain (stretch) is delayed. The delayed increase in stretch is called creep. When, stress and strain are pulsatile, as *in vivo*, strain always lags stress. Plotting strain versus stress yields a hysteresis loop. The area within the loop is the energy lost due to the viscosity of the material. When sinusoidal stress or

Fig. 10.1 Biological tissues show a stress-strain relation that is convex to the strain axis. The local slope gives the incremental Youngs modulus, E_{inc}, which increases with strain (or stress) mainly as a result of unfolding of collagen molecules

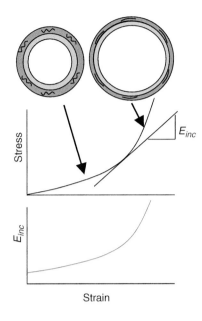

Fig. 10.2 The viscoelastic properties of biological material appear in four forms depending on the intervention and measurements. Step increases in stress and strain lead to creep and stress-relaxation, respectively. Repeated increases and decreases in stress and strain result in a hysteresis loop, area in the loop equals energy loss (hatched area). Application of sinusoidal forces and measuring strains permits the determination of the complex Young modulus in the frequency domain. The dashed, green, lines pertain to purely elastic material or the result after a steady state has been reached. Viscoelasticity also appears in a similar fashion in pressure-diameter and pressure-volume relations

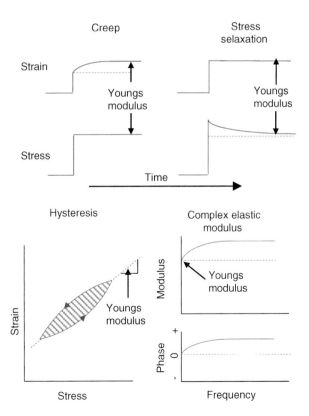

Fig. 10.3 Viscoelasticity of heart muscle requires extra pressure during filling. At velocities of stretch above one muscle length per second an additional force appears in excess of the force due to the elastic force/length curve; this effect is more obvious at large lengths. (Adapted from Ref. [1])

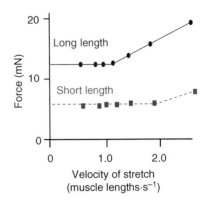

pressure is applied, the amplitude ratio and phase difference between stress and strain describe the complex elastic modulus. The complex elastic modulus depends on the frequency of oscillation. When the stress or strain is applied very slowly the viscous aspects do not become apparent and the material behaves as purely elastic.

10.1.2   Viscoelastic Models

Several models have been proposed to describe the viscoelastic properties of biological tissue (Fig. 10.4). Some of these models fall short in the sense that they do not describe all aspects of viscoelasticity. One of the examples is the Maxwell model where a spring and dash-pot or damper, are placed in series. With a constant stress this model predicts a continuous, never ending, increase in length, which is clearly not true for biological tissue. Adding another spring in parallel to the Maxwell model yields Kelvin's viscoelastic model, which is the simplest, yet realistic viscoelastic model of the vascular wall. Viscoelasticity has been implemented in arterial models [2].

10.1.3   Residual Stresses and Stress Distribution at Physiological Loads

The vascular tissue is not at a zero-stress state when all loads, i.e., transmural pressure and longitudinal tension, are removed. The same holds true for vascular and cardiac tissue. Stresses that still exist in the tissue when no external loads are applied are called residual stresses. The classical experiment to illustrate the existence of residual stress in arteries after removal of all loads is to excise a ring of artery and cut it longitudinally. The ring springs open and takes the shape of a circular arc, as shown in Fig. 10.5 on the right. The change in configuration means that stresses

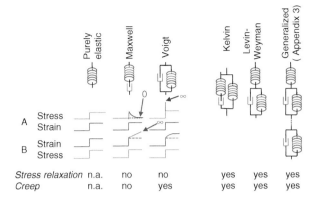

Fig. 10.4 Models of viscoelastic material in the form of springs (elastic) and dashpots (viscous – dampers). A step-change in strain (blue, experiment A) results in a stress response (green). A step change in stress (green, experiment B) gives a response in strain (blue). A purely elastic material can be described by a spring, stress and strain follow each other. The simplest two-element models (left part) represent biological material poorly, they either show stress relaxation to zero and strain that is unlimited for a step in stress (Maxwell) or show an infinite stress response to a step change in strain (Voigt). The three-element models (Kelvin and Levin-Weyman) are equivalent and qualitatively sufficient. To quantitatively describe viscoelasticity in greater detail more elements are usually required (Appendix 3)

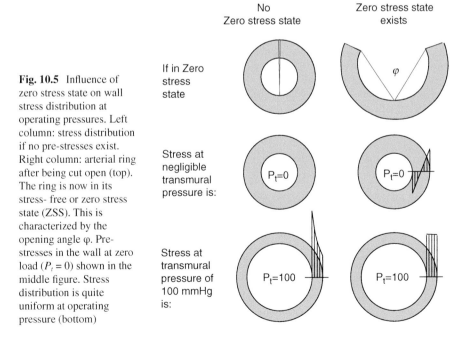

Fig. 10.5 Influence of zero stress state on wall stress distribution at operating pressures. Left column: stress distribution if no pre-stresses exist. Right column: arterial ring after being cut open (top). The ring is now in its stress- free or zero stress state (ZSS). This is characterized by the opening angle φ. Pre-stresses in the wall at zero load ($P_t = 0$) shown in the middle figure. Stress distribution is quite uniform at operating pressure (bottom)

existed within the wall before the cut. Further cuts do not seem to release more stresses, therefore we assume that the opened-up configuration after the first cut is a stress free configuration. This stress-free state or zero-stress state, ZSS, can be characterized by the 'opening angle' φ, which is the angle formed by the two ends and the midpoint of the inner arc length.

Knowledge of the ZSS is of primary importance when one wants to calculate the stress field within the arterial wall, because strains can be calculated only in reference to the ZSS. Residual stresses do play an important role in maintaining a fairly uniform stress distribution across the arterial wall at physiological transmural pressures. This can be visualized with the help of the schematic drawings shown in Fig. 10.5. The left column shows an arterial cross-section where the ZSS is a circular ring (top). This means that at $P_t = 0$ mmHg it is assumed that there are no residual stresses (middle). At a physiological transmural pressure level ($P_t = 100$ mmHg) however, significant stresses develop with a pronounced stress peak at the inner most layer of the wall (bottom). The higher stress concentration in the inner wall is a direct consequence of the fact that these layers are stretched much more during the pressure-induced inflation. The right column shows an artery where the ZSS is characterized by an opened-up configuration (top). The ZSS means that at zero load, and in a closed ring configuration (middle row of Fig. 10.5) residual stresses exist. Residual stresses are compressive in the inner part of the wall and tensile in the outer part of the wall. During inflation, the inner layers will be stretched more than the outer layers of the wall. However, because at the beginning of the inflation, $P_t = 0$ mmHg, the inner wall was under compression whereas the outer wall already was under some extension, at the physiological pressure level the degree of extension is the same in both inner and outer wall layers. The stress distribution is therefore uniform across the wall (bottom).

Knowledge of the ZSS is not required when one wants to calculate the average circumferential stress in the wall using Laplace's law.

10.2   Physiological and Clinical Relevance

Elasticity plays an important role in the circulation. All blood vessels are elastic and their elastic moduli do not differ greatly. A typical value of the incremental elastic modulus of arteries in the normal human at a pressure of 100 mmHg, is about $5 \cdot 10^6$ dyn/cm^2 or 500 kPa. With 1 kPa = 7.5 mmHg the elastic modulus is 3750 mmHg. For diastolic heart tissue the incremental elastic modulus at a filling pressure of 5 mmHg is about $4 \cdot 10^5$ dyn/cm^2 or 40 kPa. In systole these values are about 20 times larger. Thus cardiac muscle is much stiffer in systole than in diastole.

10.2.1   The Elasticity of Cardiovascular Tissue

Vascular tissue is mainly composed of elastin, vascular smooth muscle and collagen. Elastin fibers are highly extensible and even at large deformations they can be characterized by an almost constant Youngs modulus. Collagen fibers, on the other hand, are very stiff: $E_{collagen} \approx 1000\, E_{elastin}$. At lower strains, collagen fibers are wavy are bearing no load, and the elastin and smooth muscle mainly determine the wall elasticity. At larger strains collagen waviness decreases and collagen begins to bear more load leading to an increasingly stiff wall, i.e., a larger E_{inc}. The same holds for cardiac tissue.

The curved relation between stress and strain can be described in several ways. One simple relation, with only two parameters, is the equation originally suggested by Fung [3].

$$\sigma = a \cdot \left[e^{b(\varepsilon - 1)} - 1 \right]$$

This model gives fairly accurate fits of the stress-strain relations.

The nonlinear relation between stress and strain has led to much confusion. An example is in hypertension. When elastic properties of arteries are derived at the working point, i.e., the operating mean pressure of the individual patient, the vessels of hypertensive patients are found to have a higher incremental elastic modulus as compared with normal human subjects. However, this apparently increased stiffness in the hypertensive patients is mainly the result of their higher blood pressure (see Chap. 29). Thus either a stress-strain graph should be made or the incremental elastic modulus should be compared at similar stresses or strains to be able to conclude if mechanical properties have changed or not.

Elasticity of the conduit arteries stands at the basis of arterial compliance (Chap. 11). The role of arterial compliance in wave travel, and the Windkessel is discussed in (Chaps. 12 and 25, respectively).

10.2.2   Determination of the Youngs Modulus

In practice the Youngs modulus is often not measured directly, because isolated tissue samples without perfusion are not viable. Therefore, for hollow organs like heart and vessels, pressure-volume or, for vessels, pressure-diameter relations are determined. Subsequent use of the law of Laplace, and accounting for geometry, the calculation of the Youngs modulus is feasible (Chaps. 9 and 11).

References

1. Noble MIM. The diastolic viscous properties of cat papillary muscle. Circ Res. 1977;40:287–92.
2. Westerhof N, Noordergraaf A. Arterial elasticity: a generalized model. Effect on input impedance and wave travel in the systemic arterial tree. J Biomech. 1970;3:357–79.
3. Fung YC. Elasticity of soft tissues in simple elongation. Am J Phys. 1967;28:1532–44.

Chapter 11
Compliance

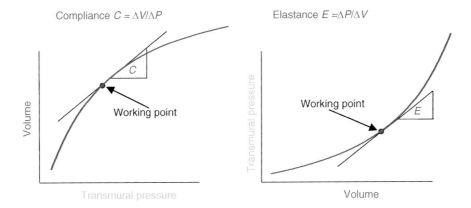

Compliance quantifies a pressure-volume relation. When the transmural or distending pressure is increased, the volume increases (left figure, as customary in arterial research). When volume is increased pressure increases (right figure, customary in cardiac research, and now gaining more attention in vascular research). For biological organs the relation is, in general, not straight but convex to the volume axis, implying that both slopes, Compliance $C = \Delta V/\Delta P$, and Elastance $E = \Delta P/\Delta V$, depend on pressure or volume. Elastance and compliance are the inverse of each other: $E = 1/C$. When organs of different size are to be compared we can normalize both E and C with respect to volume. These normalized descriptions are distensibility, $C/V = (\Delta V/\Delta P)/V$, and bulk modulus or volume elasticity, $EV = V\Delta P/\Delta V$, respectively. When cross-sectional area is measured, as is often done in blood vessels, we derive 'area compliance' and 'area elastance', where luminal area A replaces volume V. When diameters or radii are measured the relations are called diameter and radius compliance and elastance, respectively. The rules for addition of compliances and elastances are discussed. The equivalent of the bulk modulus is the

N. Westerhof et al., *Snapshots of Hemodynamics*,
https://doi.org/10.1007/978-3-319-91932-4_11

'pressure-strain' or 'Peterson's modulus', $E_p = r\Delta P/\Delta r$. Compliance and elastance are not material parameters, but structural parameters, they can be derived from the material properties, i.e., elastic modulus, and the geometry, e.g., diameter, wall thickness, etc.

11.1 Description

The advantage of the pressure-volume (or -diameter and -radius) relation (Figures in the Box) is that *in vivo* compliance can be determined. It is important to note that pressure-volume relations do not characterize the material alone but include the structure of the organ as a whole.

If the pressure-volume relations were straight and going through the origin, the slope, compliance or elastance would give the full characterization of the organ by a single quantity. However, in biology the pressure-volume relations are never straight. For a small change around a chosen working point, the curve is approximately straight, and the tangent of the pressure-volume curve can be used. We can determine compliance in the 'working point' as $C = \Delta V/\Delta P$. The elastance, the inverse of compliance is $E = \Delta P/\Delta V$. Of course, these local slopes depend on the pressure or volume chosen. Thus, when comparing compliance or elastance data one should report the chosen working point, i.e., the pressure at which compliance or elastance was determined. For instance, when the elastance of a heart in diastole is studied and appears increased, the increase can result from either a higher filling pressure but otherwise normal heart, or a normal filling pressure but a hypertrophied heart with thicker wall (Fig. 11.1).

The curvature of the pressure-volume relation is mainly the result of the fact that Youngs modulus increases with stretch, therefore C decreases and E increases, with volume.

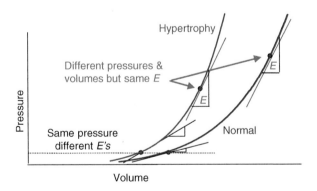

Fig. 11.1 Examples of diastolic pressure-volume relations of a normal and hypertrophied heart. If only the similar elastance values are reported without further information on pressure or volume, it cannot be decided if the heart is normal and overfilled, or hypertrophied and under-filled, since both have the same E. At similar pressure the hypertrophied heart is stiffer (larger E). The full graph is required to give the complete information

11.1.1 Measurement of Elastance and Compliance

Elastance is customarily used for the heart, while compliance was mostly used to describe blood vessels, but the term stiffness is (meaning elastance) is now more and more used in vascular research as well.

Ventricular elastance is best determined by the measurement of pressure and volume. A number of noninvasive techniques are now available to determine ventricular volumes, such as Computed Tomography, Magnetic Resonance Imaging, Ultrasound Echo, while the Pressure-Volume catheter allows for determination of elastance in experimental situations [1]. Cardiac elastance determination requires volume and pressure measurements in systole and diastole, because of the varying properties of the cardiac muscle. Diameter as estimate of volume is inaccurate.

Compliance used in vascular studies can be based on cross-sectional area or on diameter (Fig. 11.2). Diameter changes can be measured by wall-tracking [2] and for large vessels like the aorta by MRI. From the local diameter the cross-sectional area is calculated assuming a circular cross-section. When area and pressure are related the term area compliance, $C_A = \Delta A/\Delta P$, is used to distinguish it from (volume) compliance. For instance, the systolic-diastolic differences in vessel area, ΔA, and pressure, ΔP, i.e., Pulse Pressure, when measured *in vivo*, can be used to obtain the area compliance. With modern echo-tracking techniques it is possible to determine vessel diameter noninvasively. In that case it is customary to report diameter compliance, $C_D = \Delta D/\Delta P$. The area compliance, C_A, and diameter compliance, C_D, are related by: $C_A = \pi \cdot D \cdot C_D/2$. The relations between the different expressions of compliance are given in Table 11.1.

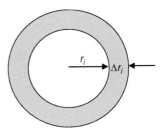

Fig. 11.2 For geometrically simple shapes, like blood vessels, measurement of changes in internal radius or diameter is sufficient to obtain (radial or diameter) compliance. In complex geometries as that of the heart this cannot be done

Table 11.1 Summary of structural[a] parameters of elasticity of blood vessels (length assumed constant)

	Volume	Area	Diameter	Radius
Compliance, C	$\Delta V/\Delta P$	$\Delta A/\Delta P = C_A$	$\tfrac{1}{2}\pi D \cdot (\Delta D/\Delta P) = \tfrac{1}{2}\pi D\, C_D$	$2\pi r \cdot (\Delta r/\Delta P) = 2\pi r\, C_r$
Elastance (stiffness), E	$\Delta P/\Delta V$	$\Delta P/\Delta A$	$(2/\pi D)(\Delta P/\Delta D)$	$(1/2\pi r)\cdot(\Delta P/\Delta r)$
Distensibility, K	$(\Delta V/\Delta P)/V$	$(\Delta A/\Delta P)/A$	$2\cdot(\Delta D/\Delta P)/D$	$2\cdot(\Delta r/\Delta P)/r$
Bulk Modulus, BM^b	$V\cdot\Delta P/\Delta V$	$A\cdot\Delta P/\Delta A$	$\tfrac{1}{2}D\cdot(\Delta P/\Delta D)$	$(\tfrac{1}{2}r)\cdot(\Delta P/\Delta r)^c$

$P, V, A, D,$ and r are pressure, volume, area, diameter and radius, respectively
[a]*Structural: parameters depend on organ geometry and material properties*
[b]*Bulk modulus or Volume elasticity*
[c]*The Pressure-Strain modulus or Peterson's modulus, $E_p = r_0 \cdot \Delta P/\Delta r_0 \approx 2/K \approx 2 \cdot BM$; where outer radius is used. In all other relations internal diameter or radius is used*

11.1.2   Distensibility and Bulk Modulus

Compliance and elastance depend on the size of the organ under study. To compare properties of blood vessels, or hearts from different animal species we can normalize compliance and elastance with respect to the volume of the organ. We use $C/V = (\Delta V/\Delta P)/V$, called distensibility, and the inverse, $E \cdot V = (\Delta P/\Delta V) \cdot V$, called bulk modulus or volume elasticity. Area and diameter distensibilities are also used, area distensibility is $(\Delta A/A)/\Delta P$ and diameter distensibility is $2 \cdot (\Delta D/D)/\Delta P$.

11.1.3   The Pressure-Strain Elastic Modulus

Peterson [3] introduced the pressure-strain elastic modulus in blood vessel research. This measure of blood vessel elasticity requires the measurement of diameter and pressure only, and can be used to compare vessels of different size. The pressure-strain elastic modulus, or Peterson modulus [3], is defined as $E_p = \Delta P/(\Delta r_o/r_o)$, where usually external radius, r_o, instead of the internal radius r_i is used. The E_p compares to the bulk modulus.

11.1.4   The Stiffness Index β

Compliance, distensibility and Peterson's modulus depend strongly on pressure. To describe the nonlinearity with a minimal number of parameters Hayashi et al. [4] introduced the stiffness index (or parameter) β, defined by the following relation

$$\ln(P/P_o) = \beta \cdot (D/D_0 - 1)$$

where P_o is a reference pressure (working point), typically mean pressure or 100 mmHg and D_0 is the outer diameter at that pressure. Basic research and also several clinical studies have shown that the stiffness parameter β does not depend on pressure within the physiological pressure range. However, outside the physiological pressure range, and for pressures far from the reference pressure P_o, the β-stiffness index is not pressure-independent anymore. A recent study by Spronck et al. showed that a correction can reduce the pressure dependency [5].

11.1.5   Describing the Pressure-Area or Pressure-Diameter Relation of Blood Vessels

The pressure-area and pressure-diameter relations of blood vessels have been described in a number of ways. At a working pressure the slope of the relation gives compliance. However, description of the relation over a range of pressures and

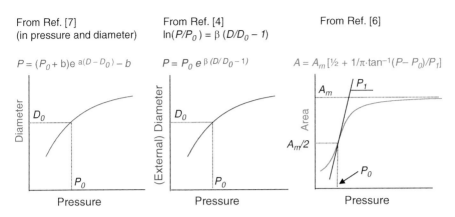

From Ref. [7]
(in pressure and diameter)

$P = (P_0 + b)e^{\,a(D - D_0)} - b$

From Ref. [4]
$\ln(P/P_0) = \beta\,(D/D_0 - 1)$

$P = P_0\,e^{\,\beta\,(D/D_0 - 1)}$

From Ref. [6]

$A = A_m[\tfrac{1}{2} + 1/\pi \cdot \tan^{-1}(P - P_0)/P_1]$

Fig. 11.3 Mathematical models of pressure-diameter and pressure-area relations

volumes gives more insight. Although these descriptions are phenomenological, we mention them here because of their general utility in arterial mechanics (Fig. 11.3).

The relation proposed by Langewouters et al. [6], describes the pressure-area relation over the widest range of pressures, i.e., from 0 to 200 mmHg. The relations of Fung [7] and Hayashi [4] can be applied over the physiological range of pressures. The D_0 and P_0 are reference values for the relations of Fung [7] and Hayashi [4]. In the relation by Langewouters $A_m/2$ and P_0 designate the inflection point and P_1 relates to the slope at the inflection point; A_m is the maximal, asymptotic, vessel area. The relations can also be presented in terms of volumes.

11.1.6 Addition of Compliances and Elastances

Let us consider the compliance of the entire aorta (Fig. 11.4), the individual compliances of three sections of the aorta are shown. In all sections the pressure is virtually equal. This implies that

$$C_1 + C_2 + C_3 = \Delta V_1\,/\,\Delta P + \Delta V_2\,/\,\Delta P + \Delta V_3\,/\,\Delta P$$
$$= \left(\Delta V_1 + \Delta V_2 + \Delta V_3\right)/\,\Delta P = \Delta V_{total}\,/\,\Delta P$$

or

$$C_1 + C_2 + C_3 = C_{total}$$

Thus, simple addition of compliances is allowed and the total compliance is their sum and is therefore larger than the individual compliances. For vessels in parallel compliances may also be added. Thus for the entire systemic circulation the total arterial compliance is the sum of all local compliances.

Fig. 11.4 Addition of
compliances. Note the
choice of axes. The
compliances of different
sections can be added to
obtain total aortic
compliance. The whole
graphs may also be
summed, by adding
volumes at similar
pressures (dashed lines).
The aa, da, and ab are
ascending, descending, and
abdominal aorta

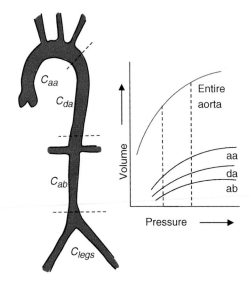

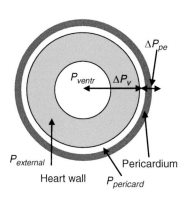

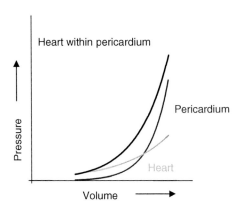

Fig. 11.5 Addition of elastances. Note the choice of axes. Heart and pericardium have their individual elastances and the total elastance of the heart in pericardium can be obtained directly from
addition of their individual elastances. Addition of the whole graphs is also allowed at similar
volumes. Thus, for structures within each other the elastances can be added directly to obtain overall elastance. Transmural pressure over the ventricular wall is $\Delta P_v = P_{ventr} - P_{pericard}$ and transmural
pressure of the pericardium is $\Delta P_{pe} = P_{pericard} - P_{external}$

If an organ with compliance C_1 is enveloped with an organ with compliance C_2,
the total volume change equals the individual volume changes (Fig. 11.5). In that
case the pressures need to be added. The distending pressure of the inner organ is
the luminal pressure minus the pressure in between the organs. The distending pressure of the outer organ is the pressure between the organs minus the pressure of the
environment. Thus, the distending pressure acting on the two organs combined, i.e.,

the luminal pressure minus the external pressure is the sum of the distending pressures of the individual organs.

$$1/C_{total} = 1/C_1 + 1/C_2$$

In this situation addition of the elastances is easier. As an example, we use the heart with pericardium. When the transmural pressure over the ventricular wall is ΔP_v and over the pericardium is ΔP_{pe}, for the heart inside the pericardium the transmural pressure equals $\Delta P_{total} = \Delta P_v + \Delta P_{pe}$. Therefore

$$E_{total} = \Delta P_{total} / \Delta V = \left(\Delta P_v + \Delta P_{pe}\right)/\Delta V = \Delta P_v / \Delta V + \Delta P_{pe} / \Delta V = E_v + E_{pe}$$

with E_v, and E_{pe} the ventricular elastance and pericardial elastance, respectively. The implicit assumption is that the intra-pericardial pressure, ΔP_{pe}, is the same at all locations. There are indications that the actual situation is more complex.

11.1.7   *Relating Compliance to Youngs Modulus*

The measurement of pressure-volume or pressure-radius relationships in arteries allows for derivation of compliance. However, as discussed in Chap. 9, estimation of Youngs modulus or incremental elastic modulus requires, in addition to radius and pressure, the measurement of wall thickness.

An accurate relation between the Youngs modulus and compliance, for a cylindrical vessel, is given by Love [8], and is used to model transverse impedance of an arterial segment (Appendix 3):

$$C_A = 3\pi \cdot r_i^2 \left(r_i + h\right)^2 / E_{inc}\left(2r_i + h\right)h = 3\pi \cdot r_i^2 \left(a + 1\right)^2 / E_{inc}\left(2a + 1\right), \text{with } a = r_i / h$$

For thin-walled vessels the equation reduces to:

$$C_A \approx k\left(\pi \cdot r_i^3\right)/\left(E_{inc} \cdot h\right), \text{with } k = 1.5$$

Sometimes $k = 2$ instead of 1.5 is used.

(Area) compliance, being a structural property, should be plotted against distending pressure. The incremental elastic modulus, being a material property, should be plotted against stress or strain. Plotting E_{inc} against pressure, as is often done, leads to misinterpretation of vessel properties.

An example where the structural aspect of compliance can be seen, is the comparison of the elastic properties of veins and arteries. The main reason why pressure-volume relations of veins differ from those of arteries is not the difference in wall material properties but their difference in wall thickness. More accurately stated, the ratio of wall thickness to radius is much smaller in veins than in arteries.

11.2   Physiological and Clinical Relevance

Compliance or elastance gives a quantitative measure of the mechanical and structural properties of an organ. Changes with disease and aging can be quantitatively investigated.

Arterial compliance decreases with age, and thus elastance (stiffness) increases with age and this is the main reason why arterial Pulse Pressure, Systolic minus Diastolic pressure, increases with age. The concomitant increase in systolic pressure is an extra load on the heart possibly leading to (concentric) hypertrophy. Concentric hypertrophy increases the elastance of the left ventricle in both diastole and systole. The increase in diastolic elastance results in decreased filling and filling volume can only return to near normal values with an increase in diastolic filling pressure (Fig. 11.6), which in turn may lead to increased pressure in the pulmonary veins and pulmonary edema.

With the now available wall-track technique arterial diameters can be measured noninvasively in superficial arteries and if pressure is determined simultaneously as well, diameter compliance can be derived in large groups of patients [2]. However, we should realize that this is the local area compliance of a single, often peripheral, artery, such as the carotid or radial artery, and may not be a good measure of aortic compliance or total arterial compliance (see below and Chap. 25).

Compliance and elastance depend on volume and pressure. Comparison should thus be carried out at similar pressure. However, compliance and elastance, in contrast to the Youngs modulus, also depend on the size of the organ. Distensibility and volume elasticity account for vessel size and are often used for comparisons of groups.

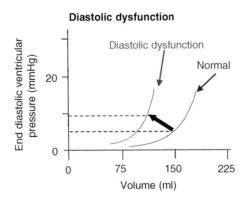

Fig. 11.6 Loss of diastolic ventricular compliance, i.e., increased diastolic elastance means that distension (filling) of the left ventricle in diastole becomes more difficult. Even a higher filling pressure is not capable to reach sufficient end-diastolic volume. An increase in diastolic filling pressure implies an increase in the pulmonary venous pressure, leading to pulmonary edema

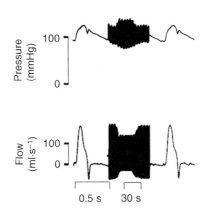

Fig. 11.7 Aortic pressure and flow in the intact dog during an acute decrease in aortic compliance, but unaltered peripheral resistance. The decreased compliance causes an increase in pulse pressure and decrease in flow. (Adapted from Ref. [9], by permission)

11.2.1 Buffering Function of Arterial Compliance

Arterial compliance is the buffering element for pressure so that the oscillations in pressure during the cardiac cycle are limited (Chap. 25). The Pulse Pressure in the aorta, the difference between systolic and diastolic aortic pressure, is about 40 mmHg in the young healthy adult. It was shown by Randall et al. [9], *in vivo*, that an acute reduction of total arterial compliance results in a considerable increase in Pulse Pressure (Fig. 11.7). The effect of long term, i.e., ~60 days reduction of aortic compliance to 60%, increased systolic pressure by 31 mmHg and diastolic pressure by 10 mmHg without affecting Cardiac Output and peripheral resistance [10].

It is now accepted knowledge that increased Pulse Pressure is the strongest pressure-based indicator of cardiac mortality and morbidity [11, 12]. It has also been reported that cardiac elastance is affected when arterial compliance is decreased [13]. The scientific community is becoming more and more convinced that decreased compliance plays a major role in hypertension. In Chap. 25 it is shown that the change in compliance, with age, is considerable and contributes importantly to Pulse Pressure.

References

1. Baan J, van der Velde ET, de Bruin HG, Smeenk GJ, Koops J, van Dijk AD, et al. Continuous measurement of left ventricular volume in animals and humans by conductance catheter. Circulation. 1984;70:812–23.
2. Hoeks AP, Brands PJ, Reneman RS. Assessment of the arterial distension waveform using Doppler signal processing. J Hypertens Suppl. 1992;10:S19–22.
3. Peterson LH, Jensen RE, Parnell J. Mechanical properties of arteries in vivo. Circ Res. 1960;8:622–39.
4. Hayashi K, Handa H, Nagasawa S, Okumura A, Moritake K. Stiffness and elastic behavior of human intracranial and extracranial arteries. J Biomech. 1980;13:175–84.

5. Spronck B, Avolio AP, Tan I, Butlin M, Reesink KD, Delhaas T. Arterial stiffness index beta and cardio-ankle vascular index inherently depend on blood pressure but can be readily corrected. J Hypertens. 2017;35:98–104.
6. Langewouters GJ, Wesseling KH, Goedhard WJ. The static elastic properties of 45 human thoracic and 20 abdominal aortas in vitro and the parameters of a new model. J Biomech. 1984;17:425–35.
7. Fung YC. Biomechanics. mechanical properties of living tissues. New York & Heidelberg: Springer; 1981.
8. Love AEH. A treatise on the mathematical theory of elasticity. 4th ed. Cambridge: Cambridge University Press; 1952.
9. Randall OS, van den Bos GC, Westerhof N. Systemic compliance: does it play a role in the genesis of essential hypertension? Cardiovasc Res. 1984;18:455–62.
10. Ioannou CV, Morel DR, Katsamouris AN, Katranitsa S, Startchik I, Kalangos A, et al. Left ventricular hypertrophy induced by reduced aortic compliance. J Vasc Res. 2009;46:417–25.
11. Benetos A, Safar M, Rudnichi A, Smulyan H, Richard JL, Ducimetieere P, et al. Pulse pressure: a predictor of long-term cardiovascular mortality in a French male population. Hypertension. 1997;30:1410–5.
12. Mitchell GF, Moye LA, Braunwald E, Rouleau JL, Bernstein V, Geltman EM, et al. Sphygmomanometrically determined pulse pressure is a powerful independent predictor of recurrent events after myocardial infarction in patients with impaired left ventricular function. Circulation. 1997;96:4254–60.
13. Kawaguchi M, Hay I, Fetics B, Kass DA. Combined ventricular systolic and arterial stiffening in patients with heart failure and preserved ejection fraction: implications for systolic and diastolic reserve limitations. Circulation. 2003;107:714–20.

Chapter 12
Wave Travel and Reflection

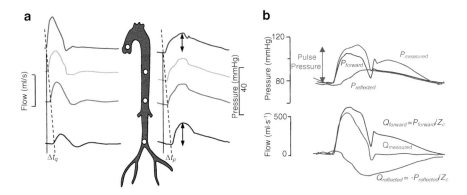

Panel A. Schematic presentation of pressure and flow along the aorta. Flow velocity is depicted to make the amplitude comparable at the different locations. Volume flow equals velocity times cross-sectional area. Both pressure and flow are travelling waves: they vary in time over the cardiac cycle and depend on location. The time delay in flow Δt_q or pressure Δt_p allows calculation of Pulse Wave Velocity, PWV = distance/Δt. The increase in pulse pressure towards the periphery, called amplification, results from wave reflections. The different wave shapes of pressure and flow also result from wave reflection. Reflections occur at all changes in arterial size, bifurcations, and changes in wall properties. Panel B shows the separation of proximal aortic pressure and flow in their forward and reflected components. Reflections of pressure and flow are equal in magnitude but 'inversed': when positive for pressure, they are negative for flow. The forward pressure and flow are related by characteristic impedance and the reflected pressure and flow are also related by characteristic impedance but they are 'inversed'.

© Springer International Publishing AG, part of Springer Nature 2019
N. Westerhof et al., *Snapshots of Hemodynamics*,
https://doi.org/10.1007/978-3-319-91932-4_12

12.1 Description

Pressure and flow are waves by definition, they change in time and travel over the vascular system. Both pressure and flow waves are reflected at all locations where geometry and vascular (wall) properties change, such as bifurcations and changes in vessel diameter and wall stiffness. Wave travel and reflection give information on the arterial system.

Characteristic impedance, Z_c, and wave speed, c, are two important vessel parameters describing wave transmission and reflection. Both Z_c, and c depend on vessel properties (Appendix 3), and can be derived using so-called wave transmission theory, in analogy to what happens in telegraph lines or antenna cables for the transmission of electromagnetic waves.

The characteristic impedance equals $Z_c = \sqrt{Z_l' \cdot Z_t'}$, with Z_l' and Z_t' the longitudinal and transverse impedance per unit length as given in Appendix 3 and shown in Fig. 12.1. Inserting the relations for *large* vessels (large cross-sectional area and large Womersley's α, Chap. 8), $Z_l' \approx i\omega L' \approx i\omega\rho/A$, since $R' \approx 0$ (Poiseuille's law). Also in large vessels, the wall is close to purely elastic (Appendix 3) and $Z_t' \approx 1/i\omega C' = 1/i\omega C_A$ with $C_A = \Delta A/\Delta P$ (Appendix 3) and

$$Z_c = \sqrt{Z_l' \cdot Z_t'} \approx \sqrt{L'/C_A} = \sqrt{\rho\Delta P/(\Delta A \cdot A)}$$

Vessel segment

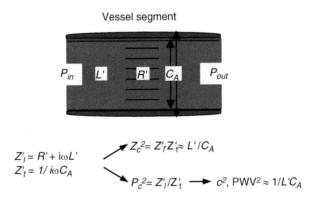

$$Z_l' = R' + i\omega L'$$
$$Z_t' = 1/i\omega C_A$$

$$Z_c^2 = Z_l' Z_t' \approx L'/C_A$$

$$P_c^2 = Z_l'/Z_t' \longrightarrow c^2,\ PWV^2 \approx 1/L'C_A$$

Fig. 12.1 The arterial segment is a short and supposedly uniform part of a blood vessel. The segment stands at the basis of pressure-flow relations (characteristic impedance) and pressure-pressure and flow-flow relations (wave speed) when no reflections are present. The longitudinal and transverse impedances per unit length Z_l' and Z_t' are frequency dependent. (see text and Appendix 3), and they determine the vessel's characteristic impedance $Z_c^2 = Z_l' Z_t'$ and wave propagation (speed and damping) $P_c^2 = Z_l'/Z_t'$, with wave speed $c = i\omega/\text{im}[P_c]$ called phase velocity. In large arteries $Z_l' = i\omega\rho/A = i\omega L'$, with L' inertia, and $Z_t' = 1/i\omega C' = 1/i\omega C_A$, with C' compliance per length. The Z_c and c are then frequency independent with $Z_c^2 = L'/C_A$ and $c^2 = 1/L'C_A$. Thus, the foot-foot Pulse Wave Velocity, which is minimally affected by reflections, equals c

Thus, for large vessels Z_c is a (mathematically) real number and independent of frequency. Characteristic impedance accounts for the combined effect of the accelerating blood mass (inertia) and the vessel compliance vessel storing blood.

The wave propagation constant $P_c = \sqrt{Z_l'/Z_t'}$ describes transmission of waves. The propagation constant consists of a real part (wave damping) and imaginary part, $\mathrm{im}[P_c]$, the wave speed. Since wave propagation is virtually always determined in large vessels (large α) we can insert the above relations of Z_l' and Z_t', and $P_c = \sqrt{Z_l'/Z_t'} \approx i\omega \cdot \sqrt{L' C_A}$. The wave speed, called phase velocity, $c = i\omega/\mathrm{im}[P_c] = i\omega/[i\omega \cdot \sqrt{L' C_A}] = 1/\sqrt{L' C_A}$. The phase velocity holds when no reflections are present and depends on local vessel properties only. Inserting the values of large vessels, as above results in

$$c = \sqrt{A / \rho \cdot C_A} = \sqrt{A \cdot \Delta P / \Delta A \cdot \rho}$$

The $c = \sqrt{A/\rho \cdot C_A}$ is the equation for Pulse Wave Velocity as introduced by Frank and later by Bramwell-Hill (Chap. 21). The wave speed can also be written as $c = \sqrt{V \Delta P/\Delta V \cdot \rho} = \sqrt{K/\rho}$ with $K = A\Delta P/\Delta A = V\Delta P/\Delta V$ the bulk modulus (Chap. 11).

Using $A = \pi r_i^2$ and thus $\Delta A = 2\pi r_i \cdot \Delta r_i$, we arrive at $c = \sqrt{r_i \cdot \Delta P/2\Delta r_i \cdot \rho}$. Using $C_A \approx 3\pi \cdot r_i^3/2E_{inc} \cdot h$ (Chap. 11) and from Womersley's theory $L' = 4\rho/3\pi \cdot r_i^2$ (Appendix 3), gives

$$\mathrm{PWV} = 1/\sqrt{C_A L'} = \sqrt{E_{inc} \cdot h / 2r_i \cdot \rho}$$

Using $\Delta P/\Delta r_i = h/r_i \cdot (\Delta\sigma/\Delta r_i)$ also gives $c = \sqrt{E_{inc} \cdot h/2r_i\rho}$. This is the Moens-Korteweg equation for Pulse Wave Velocity (Chap. 21). Sometimes $L' = \rho/\pi \cdot r_i^2$ is used instead of $L' = 4\rho/3\pi \cdot r_i^2$, which leads to $c = \sqrt{2E_{inc} \cdot h/3r_i\rho}$. The difference in the square root of 2/3 and 1/2 is about 15%.

The choice of the formula of wave speed depends on the information desired. If local compliance is to be derived, the Frank/Bramwell-Hill equation is preferred. If the material constant, E_{inc}, is to be obtained the Moens-Korteweg equation is used.

It should be emphasized that the derivations of Z_c and PWV pertain to large uniform vessels, without reflected waves. If reflections contribute to the pressure or flow waves the apparent wave velocity, c_{app}, is found which may differ considerably from the phase velocity, c. This is the reason that PWV is measured from the foot of the waves since the foot is mainly determined by the higher frequencies and assumed to be little affected by reflections [1, 2].

It can be seen that $c/Z_c = A/\rho$, and in the cgs system with $\rho \sim 1$ g·cm^{-3} it holds that $c/Z_c \approx A$. When flow velocity (Q/A) rather than volume flow is used $c = Z_c$ $/\rho \approx Z_c$.

12.1.1 Reflection of Waves

Reflections pertain to waves only (not mean pressure and flow) and occur at all discontinuities. If no reflections exist the measured pressure and flow would have the same wave shape, and are related by characteristic impedance as '$Q_{measured}$' = '$P_{measured}$'$/Z_c$. The difference in wave shape of measured pressure and flow results from wave reflection.

We can quantify the amount of reflection by the reflection coefficient (Fig. 12.2). The *local* pressure reflection coefficient for pressure, Γ_p, is calculated from the distal and proximal characteristic impedances

$$\Gamma_{p,l}(\omega) = \left(Z_{c,distal}(\omega) - Z_{c,proximal}(\omega)\right) / \left(Z_{c,distal}(\omega) + Z_{c,proximal}(\omega)\right)$$
$$\approx \left(Z_{c,distal} - Z_{c,proximal}\right) / \left(Z_{c,distal} + Z_{c,proximal}\right)$$

In large arteries, the characteristic impedances are practically frequency independent and $\Gamma_{p,l}(\omega) \approx \Gamma_{p,l}$, thus also frequency independent. Flow waves are reflected as well and the local reflection coefficient for flow is:

$$\Gamma_{q,l} = -\Gamma_{p,l}$$

The *global* reflection coefficient depends on the whole distal load of the segment, $Z_{load}(\omega)$, which is the input impedance of the distal vasculature, and is frequency dependent (Fig. 12.2).

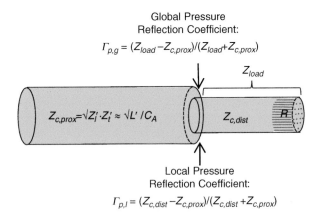

Global Pressure
Reflection Coefficient:

$\Gamma_{p,g} = (Z_{load} - Z_{c,prox}) / (Z_{load} + Z_{c,prox})$

Z_{load}

$Z_{c,prox} = \sqrt{Z'_l \cdot Z'_t} \approx \sqrt{L' / C_A}$

$Z_{c,dist}$

R

Local Pressure
Reflection Coefficient:

$\Gamma_{p,l} = (Z_{c,dist} - Z_{c,prox}) / (Z_{c,dist} + Z_{c,prox})$

Fig. 12.2 Reflections are due to discontinuities. The local reflection depends on local vessel properties: the characteristic impedances, proximal and distal of the discontinuity. The overall or global reflection coefficient depends on the characteristic impedance of the proximal vessel and load impedance, i.e., the input impedance of the distal vascular bed. The local and the global reflection coefficient for flow equal $\Gamma_q = -\Gamma_p$. When the distal vessel is larger in diameter the $\Gamma_{p,l}$ becomes negative and the $\Gamma_{q,l}$ is positive. See also Fig. 12.3

$$\Gamma_{p,g}(\omega) = \left(Z_{load}(\omega) - Z_c\right) / \left(Z_{load}(\omega) + Z_c\right)$$

and again

$$\Gamma_{q,g}(\omega) = -\Gamma_{p,g}(\omega)$$

The global reflection coefficient quantifies the reflection at a certain location due to the total system distal to the segment under study and is always frequency dependent. The global reflection coefficient should be calculated for each harmonic obtained by Fourier Analysis of pressure and flow (Appendix 1). At more distal locations with smaller vessels the Z_c is not frequency-independent either and $Z_c(\omega)$ requires longitudinal impedance (Oscillatory flow theory, Chap. 8, Appendix 3) and transverse impedance (frequency dependent Youngs modulus (Chap. 10 and Appendix 3). Calculations are to be performed for each frequency of the $Z_{load}(\omega)$ and the $Z_c(\omega)$.

To calculate the local reflection coefficient at a bifurcation, a mother vessel, $Z_{c,m}$, with two daughter vessels, the distal characteristic impedance is the inversed sum of the two characteristic impedances (see Chap. 6), i.e., distal characteristic impedance equals $1/Z_{c,distal} = 1/Z_{c,d1} + 1/Z_{c,d2}$, with $Z_{c,d}$ characteristic impedances of the daughters. For two equal daughters total $Z_{c,distal} = \frac{1}{2} \cdot Z_{c,d}$. For large vessels (large Womersley's α), characteristic impedance can calculated from $L' = 4\rho/3A$ and $C_A = 3\pi \cdot r_i^2(r_i + h)^2/E_{inc} \cdot (2r_i + h)h$ with $a = r_i/h$ (Chap. 11). Further assuming that the wall thickness to radius ratio (h/r_i) and Youngs modulus (E_{inc}) of mother and daughters are equal leads to a characteristic impedance inversely proportional to area, $Z_c = k/A$. The local pressure reflection coefficient is $\Gamma_{p,l} = (\frac{1}{2} \cdot Z_{c,d} - Z_{c,m})/(\frac{1}{2} \cdot Z_{c,d} + Z_{c,m}) = (1 - 2A_d/A_m)/(1 + 2A_d/A_m)$. Thus, when the summed area of both daughters $2A_d$ equals the area of the mother vessel A_m, the reflection coefficient would be zero (Fig. 12.3). When the summed area of the daughters is larger than that of the mother the pressure reflection coefficient is negative, and the flow reflection coefficient positive.

Womersley used for two equal daughters $Z_m/Z_d = 2r_{i,d}^2 c_m/r_{i,m}^2 c_d$ with c wave speed, with an extra assumption that $c_m/c_d = \sqrt{r_{i,d}/r_{i,m}}$. This leads to $Z_m/Z_d = 2r_{i,d}^2 r_{i,d}^{0.5}/r_{i,m}^2 r_{i,m}^{0.5} = 2r_{i,d}^{2.5}/r_{i,m}^{2.5}$. The local pressure reflection coefficient is then $\Gamma_{p,l} = (1 - Z_m/Z_d)/(1 + Z_m/Z_d) = (1 - 2r_{i,d}^{2.5}/r_{i,m}^{2.5})/(1 + 2r_{i,d}^{2.5}/r_{i,m}^{2.5})$ and the $\Gamma_{p,l} = 0$ for $2r_{i,d}^{2.5}/r_{i,m}^{2.5} = 1$ which corresponds with an area ratio for $2\pi r_{i,d}^2/\pi r_{i,m}^2 \approx 1.15$ (Fig. 12.3). In smaller vessels, when Womersley's α is not large the calculation of the local reflection coefficient requires information of $Z_l(\omega)$ and $Z_t(\omega)$ (Appendix 3) and the minimum of the reflection coefficient is found at larger area ratios and depends on α [3]. Murray's law (Chap. 2) predicts similar ratios.

In summary, both the modulus of the local and the global reflection coefficient are the same for pressure and flow (same magnitude of reflection) but the phase angle of the reflection coefficients of pressure and flow differ by 180 degrees ('upside down') [4]. This implies that the reflected pressure and flow waves are inversed with respect to each other.

Fig. 12.3 Local reflection coefficients at a symmetrical bifurcation: a mother vessel with cross-sectional area A_m and two equal daughters each with areas A_d. When no losses are present, and characteristic impedances are real numbers, an area ratio $2A_d/A_m = 1$ implies that the reflection coefficient is zero. For area ratio < 1 the pressure reflection coefficient is positive, $\Gamma_{p,l} > 0$. For an area ratio > 1 reflection is negative $\Gamma_{p,l} > 0$ (see phase angle). Womersley based the calculation on oscillatory flow theory and found that the reflection coefficient depends on parameter α. See text for details

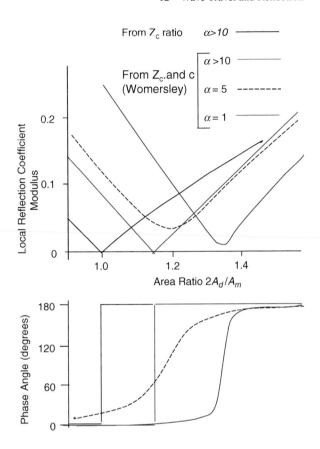

In reality, reflected waves result from many local reflections, by summation giving a compound reflected wave. However, calculation of such a sum, consisting of forward, reflected and re-reflected waves is not feasible and the compound reflected wave is best obtained by the calculation of the global reflection coefficient. Since the global reflection coefficient is frequency dependent the (compound) reflected wave is out of phase with the forward wave. The phase difference relates to a time shift, and the time shift may suggest that the reflected wave appears to reflect from a certain distance. The time shift, thus the apparent distance, can depend on location but does not systematically decrease towards the periphery. Thus at more distal locations a time shift remains resulting in an elusive reflection site or 'horizon effect' [5–7].

12.1.2   Transmission of Waves

Next to reflections, also transmission of waves (Fig. 12.4) occurs at discontinuities. The pressure transmission coefficient is $1 + \Gamma_p$ since the measured and also the transmitted pressure wave is the sum of the forward and reflected pressure wave.

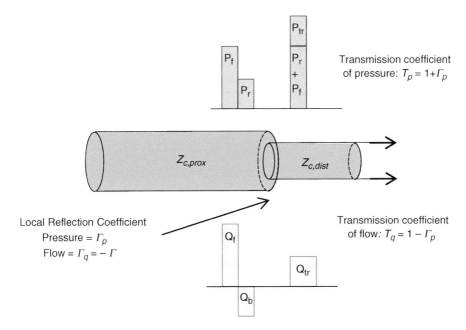

Fig. 12.4 Pressure and flow waves are reflected and transmitted at discontinuities. The local reflection coefficient depends om distal and proximal characteristic impedance. The local reflection coefficients of pressure $\Gamma_{p,l}$ and flow $\Gamma_{q,l} = -\Gamma_{p,l}$ are similar in magnitude but opposite in phase. Transmission of pressure is $T_{p,l} = 1 + \Gamma_{p,l}$, i.e., $P_{transmitted} = (1 + \Gamma_{p,l}) \cdot P_f = P_f + P_r$, with P_f and P_r forward and reflected pressure. Flow transmission equals $Q_{transmitted} = (1 + \Gamma_q) \cdot Q_f = Q_f(1 - \Gamma_p) = Q_f - Q_r$. Local reflection, with $Z_{c,dist} > Z_{c,prox}$, results in a $\Gamma_p > 0$ thus increased transmitted pressure waves, but the transmitted flow amplitude decreases. When $Z_{c,dist} < Z_{c,prox}$ the transmitted pressure is decreased but flow increased

With a local reflection coefficient of $\Gamma_p = 0.1$ the reflected pressure wave is 10% of the forward wave and the transmitted wave is $1 + \Gamma_p = 1.1$ times the forward pressure wave. For flow the transmission coefficient is $1 + \Gamma_q = 1 - \Gamma_p$ and the transmitted flow wave is thus 90%. With reflection at a bifurcation this total transmitted flow is further divided between the two daughters, for instance with two equal daughters the transmitted flow wave in each daughter is 45%.

12.1.3   Derivation of Characteristic Impedance

In the calculation of local reflection, the proximal and distal characteristic impedances need to be known. To calculate the global reflection the proximal characteristic impedance and distal input impedance are required. Since, for high frequencies, corresponding to short time scales, the arterial tree approaches a reflection-less system, the input impedance at high frequencies is close to the characteristic impedance of the vessel where the impedance is determined (Chap. 24). This allows for an

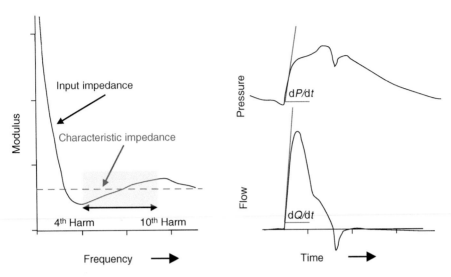

Fig. 12.5 The characteristic impedance can be estimated from the input impedance modulus at high frequencies: Z_c = averaged $|Z_{in}|$ for harmonics 4–10 (colored section). Characteristic impedance can also be estimated from the slope of the pressure and flow during their initial increase: $Z_c = dP/dt/dQ/dt = dP/dQ$. Both methods assume reflections to be negligible

estimation of characteristic impedance from the modulus of the input impedance at high frequencies (Fig. 12.5, left). In practice, the averaged impedance modulus between the fourth to tenth harmonic is used [1].

It is also assumed that during the early increase of pressure and flow reflections play a minor role, and that pressure and flow are related through the characteristic impedance [1, 8]. This allows calculation of characteristic impedance from the ratio of the slopes of (aortic) pressure and flow (Fig. 12.5, right).

12.1.4   Forward and Reflected Waves

The measured pressure and flow are not similar in shape since they consist of forward and reflected components (Fig. 12.6 panels a and b), and their sum is the actually measured wave (Fig. 12.6, panel c). Measured pressure and flow, P_m and Q_m are both the sum of a forward and reflected (reflected) waves, P_f, P_r, Q_f, Q_b.

$$P_m = P_f + P_r \text{ and } Q_m = Q_f + Q_r$$

The (local) characteristic impedance gives the relation between pressure and flow of a vessel without reflections with $P_f = Z_c \cdot Q_f$, and $P_r = -Z_c \cdot Q_r$. The minus sign results from the fact that flow is reflected 'upside down' in comparison with pressure. For

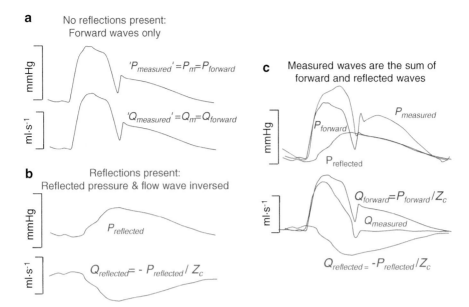

Fig. 12.6 Panel **a**: If a (large) tube is reflection-less the pressure and flow wave have the same wave shape and the pressure and flow only consist of forward waves, with $P_{measured} = P_{forward} = Z_c \cdot Q_{forward}$, with Z_c characteristic impedance of the tube. Panel **b**: With reflections present the reflected pressure and flow waves are similar in shape but they are inversed with respect to each other. It holds that $P_{forward} = Z_c \cdot Q_{forward}$, and $P_{reflected} = -Z_c \cdot Q_{reflected}$. Panel **c**: The measured pressure and flow waves are the sum of forward and reflected waves. The reflected waves are compound waves originating from many reflection sites in the arterial system

large arteries, when Z_c is real the calculations can be performed in the time domain. Substituting Q_f and Q_r into the above equations leads to [4]:

$$P_f(t) = Z_c \cdot Q_f(t) = \left(P_m(t) + Z_c \cdot Q_m(t) \right)/2$$
and
$$P_r(t) = -Z_c \cdot Q_r(t) = \left(P_m(t) - Z_c \cdot Q_m(t) \right)/2$$

In smaller vessels, the characteristic impedance is a frequency-dependent quantity (real and imaginary part, see Appendix 3). In that case the analysis should be done in the frequency domain, requiring Fourier analysis (Appendix 1) of the measured pressure and flow waves, and subsequent application of the above relations for each harmonic and $Z_c(\omega)$, and finally inverse Fourier to reconstruct the time functions of the pressure and flow waves (Appendix 1).

The above relations form the basis of wave separation (Chap. 22). Forward and reflected wave analysis pertains to the pulsatile part of pressure and flow. The question how mean pressure and flow can be separated in their forward and reflected components was recently solved by Mynard et al. [9]. A simple easy approximate approach is to assume that for very low frequencies all local pressure variations occur simultaneously and arterial system can be seen as a very short piece of aorta, with characteristic impedance Z_c, loaded with the peripheral resistance, R_p. The reflection coefficient then can be estimated as $\Gamma_p = (R_p - Z_c)/(R_p + Z_c)$. With R_p about 15 times Z_c the $\Gamma_p \approx 0.87 = P_r/P_f$, and with $P_m = P_f + P_r = P_f + 0.87 \cdot P_f = 1.87 \cdot P_f$, thus $P_f = 1/1.87 \cdot P_m = 0.53 \cdot P_m$ and $P_r = 0.47 \cdot P_m$, values close to those reported by Maynard [10].

In Wave Intensity Analysis the forward and reflected waves can be calculated as well. Separation of dP/dt and dQ/dt as given above into their forward and reflected components dP_+/dt, dP_-/dt, dQ_+/dt, and dQ_-/dt, and subsequent integration leads to the forward and reflected waves of pressure and flow (see Chap. 23).

In diastole and aortic valves without insufficiency, measured aortic flow is essentially zero: forward and reflected flow waves 'self-cancel'. This 'cancelling' was assumed by some to be impossible [11]. However, self-cancelling waves are perfectly in line with wave theory, since the compound forward and compound reflected *flow* waves cancel when reflecting against a closed valve. Compare a single tube, where at the closed end measured pressure is large but measured flow is zero: the forward and reflected flow waves are 'self-cancelling'.

12.1.5 Amplification of Pressure, and Form Factor

The systolic and Pulse Pressure increase in amplitude while travelling towards the periphery. This phenomenon is called amplification. Diastolic pressure decreases little. Pressure amplification was first shown by Hamilton [12]. Luchsinger and Latham [13, 14] showed using Fourier analysis that the lower harmonics of pressure all increase in amplitude while travelling towards the periphery. Not only reflections at the periphery (peripheral resistance) determine wave amplification but vessel compliance also plays a role. This is exemplified by the data of Latham et al. [14] who measured pressures between aortic arch and iliac artery, during the Valsalva maneuver. They found that pulse wave velocity decreased from 5.63 m/s to 3.85 m/s, i.e. aortic compliance increased and amplification increased from 9% to 18%. O'Rourke et al. [15] showed that amplification decreases with increased aortic stiffness (PWV) and with age (increased PWV), see Fig. 12.7. These findings suggest that amplification is mainly determined by arterial elasticity.

The so-called form factor of pressure relates systolic and diastolic pressure with mean blood pressure as follows: $P_{mean} = ff \cdot PP + P_{diastolic}$, with PP Pulse Pressure. The pressure form factor in large arteries (brachial artery) is about 1/3 (or 2/5, [16]) and in the aorta it is about ½. Thus, in the brachial artery, with $ff = 1/3$, we find: $P_{mean,bra} = (P_{systolic,bra} - P_{diastolic,bra})/3 + P_{diastolic,bra} = (P_{systolic,bra} + 2P_{diastolic,bra})/3$. For the aorta with ff about ½ the $P_{mean,ao} = (P_{systolic,ao} + P_{diastolic,ao})/2$ [17].

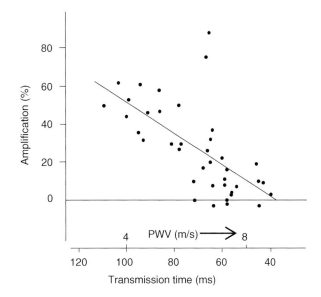

Fig. 12.7 Relation between pressure amplification (%) and PWV (aortic stiffness) expressed as travel time from aortic arch to iliac artery. Increased stiffness, as in aging, causes a decrease in pressure amplification. (Based on data from Ref. [15])

It has been shown that mean and diastolic pressure are similar in brachial artery and aorta. This allows for estimation of systolic pressure in the aorta.

$$P_{systolic,ao} = 2P_{mean,ao} - P_{diastolic,ao} = 2P_{mean,bra} - P_{diastolic,bra}$$

with systolic and diastolic brachial artery pressures 120 mmHg and 80 mmHg, $P_{mean,bra} = 93$ mmHg. The systolic pressure in the aorta is now $P_{systolic,\ aorta} = 2 \cdot 93 - 80 = 106$ mmHg. Thus, using the form factors it is possible to derive values for aortic systolic and diastolic pressures from calibrated peripheral (e.g., brachial) pressure.

With the mean and diastolic pressures the same in brachial artery and aorta it holds that aortic $PP_{ao} = (P_{mean,ao} - P_{diastole,ao})/ff_{ao} = (P_{mean,bra} - P_{diastole,bra})/ff_{ao}$ and $PP_{brach} = (P_{mean,bra} - P_{diastole,bra})/ff_{bra}$ and thus $PP_{ao} \cdot ff_{ao} = PP_{bra} \cdot ff_{bra}$, or $PP_{brach}/PP_{ao} = ff_{ao}/ff_{bra} = (1/2)/(1/3) = 1.5$. Thus Pulse Pressure amplification is 50%. It should be realized that amplification decreases with arterial stiffness (age) implying that the form factor changes as well.

12.2 Physiological and Clinical Relevance

When the heart ejects, it has to accelerate the blood into a compliant aorta. Thus, what the heart encounters first during ejection is the combination of the effects of compliance and inertance. Inertance increases the load but compliance makes it

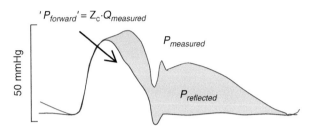

Fig. 12.8 Up till about the 1970 it was assumed that only pressures reflect while flow was unaffected by reflections, The reflected pressure wave was erroneously assumed to be the difference between measured pressure and measured flow times characteristic impedance ('$P_{forward}$')

easier to eject. The combined effect is given by the characteristic impedance $Z_c = \sqrt{L'/C_A}$, with L' inertia (Chap. 7) and C_A area compliance (Chap. 11). The Z_c is called characteristic impedance because it is characteristic for the vessel under study and gives the relation between pressure and flow when reflections are absent. Z_c for large vessels is a (mathematical) real number independent of frequency. If we take the proximal aorta as an example, the ventricle encounters, during the initial phase of ejection, an impedance to flow that is the characteristic impedance of the proximal aorta. If the heart were loaded with the peripheral resistance the load would be much higher, because the systemic peripheral resistance is about 15 times higher than aortic characteristic impedance.

For an infinitely long aorta or a reflection-less arterial system measured pressure and flow would have similar shape with $P(t) = Z_c \cdot Q(t)$. Up till about 1970 it was assumed that only pressure wave was subject to reflections, see Fig. 12.8 [4, 18]. However, now we know that both pressure and flow waves consist of forward and reflected components, and in large arteries the separation into forward and reflected waves is simple (see above).

12.2.1 Wave Speed and Reflection

In large vessels where the wave speed is usually studied (aorta, carotid artery, and large leg and arm arteries, large Womersley's α) the viscous properties of blood and the viscosity of the wall are small so that damping of the waves plays only a small role. In these arteries, the compliance and inertance together determine the wave speed and the characteristic impedance. When smaller vessels are studied the situation gets much more complex, the wave is not only transmitted but damped as well.

The phase velocity in large vessels is $c = 1/\sqrt{L'C_A}$. The PWV is equal to c when no reflections are present. Since, for high frequencies, corresponding to short time scales, the arterial tree approaches a reflection-less system (Fig. 12.5), rapid changes in the signals may be assumed not affected by reflections and PWV equals the phase velocity c. This is why the foot of the pressure or flow wave should be used in the measurement of PWV. PWV can be written as PWV $= \sqrt{A/\rho \cdot C_A} = \sqrt{A \cdot \Delta P/\Delta A \cdot \rho}$ (Frank/Bramwell-Hill) or PWV $= \sqrt{E_{inc} \cdot h/2r_i \cdot \rho}$ (Moens-Korteweg). PWV can be measured (noninvasively) using pressures, flows (Figure in the Box), or diameter signals at two locations, and can give information on vessel compliance, C_A, a structural property, and on E_{inc}, a material property. However, it should be remembered that when aortic PWV is measured it is assumed that the aorta is uniform, i.e., the same diameter and wall properties.

A decrease in aortic compliance with age by a factor of 4 increases the pulse wave velocity by about a factor 2, assuming constant radius of the vessel. Decreased aortic compliance also results in increased characteristic impedance, which affects early ejection [19] and reflections. Both the decrease in compliance and the increase in characteristic impedance lead to a higher Pulse Pressure if ejection flow is unaltered.

In the aorta and conduit arteries the local pressure reflection coefficients are typically about 0.1 [2, 3], but both positive and negative values have been reported. The increase in pressure amplitude towards the periphery, called pressure amplification, may, in part, be the result from many small local reflections, but data are missing to quantify this effect.

To explain reflections on the basis of the many local reflection sites is extremely complex, therefore the global reflection coefficient is a better parameter to understand reflections.

Amplification of the pulse pressure appears to inversely associate with age and (mean) pressure, while reflections are increased. Amplification depends not only on the magnitude of the reflected waves but also on their timing thus on wave speed. Increased stiffness with age results in increased wave speed and increased reflections (Chap. 22), but microvascular resistance and arterial geometry change little.

The systemic arterial tree has often been modeled with a uniform tube (the aorta) with a resistor or Windkessel at its distal end (Chap. 26). However, reflections occur at every bifurcation and discontinuity. Therefore, the reflected wave is a compound wave consisting of many individually reflected and re-reflected waves and a single reflection site is elusive [6]. This limits the single tube as model of the systemic arterial system. Tube models are discussed in Chap. 26. The Windkessel, is a lumped arterial model, and wave reflections are nonexistent.

It should be realized that the hemodynamic approach above does not take into account flow profile disturbance such as eddies and energy losses [20].

References

1. Nichols WW, O'Rourke MF, Charalambos Vlachopoulos C. McDonald's blood flow in arteries. 6th ed. Boca Raton: CRC Press Taylor & Francis; 2011.
2. Milnor WR. Hemodynamics. 2nd ed. Baltimore & London: Williams & Wilkins.; 1989.
3. Womersley JR. Oscillatory flow in arteries. II. The reflection of the pulse wave at junctions and rigid inserts in the arterial system. Phys Med Biol. 1958;2:313–23.

4. Westerhof N, Sipkema P, van den Bos GC, Elzinga G. Forward and backward waves in the arterial system. Cardiovasc Res. 1972;6:648–56.
5. Sipkema P, Westerhof N. Effective length of the arterial system. Ann Biomed Eng. 1975;3:296–307.
6. Westerhof BE, van den Wijngaard JP, Murgo JP, Westerhof N. Location of a reflection site is elusive: consequences for the calculation of aortic pulse wave velocity. Hypertension. 2008;52:478–83.
7. Davies JE, Alastruey J, Francis DP, Hadjiloizou N, Whinnett ZI, Manisty CH, et al. Attenuation of wave reflection by wave entrapment creates a "horizon effect" in the human aorta. Hypertension. 2012;60:778–85.
8. Dujardin JP, Stone DN. Characteristic impedance of the proximal aorta determined in the time and frequency domain: a comparison. Med Biol Eng Comput. 1981;19:565–8.
9. Mynard JP, Smolich JJ. Wave potential and the one-dimensional windkessel as a wave-based paradigm of diastolic arterial hemodynamics. Am J Physiol Heart Circ Physiol. 2014;307:H307–18.
10. Mynard JP, Smolich JJ. Novel wave power analysis linking pressure-flow waves, wave potential, and the forward and backward components of hydraulic power. Am J Physiol Heart Circ Physiol. 2016;310:H1026–38.
11. Davies JE, Baksi J, Francis DP, Hadjiloizou N, Whinnett ZI, Manisty CH, et al. The arterial reservoir pressure increases with aging and is the major determinant of the aortic augmentation index. Am J Physiol Heart Circ Physiol. 2010;298:H580–6.
12. Hamilton WF, Dow P. An experimental study of the standing waves in the pulse propagated through the aorta. Am J Phys. 1939;125:48–59.
13. Luchsinger PC, Snell RE, Patel DJ, Fry DL. Instantaneous pressure distribution along the human aorta. Circ Res. 1964;15:503–10.
14. Latham RD, Westerhof N, Sipkema P, Rubal BJ, Reuderink P, Murgo JP. Regional wave travel and reflections along the human aorta: a study with six simultaneous micromanometric pressures. Circulation. 1985;72:1257–69.
15. O'Rourke MF, Blazek JV, Morreels CL Jr, Krovetz LJ. Pressure wave transmission along the human aorta. Changes with age and in arterial degenerative disease. Circ Res. 1968;23:567–79.
16. Bos WJ, Verrij E, Vincent HH, Westerhof BE, Parati G, van Montfrans GA. How to assess mean blood pressure properly at the brachial artery level. J Hypertens. 2007;25:751–5.
17. Kelly R, Fitchett D. Noninvasive determination of aortic input impedance and external left ventricular power output: a validation and repeatability study of a new technique. J Am Coll Cardiol. 1992;20:952–63.
18. Kouchoukos NT, Sheppard LC, McDonald DA. Estimation of stroke volume in the dog by a pulse contour method. Circ Res. 1970;26:611–23.
19. Mitchell GF, Lacourcière Y, Ouellet JP, Izzo JL Jr, Neutel J, Kerwin LJ, et al. Determinants of elevated pulse pressure in middle-aged and older subjects with uncomplicated systolic hypertension: the role of proximal aortic diameter and the aortic pressure-flow relationship. Circulation. 2003;108:1592–8.
20. Perktold K, Rappitsch G. Computer simulation of local blood flow and vessel mechanics in a compliant carotid artery bifurcation model. J Biomech. 1995;28:845–56.

Part II
Cardiac Hemodynamics

Chapter 13
Cardiac Muscle Mechanics

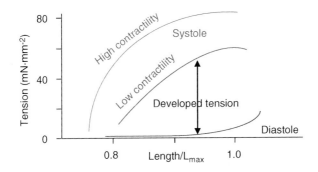

Relations between force and length in the relaxed state, diastole, and in two active states, systoles, of an isolated cardiac muscle. A low and high contractile state can be obtained by, for instance, changing the Calcium concentration in the extracellular medium and thus intra-cellular as well. During contraction a family of force-length relations is traversed, but here only the diastolic and the maximal or systolic relations are shown. The difference between the systolic and diastolic force is developed force. Force is expressed relative to cross-sectional area of the muscle and called tension (stress would be a better term). The length is normalized with respect to L_{max}, the length where developed force is maximal. The force-length relation forms the basis of the pressure-volume relation. Other important relations are:

- The force-velocity relation, showing that velocity of contraction decreases when force increases.
- The relation between intracellular calcium and force, showing that an increase in Calcium results in increased force.

© Springer International Publishing AG, part of Springer Nature 2019
N Westerhof et al., *Snapshots of Hemodynamics*,
https://doi.org/10.1007/978-3-319-91932-4_13

13.1   Description

The cardiac muscle cells, or fibers, branch and interdigitate. They are typically 40 μm long and about 10 μm in diameter; the fibers contain fibrils that are built up by the basic contractile units the sarcomere (Fig. 13.1). Each sarcomere is bounded at the ends by Z-discs about 2 μm apart. The thin actin filaments about 1 μm long, are attached to the Z-discs, and extend towards the center of the sarcomere. They can either meet in the center, when sarcomere length is short, i.e., about 2.0 μm, overlap each other when sarcomere length is <2.0 μm, or not quite reach each other when sarcomere length >2.0 μm. Spanning the center of the sarcomere length are the thick myosin filaments, 1.6 μm long, which interdigitate with the thin filaments. They are connected to the Z-discs with a titin molecule, the third filament. The titin filament contains several spring sections, each with their own stiffness. The titin is the main determinant of muscle stiffness in diastole [1]. Changes in sarcomere length are achieved by sliding of thin between thick filaments; the sliding filament model. This sliding is caused by the action of the active, heavy meromyosin ATPase, i.e., ATP consuming unit, the 'cross-bridge'. The cross-bridges project sideways from the thick filaments, apart from a 'bare area' in the central zone of approximately 0.2 μm in length. The physiological range of sarcomere lengths (SL) is 1.6–2.3 μm, so that the number of cross-bridges in apposition to thin filaments is (approximately) constant.

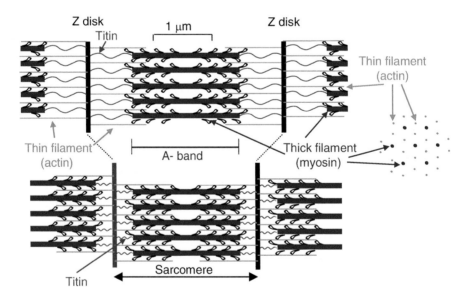

Fig. 13.1 The contractile unit of cardiac muscle is the sarcomere. The basic mechanical elements are presented here at two muscle lengths in the longitudinal direction. On the right hand side the cross section at overlap of thin and thick filaments is shown. Only one (instead of 6) titin molecule per half thick filament is shown for simplicity

13.1.1   Calcium

Depolarization of the cardiac muscle cell membrane causes influx of calcium ions, Ca^{2+}, over the cell membrane. This increase in Ca causes a further and larger release of calcium ions from the Sarcoplasmatic Reticulum, SR, the so-called calcium-induced calcium release. Calcium reacts with myosin ATPase to produce a contraction. The magnitude of the force of contraction produced when the sarcomere is prevented from shortening, i.e., isometric sarcomeres, is a function of sarcomere length and of intracellular calcium ion concentration, $[Ca]_i$.

The interrelationships between this isometric force, F_0, with sarcomere length, SL, and the $[Ca]_i$ are sigmoidal (Fig. 13.2). On the up-sloping part of this curve, an increase in $[Ca]_i$ resulting from increased Ca^{2+} release, causes an increase in F_0, called an increase in contractility, or positive inotropic effect. This must be distinguished from an increase of F_0 due to increase in sarcomere length, which is due to increased sensitivity of the contractile filaments to Ca^{2+}. Increased sensitivity implies an upward and leftward shift of the F_0-$[Ca]_i$ curve. This effect forms the basis of the Frank-Starling Law that states that 'the energy of contraction is a function of initial fiber length'. This effect is brought about by the presence of regulatory proteins on the thin filaments, namely the tropomyosin and the troponin complex. Other proteins and factors also play a role, e.g., Titin and lattice spacing.

The curvilinear shapes of the tension (force per area) versus (normalized) muscle length vary with the level of $[Ca]_i$, as shown in the Figure in the Box.

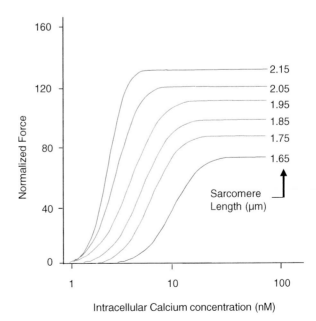

Fig. 13.2 Relation between intracellular Calcium ion concentration and isometric force. Normalization is with respect to isometric force at a sarcomere length of 1.85 μm. (Adapted from Ref. [2], used by permission)

13.1.2   The Force-length Relation

The force-length relation of cardiac muscle (see Figure in Box) forms the basis of the ventricular pressure-volume relation. The relation between pressure and (local) tension can in principle be obtained by Laplace's law, but more sophisticated approaches are advised. Many models have been proposed with varying success. The main problems are:

(Local) wall stress cannot be measured in the intact heart, so that verification of models is not yet possible [3]. Subendocardial shortening is larger than subepicardial shortening, but forces may or may not be different.

Cardiac geometry is complex. Cylindrical or ellipsoidal heart models are only rough approximations of reality.

Relations between ventricular volume and (local) fiber length, as well as between volume changes and changes in fiber length also suffer from heterogeneity and geometric complexity. The simplest approach is to assume that the heart is a cylinder, with the volume proportional to fiber length squared, or a sphere, with volume proportional to fiber length to the third power.

The force-length relation of the muscle therefore only qualitatively relates to the pressure-volume relation of the heart.

13.1.3   The Force-Velocity Relation

Another basic property of cardiac muscle is that for larger force the velocity of shortening is smaller (Fig. 13.3). This inverse relation between force and velocity is called the force-velocity relation (*F-v* relation). *In vivo*, cardiac muscle shortens against a force *F* that is less than the isometric force, F_0; these forces (stresses) are also called 'loads'. The *F-v* relation can be described by a hyperbola with the Hill equation:

$$\left(F_0 - F\right) \cdot b = \left(F + a\right) \cdot v$$

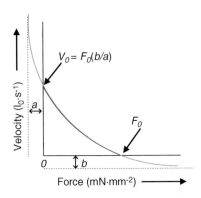

Fig. 13.3 Force-velocity relation of cardiac muscle. The hyperbola can be described by the Hill equation given in the text

Fig. 13.4 Force-sarcomere shortening velocity relations are influenced by muscle length and contractility. Two lengths and two levels of contractility are depicted. (Adapted from Ref. [4], used by permission)

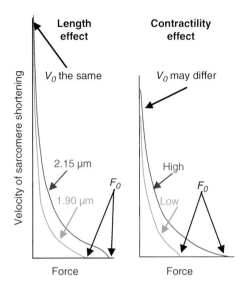

The maximal velocity, v_0, depends on the maximum velocity of ATP splitting by the myosin ATPase.

In Fig. 13.4, two sets of F-v relations are given. The F-v curves are hyperbolic except near F_0. The left hand side presents F-v relations for two sarcomere lengths, 1.90 and 2.15 μm. It shows that the increase in F_0 is not accompanied by an increase in the maximum velocity of sarcomere shortening, v_0, at zero force. This phenomenon depends on muscle length and disappears at short lengths. The right hand part of Fig. 13.3 shows the F-v relation for two contractility levels, or two levels of intracellular Calcium, $[Ca]_i$. With an increasing level of $[Ca]_i$ the v_0 increases until a saturation level is reached. In the rat this level is below the physiological $[Ca]_i$ so that v_0 will then not increase with increased contractility of increased intracellular Calcium. In the human there exists a range of Calcium concentrations where v_0 will increase.

13.1.4 The F-v Relation and Pump Function

F and v relate, through geometric transformations (Laplace) with pressure, e.g., pressure in the left ventricle, and (velocity to volume change) to flow. The F-v curves above refer to an instant in time within a contraction, whereas CO is a time-integrated quantity and not directly related. In other words, during the cardiac cycle the F-v relation is not constant but rises from one at the end of diastole, to one in systole and subsequently wanes down to the diastolic one again. This waxing and waning is not simply a 'parallel' shift because the time course of v_0 is more rapid than that of F_0. A greater duration of contraction results in a higher Stroke Volume,

SV, which is related to the average velocity. It is considered by some that the relevant F-v curve for the intact heart is the relationship between average F and average v, which is equivalent to the pump function graph relating average LVP to CO (see Chap. 15).

13.1.5   Experimental Problems

Studies on cardiac muscle are usually performed on isolated muscle strips, papillary muscle or trabeculae. These preparations are generally not perfused and therefore conditions have to be chosen such that a so-called anoxic core is avoided. These conditions are low temperature, low frequency, high P_{O2} of the superfusion fluid etc. If in vivo conditions are desired, such as 37 °C and physiological rate of contraction, a perfused preparation is required. Single skinned (permeable outer membrane) myocytes have been studied in terms of length and tension and calcium sensitivity, and very recently data on intact single myocytes have been reported [5].

Isolated cardiac muscle allows for studies of basic phenomena, such as tension development, calcium handling, effects of drugs, disease, etc. The advantage is that the muscle can be studied without the confounding effects of changes in cardiac loading. The disadvantage is that conditions are not physiological.

Determination of maximal isometric force requires that one stretches the preparation during contraction to prevent the sarcomeres from shortening because of compliant attachments of the preparation to the apparatus. This requires feedback control of the stretching apparatus keeping sarcomere length constant. The, average, sarcomere length can be derived from light diffraction provided the preparation is sufficiently thin. The method is used successfully in trabeculae, which are fine muscle bundles from the inside of the heart cavity, usually taken from the right ventricle.

In most cell cultures cell shortening is used as a measure of function. Unfortunately the shortening depends on the adherence of the cells to the substrate, and this adherence is not known. Also the amount of shortening cannot be related to the force.

13.1.6   Nomenclature Problems

Another term for v_0, used in the past was v_{max}, but this is now avoided because of erroneous attempts to calculate it in intact hearts. Traditionally, isolated muscle experiments were arranged so that the force was constant during systole and early relaxation, whereas in life, force decreases during systole and falls to about zero in early relaxation (before diastolic lengthening). This force during systole and early relaxation was called 'afterload', a term which is clearly inappropriate to use in the intact heart. Before it was possible to measure sarcomere length throughout an experiment, the muscle was hung vertically and its initial length was set with variable weights; these weights were called 'preloads'. This term is no longer appropriate because the fundamental independent variable, sarcomere length, can now be measured. It is unwise to apply terms derived from cardiac muscle mechanical studies, which are one- dimensional, to the intact heart, which is three-dimensional.

13.1.7   Limitations of the Sliding Filament Model

Students of cardiac muscle have traditionally tried to relate their findings to thinking arising from skeletal muscle studies, and the latter has been dominated by the idea that the cross-bridges attach mechanically to the thin filaments. Herzog et al. review one of the phenomena that are not compatible with the theory that the cross-bridges attach mechanically to the thin filaments [6]. Liu and Pollack provide evidence that filaments slide in steps of integers of 2.7 nm [7], called step-wise shortening, and Kishino et al. [8] show myosin heads alone, attached to glass can exert full ATP-dependent force. Finally Holohan and Marston [9] show that immobilized myosin in a motility assay can induce full bead-tailed actin filament force-velocity characteristics, when an electromagnetic field is applied in the presence of ATP.

Currently there is no sign of such critiques in the cardiac muscle literature, although it was shown in cardiac muscle that myosin binding can switch on actin filaments in rigor conditions but it does not contribute significantly under physiological conditions. The physiological mechanism of co-operative Ca^{2+} regulation of cardiac contractility must therefore be intrinsic to the thin filaments [10]. Rigor is a pathological condition characterized by cross-bridge attachment to filaments caused by ATP depletion. Physiological contraction takes place in the presence of ATP, which ensures absence of cross-bridge attachment to thin filaments and catalyzes contraction through an electromagnetic or electrostatic mechanism.

13.1.8   Diastolic Properties

The passive muscle stiffness determines the diastolic pressure-volume relation. Passive stiffness is mainly determined by changes in extracellular matrix and the titin molecule [1, 11] and to the speed of relaxation (Calcium reuptake in the Sarcoplasmatic Reticulum and extracellular transport).

13.2   Physiological and Clinical Relevance

The maintenance of the circulation requires that the cardiac muscles have a sufficiently high F-v relation and duration of active state. Failure of these, as for example due to reduced contractility, will lead to clinical heart failure. Clinical heart failure can also occur due to damage of part of the heart, e.g. myocardial infarction. More complex dysfunction is associated with heterogeneity, i.e., site variation of contractile function, sometimes referred to as hibernating myocardium which some claim to be improved by removing atheromatous stenoses. Hypertrophy, as a result of hypertension or valve disease also increases the demand for coronary blood flow and with limited supply induces dysfunction. Stimulation of contractility may be necessary in the treatment of acute heart failure, using positively inotropic drugs. Unfortunately, this seemingly logical treatment is contra-indicated in chronic heart failure because it causes earlier death, presumably because increased oxygen is required by the cardiac muscle sometimes in excess of possible supply rate; positively inotropic drugs mostly work by increasing $[Ca]_i$ which can also cause (possibly fatal) arrhythmia. However, an increase of Ca-sensitivity seems an option [12].

A different approach has recently been introduced in which the authors suggest that from an engineering perspective, many forms of heart disease can be thought of as a reduction in biomaterial performance, in which the biomaterial is the tissue comprising the ventricular wall [13]. These authors favor materials science in which the structure and properties of a material are recognized to be interconnected with performance.

In diastolic heart failure with preserved ejection fraction the increased passive stiffness of the ventricle is both the result of increased titin stiffness and extracellular matrix stiffness [14].

References

1. Fukuda N, Granzier HL. Titin/connectin-based modulation of the Frank-Starling mechanism of the heart. J Muscle Res Cell Motil. 2005;26:319–23. Review.
2. Kentish JC, ter Keurs HEDJ, Ricciardi L, Bucx JJJ, Noble MIM. Cardiac muscle mechanics: comparison between the sarcomere length-force relations of intact and skinned trabeculae from rat right ventricle. Circ Res. 1986;58:755–68.
3. Huisman RM, Elzinga G, Westerhof N, Sipkema P. Comparison of models used to calculate left ventricular wall force. Cardiovasc Res. 1980;14:142–53.
4. Daniels M, Noble MIM, ter Keurs HEDJ, Wohlfart B. Force and velocity of sarcomere shortening in rat cardiac muscle: relationship of force, sarcomere length, Ca^{++} and time. J Physiol. 1984;355:367–81.
5. van der Velden J, Klein LJ, van der Bijl M, Huybregts MA, Stooker W, Witkop J, et al. Isometric tension development and its calcium sensitivity in skinned myocyte-sized preparations from different regions of the human heart. Cardiovasc Res. 1999;42:706–19.
6. Herzog W, Lee EJ, Rassier DE. Residual force enhancement in skeletal muscle. J Physiol. 2007;578:613–5. Holohan SJ, Marston SB. IEEE Proc Nanobiotechnol 2005;152:113–20
7. Liu X, Pollack GH. Stepwise sliding of single actin and myosin filaments. Biophys J. 2004;86:353–8.
8. Kishino A, Yanagida T. Force measurements by micromanipulation of a single actin filament by glass needles. Nature. 1988;334(6177):74–6.
9. Holohan SJ, Marston SB. Force-velocity relationship of single actin filament interacting with immobilised myosin measured by electromagnetic technique. IEEE Proc Nanobiotechnol. 2005;152:113–20.
10. Sun YB, Lou F, Irving M. Calcium- and myosin-dependent changes in troponin structure during activation of heart muscle. J Physiol. 2009;587(Pt 1):155–63.

11. Granzier HL, Irving TC. Passive tension in cardiac muscle: contribution of collagen, titin, microtubules, and intermediate filaments. Biophys J. 1995;68:1027–44.
12. Drake-Holland AJ, Lee JA, Hynd J, Clarke SB, Noble MI. Beneficial effect of the calcium-sensitizing drug EMD 57033 in a canine model of dilated heart failure. Clin Sci (Lond). 1997;93:213–8.
13. Golob M, Moss RL, Chesler NC. Cardiac tissue structure, properties, and performance: a materials science perspective. Ann Biomed Eng. 2014;42:2003–13.
14. Zile MR, Baicu CF, Ikonomidis JS, Stroud RE, Nietert PJ, Bradshaw AD, et al. Myocardial stiffness in patients with heart failure and a preserved ejection fraction: contributions of collagen and titin. Circulation. 2015;131:1247–59.

Chapter 14
The Pressure-Volume Relation

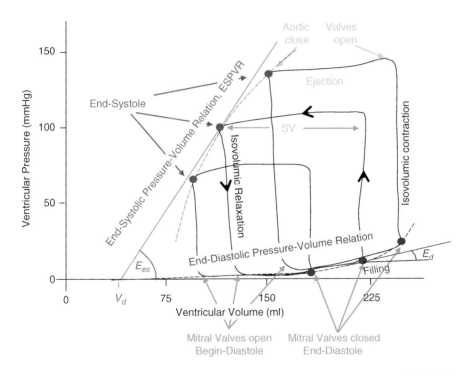

The ventricular pressure-volume relation, is an important presentation of global cardiac pump function. With every heart beat a full loop is described. Starting at End-Diastole, the first part of the loop is the isovolumic contraction phase (valves closed). When the (aortic) valves open, ejection begins and during this period ventricular volume decreases while pressure changes relatively little. Stroke Volume, SV, is indicated. After valve closure (End-Systole) isovolumic relaxation follows.

N. Westerhof et al., *Snapshots of Hemodynamics*,
https://doi.org/10.1007/978-3-319-91932-4_14

When the mitral valves open, the filling phase starts and volume increases with a small increase in ventricular pressure until the End-Diastolic volume is reached at the start of muscle contraction. When ventricular filling is changed, another loop starting from a different End-Diastolic Pressure and End-Diastolic Volume is described. The left top corners of the pressure-volume loops, i.e., the End-Systolic points, when interconnected, and approximated with a straight line, give the End-Systolic Pressure-Volume relation, ESPVR. The slope of this line, End-Systolic Elastance, E_{es}, is load-independent and is determined by systolic muscle properties (contractility) and wall mass. The Diastolic Pressure-Volume Relation is found by connecting the End-Diastolic Pressure and Volume points. The relation depends on diastolic muscle properties and wall thickness; it has considerable curvature leading to large errors when assumed straight. The local slope of the Diastolic Pressure-Volume relation at end-diastole is the End-Diastolic Elastance, E_d. Filling changes in vivo can be obtained by partial vena cava occlusions.

14.1 Description

Otto Frank studied pressure-volume relations in the isolated frog heart. He found different End-Systolic Pressure-Volume Relations, ESPVR's, for the ejecting heart and the isovolumically contracting heart. In other words, a single unique End-Systolic Pressure-Volume Relation did not appear to exist. More recent translations of his lectures given in high German (difficult for present German colleagues to understand) are being translated, so far revealing how far Frank got to the modern concept presented in this Chapter. He was certainly able to inscribe pressure-volume loops on photographic paper from mirror galvanometers connected to a pressure transducer and piston volume measuring device. These methods were inadequate, but the ideas were modern.

Measurements in the isolated blood perfused dog heart, where volume was accurately measured with a water-filled balloon, showed that the End-Systolic Pressure-Volume Relation was the same for ejecting beats and isovolumic beats. The original results suggested a linear ESPVR with an intercept with the volume axis, V_d [1]. The linear relation implies that the slope of the ESPVR, the E_{es}, with the dimension of pressure over volume (mmHg/ml), can be determined. Increased contractility, (Fig. 14.1) as obtained with epinephrine, increased the slope of the ESPVR but left the intercept volume, V_d, unchanged [1]. Therefore, the E_{es} could quantify cardiac muscle contractility. Later it turned out that both the diastolic pressure-volume relation and the ESPVR are not linear. This implies that the slope depends on the pressure and volume chosen and when approximating this locally with a straight line a virtual intercept volume is obtained, which may be positive or negative. The curvature results from failure to reach the isovolumic end-systolic pressure during ejection observed at very high systolic pressure, attributed to the longer duration of systole and limitation to maintain the active state long enough. The ESPVR, and its slope E_{es}, were shown to be only little dependent on the arterial load, hence the term

Fig. 14.1 The slope (E$_{es}$) of the linearized End-Systolic Pressure-Volume Relation (ESPVR) is a measure of cardiac contractility. An increased slope implies increased contractility. (Adapted from Ref. [1] by permission)

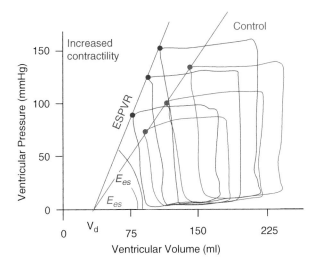

load-independence [2]. The existence of a load-independent ESPVR is of great significance in the understanding and characterization of cardiac pump function. An extensive treatment is given in [2].

14.1.1 The Varying Elastance Model

Pressure-volume loops can be analyzed by marking time points on the loop (Fig. 14.2). When different loops are obtained and the times indicated, we can connect points with the same times, and construct isochrones. The slopes of the isochrones can be determined, and the slope of an isochrone is the elastance at that moment in time. The fact that the elastance varies with time, leads to the time-varying elastance concept $E(t)$. This means that during each cardiac cycle the elastance increases from its diastolic value to its maximal value, which is close to end-systole, E_{es}, and then returns to its diastolic value again (Fig. 14.2).

This is an oversimplification in that the ESPVR lines in Fig. 14.2 are drawn straight when they are actually curved. Nevertheless, the varying elastance model is valid as demonstrated by other methods. Cardiac muscle subjected to constant amplitude oscillations of length display increased amplitude oscillations of force during contraction, i.e., dP/dl (elastance, has increased). Intact hearts subjected to constant amplitude oscillations of volume display increase amplitude oscillations of pressure during contraction, i.e., dP/dV, elastance, has increased. Elastance is a fundamental property of the contractile mechanism.

It has been shown that the $E(t)$ curve, when normalized with respect to its peak value and to the time of its peak, $E_N(t_N)$, (see Fig. 14.3), is similar for normal and diseased human hearts [3]. Similar $E_N(t_N)$ curves are found in the mouse, and dog.

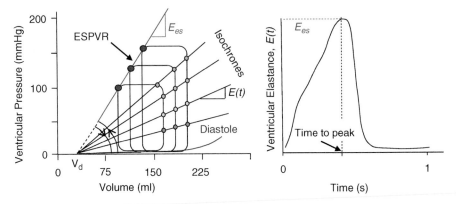

Fig. 14.2 Isochrones are lines connecting the pressures and volumes of different loops at the same moment in time. Isochrones are supposed to be straight and their slope is the instantaneous pressure-volume relation or ventricular elastance, $E(t)$, with dimension $mmHg \cdot ml^{-1}$. The line connecting the End-Systolic corners of the loops is the End-Systolic Pressure-Volume Relation, ESPVR with slope E_{es}. The ESPVR is not exactly a single isochrone. The slopes of the isochrones plotted as a function of time, the $E(t)$-curve, exemplifies the varying elastance concept (right part)

Thus there appears to exist a universal normalized $E(t)$ curve in mammals including man, which is unaltered in shape in health and disease. The only differences between hearts and state of health are in the magnitude and time of peak of the $E_N(t_N)$. This similarity of the varying $E_N(t_N)$-curve is very useful to construct lumped models of the heart [4, 5]. However, some doubt has been cast on the invariance of the $E_N(t_N)$ curve [6].

The assumed mechanism is that the cardiac muscle changes its stiffness (elastance) during the cardiac cycle (Fig. 14.4) independently of its load.

14.1.2   Determination of End Systolic Elastance

To determine E_{es} one needs to measure several pressure-volume loops and obtain a range of end-systolic pressure-volume points (see Figure in the Box). The determination should be done sufficiently rapidly to avoid changes in contractility due to the hormonal or nervous control systems. Both changes in arterial load and diastolic filling may, in principle, be used, but the former may illicit contractility changes by changes in coronary perfusion. Changes in filling are therefore preferred and are also easier to accomplish in practice. For instance, blowing up a balloon in the vena cava may decrease filling over a sufficiently wide range and can be carried out sufficiently rapidly to obtain a series of loops and an accurate ESPVR estimate. Measurement of both ventricular pressure and volume on a beat-to-beat basis can be carried out with the use of the so-called pressure-volume catheter [7].

Fig. 14.3 The $E_N(t_N)$ curve is the $E(t)$ normalized in amplitude and to time to peak, and is similar in many disease states. (Adapted from Ref. [3], by permission)

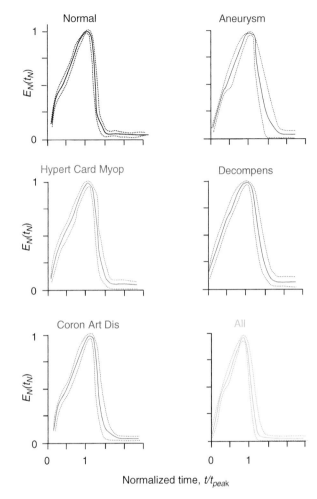

Normalized time, t/t_{peak}

Fig. 14.4 The varying elastance concept assumes that the muscle stiffness increases from diastole to systole and back. This change in stiffness, expressed as the elastance curve, $E(t)$, is assumed to be unaffected by changes in load

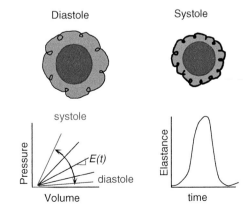

Volume also can be measured using noninvasive techniques (US-Echo, X-ray, and MRI). Pressure is preferably obtained by invasively techniques. However, aortic pressure during the cardiac ejection period can be used as an acceptable approximation of left ventricular pressure in systole to determine the systolic part of the pressure-volume loop [8, 9]. Methods allowing for the calculation of ascending aortic pressure noninvasively from peripheral pressure (Chap. 27) could, if proven sufficiently accurate, allow for a completely noninvasive determination of E_{es}.

How does one cope with the fact that most experiments show an ESPV curve that is convex to the volume axis, so that a straight line cannot be drawn? If one wants to compare contractility in an individual heart before and after an intervention, there are plenty of mathematical methods for fitting such curves and testing statistical differences between them. Alternatively, if one wants a single number for E_{es}, one can take the maximum slope of the tangent to the curve at end systole.

14.1.3 Determination of End Diastolic Elastance

The diastolic pressure-volume relation is strongly nonlinear (Figure in the Box). Therefore exponential approaches have been proposed. Klotz et al. suggested $P(t) = aV(t)^b$ with some assumptions on the intercept volume, the volume at negligible transmural pressure [10]. Rain et al. and Trip et al. used $P(t) = a \cdot (e^{b \cdot V(t)} - 1)$ [10, 11]. The curve fit of the end-diastolic pressure-volume points of the different loops is used to obtain the constants a and b. The End-Diastolic Elastance, E_d is the slope of the relation at end-diastolic volume, V_{ed}, and equals $E_d = a \cdot b \cdot e^{b \cdot Ved}$.

14.1.4 Derivation of End Systolic Elastance and End Diastolic Elastance from Single Beats

The slope of the end-systolic and end-diastolic Pressure-Volume relations E_{es} and E_d, are best obtained by filling changes, as for instance obtained by partial vena cava occlusion. However, this approach is often not feasible in clinical studies. Therefore so-called single beat approaches have been proposed to estimate E_{es} and E_d, see Fig. 14.5.

To derive the slope of the End-Systolic Pressure Volume Relation, E_{es}, from a single beat Sunagawa proposed to fit a sinewave to the isovolumic contraction and relaxation periods of measured ventricular pressure [12]. The maximum of the sinewave is then assumed to be the isovolumic pressure, 'P_{isovol}' and $E_{es} = ('P_{isovol}' - P_{es})/SV$. Senzaki used the generalized $E_N(t_N)$ curve (Fig. 14.3) and calibrated the curve using $P_{es} = 0.9 \cdot P_{ao,syst}$, with $P_{ao,syst}$ systolic aortic pressure and via t_{peak}, using an iterative approach the intercept pressure $V_{o(SB)}$ was estimated so that $E_{es} = 0.9 \cdot P_{ao,syst} / (V_{es} - V_{o(SB)})$ [3]. Other simulations of the isovolumic ventricular pressure, such as

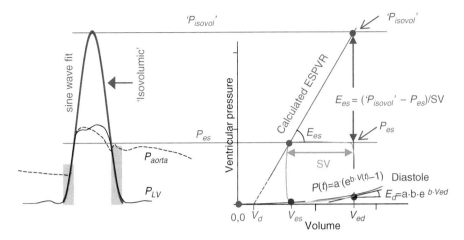

Fig. 14.5 Single beat methods to obtain the slope of the End-Systolic Pressure-Volume Relation, E_{es} and the End-Diastolic Pressure-Volume Relation, E_d. Left panel: The isovolumic contraction and relaxation phase of ventricular pressure (gray areas) are used to fit a (half) sine wave. The maximum of the sine-wave is assumed be isovolumic systolic pressure 'P_{isovol}'. Right panel: The 'P_{isovol}', and end-systolic pressure, P_{es}, together with Stroke Volume is used to calculate $E_{es} = ('P_{isovol}'-P_{es})/SV$. The diastolic pressure-volume relation can be fitted with an exponential curve using three data pressure-volume points: 0,0, begin-diastole and end-diastole. The slope at end-diastole is E_d.

by polynomials, have been suggested but the results are hardly better than the use of the sine wave.

When brachial pressure is measured the systolic aortic pressure can be derived [13], see Chap. 12. Together with noninvasive volume measurement (MRI) and using the normalized $E_N(t_N)$ curve (Fig. 14.3), the E_{es} can be derived noninvasively from a single beat [14].

To derive the End-Diastolic Pressure-Volume relation from a single beat an exponential curve between pressure and volume is assumed: $P(t) = a \cdot (e^{b \cdot V(t)} - 1)$, and fitted through the hypothetical zero pressure-zero volume point (0,0) and the pressure-volume data at beginning and end diastole as shown in Fig. 14.5 [10, 11]. The slope at end diastole then gives $E_d = a \cdot b \ e^{b \cdot Ved}$.

14.2   Physiological and Clinical Relevance

The ESPVR and E_{es} together with the diastolic pressure-volume relation, are important characterizations of cardiac pump function and they are often used in animal research; clinical use is now increasing. The $E(t)$ curve depends on heart size and thus on body size: Pressures are similar in different animals but volumes are not. Volumes are proportional to body mass (Chap. 32). Thus E_{es} should be normalized with respect to ventricular lumen volume (see Chap. 11) or to heart mass or body mass to compare mammals. Since not only muscle contractility but ventricular wall thickness and lumen also contribute to E_{es} and E_d, normalization with respect to wall thickness may help to quantify changes in muscle mass and in muscle contractility to E_{es} and E_d.

14.2.1   The Frank-Starling Law

The varying elastance concept contains both Frank's and Starling's original experimental results, as shown in Fig. 14.6. Frank studied the frog heart in both isovolumic and ejecting beats, but we show here how isovolumic contractions behave in the pressure-volume plane when diastolic volume is increased. Starling also changed diastolic filling but studied an ejecting heart that was loaded with a Starling resistor. This meant that in his experiments the aortic pressure and ventricular pressure in systole were kept constant. The increase in filling resulted in an increase in Stroke Volume and thus in Cardiac Output.

14.2.2   Systolic and Diastolic Dysfunction

It is important to realize that both diastolic and systolic properties play an important role in cardiac function (Fig. 14.7). This can be illustrated with the following example. Systolic dysfunction results in a decreased Stroke Volume, and Cardiac Output at constant Heart Rate when not compensated by increased diastolic filling. Diastolic dysfunction, with a stiffer ventricle in diastole causes decreased filling and higher

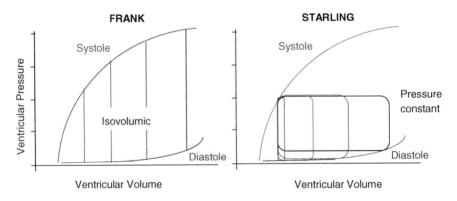

Fig. 14.6 Frank (left, isovolumic contractions) and Starling (right, ejections against constant ejection pressure) experiments to show the effect of ventricular filling in terms of pressure-volume relations. Increased filling causes increased isovolumic pressure (Frank) or increased Stroke Volume and Cardiac Output (Starling)

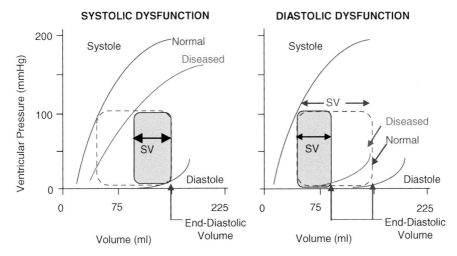

Fig. 14.7 Systolic and diastolic dysfunction are shown here by the red lines, and normal function by the blue lines. Left panel: In systolic dysfunction of failure the ESPVR is decreased and Stroke Volume, SV and Ejection Fraction, EF = SV/EDV, decrease also. Right panel: In diastolic dysfunction or failure with increased diastolic stiffness filling is decreased although filling pressure may be higher, End-Diastolic Volume and Stroke Volume are both decreased, but EF = SV/EDV may be similar: Heart Failure with Preserved Ejection Fraction, HFPEF

filling pressure and pulmonary venous pressure, the latter leading to shortness of breath. The smaller diastolic volume results in a decreased Stroke Volume and Cardiac Output.

Ejection Fraction, EF, defined as the ratio of Stroke Volume, SV, and End-Diastolic Volume, EDV, is decreased in systolic dysfunction but may be unaltered in diastolic dysfunction (Fig. 14.7). This is the case when SV and EDV decrease in the same proportion. This situation is called diastolic dysfunction or Heart Failure with Preserved Ejection Fraction, HFPEF [15], and it shows that EF is not in all situations a measure of changed cardiac pump function. Breathing difficulty is a more common feature in diastolic dysfunction because systolic dysfunction usually results in a smaller increase in filling pressure and smaller increase in pressure in the lung veins.

Since EF depends on the cardiac pump and the arterial load, the EF should be considered as a ventriculo-arterial coupling factor rather than a characterization of heart function alone (Chap. 18).

14.2.3 Concentric and Eccentric Hypertrophy

Concentric and eccentric hypertrophy are interesting examples in the context of the varying elastance concept and the pressure-volume relation (Fig. 14.8).

Fig. 14.8 Schematic drawings of pressure-volume relations in control (blue lines) and concentric hypertrophy (left) and dilatation, eccentric hypertrophy (right), red lines

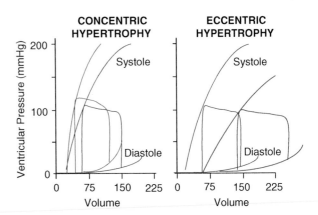

Concentric hypertrophy implies an increased wall thickness with similar lumen volume. This means a stiffer ventricle both in diastole and in systole, i.e., both E_{es} and E_d are increased. The increase in E_{es} does not necessarily imply increased contractility of the contractile apparatus of the muscle but is mainly a result of more sarcomeres in parallel, i.e., a thicker fiber and therefore increased wall thickness. Concentric hypertrophy, with its increased diastolic stiffness results in increased diastolic pressure but smaller volume in end-diastole, and higher pressure but smaller volume in systole, but similar or slightly decreased Stroke Volume. It has been suggested that the intracellular molecular events in hypertrophy may be detrimental to cardiac muscle function [16].

In eccentric hypertrophy the ventricular lumen volume is greatly increased, more sarcomeres in series, and longer cells, while the wall thickness may be unchanged or somewhat increased. The shift of the entire pressure-volume relation to larger volumes in eccentric hypertrophy implies, by virtue of the law of Laplace (Chap. 9), that wall forces are increased. It is not clear why the cardiac muscle does not respond by hypertrophy when diastolic wall stress is increased. The increased V_d in eccentric hypertrophy emphasizes that the slope of the ESPVR cannot be determined from a single pressure and volume measurement, assuming that the V_d is negligible (see below).

14.2.4   Modeling on the Basis of the Varying Elastance Concept

The finding that the normalized $E(t)$ curve appears to be quite independent of the cardiac condition (Fig. 14.3), and that it is similar in mammals (Chap. 32) allows quantitative modeling of the circulation [4, 17]. The nonlinearity of the isochrones (see below) appears of little consequence in this type of modeling [4].

14.2.5   *Limitations*

It should be emphasized that the time varying elastance concept pertains to the ventricle as a whole. It allows no distinction between underlying cardiac pathologies. For instance, asynchronous contraction, local ischemia or infarction etc., all decrease the slope of the End-Systolic Pressure-Volume Relation. Also the E_{es} depends on ventricular lumen, wall size and muscle contractility. In acute experiments cardiac contractility changes can be studied, but in long range studies as hypertrophy where muscle mass is increased both muscle mass and muscle contractility changes contribute to the changes in E_{es}. Normalization with respect to muscle mass and lumen have been suggested.

The pressure-volume relations, expressed by isochrones (Fig. 14.9), are not straight [17]. The systolic pressure-volume relations may be reasonably straight when muscle contractility is low, but become more and more convex to the pressure axis with increasing contractility. A curved relation implies that the E_{es} depends on volume and pressure. It is customary to approximate the ESPVR's in the working range by a straight line. Although this sometimes gives an acceptable approximation of reality, a virtual, often a negative, V_d is found by linear extrapolation of the ESPVR to the volume axis Fig. 14.9, left panel). A negative V_d is physically impossible.

In several studies the E_{es} has been estimated from a single pressure-volume loop assuming the intercept volume V_d to be negligible. However the lines connecting the

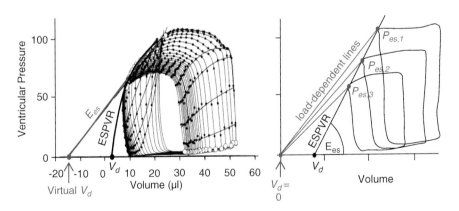

Fig. 14.9 Left Panel: Neither the isochrones nor the end-systolic pressure-volume relation is linear. Thus the linear approximation may not always be correct and may lead to a negative calculated volume intercept, the virtual V_d, which is physically impossible. The E_{es} in the working range may be approximated using the straight line. (Data of the mouse, adapted from Ref. [17], used by permission). Right panel: When the virtual volume intercept is assumed to be zero the slopes of the calculated end-systolic lines, P_{es}/V_{es}, depend on end-systolic pressure and end-systolic volume, and are not a load-independent characterization of the ventricle

end-systolic pressure-volume points with $V_d = 0$, give slopes that differ between beats and are not load-independent characterizations of the ventricle (see Fig. 14.9, right panel).

It has been shown by a number of investigators that load changes affect the End-Systolic Pressure-Volume Relation. However, the effect is rather small and may be due to the fact that, at high loads, the duration of ejection is curtailed and may not be long enough for E_{es} to be attained [2].

References

1. Suga H, Sagawa K, Shoukas A. A. Load independence of the instantaneous pressure-volume ratio of the canine left ventricle and the effect of epinephrine and heart rate on the ratio. Circ Res. 1973;32:314–22.
2. Sagawa K, Maughan WL, Suga H, Sunagawa K. Cardiac contraction and the pressure-volume relationship. NewYork/Oxford: Oxford University Press; 1988.
3. Senzaki H, Chen C-H, Kass DA. Single beat estimation of end-systolic pressure-volume relation in humans: a new method with the potential for noninvasive application. Circulation. 1996;94:2497–506.
4. Segers P, Stergiopulos N, Westerhof N. Quantification of the contribution of cardiac and arterial remodeling to hypertension. Hypertension. 2000;36:760–5.
5. Lankhaar JW, Rövekamp FA, Steendijk P, Faes TJ, Westerhof BE, Kind T, et al. Modeling the instantaneous pressure-volume relation of the left ventricle: a comparison of six models. Ann Biomed Eng. 2009;37:1710–26.
6. van der Velde ET, Burkhoff D, Steendijk P, Karsdon J, Sagawa K, Baan J. Nonlinearity and load sensitivity of end-systolic pressure-volume relation of canine left ventricle in vivo. Circulation. 1991;83:315–27.
7. Baan J, van der Velde ET, de Bruin HG, Smeenk GJ, Koops J, van Dijk AD, et al. Continuous measurement of left ventricular volume in animals and humans by conductance catheter. Circulation. 1984;70:812–23.
8. Chen CH, Nakayama M, Nevo E, Fetics BJ, Maughan WL, Kass DA. Coupled systolic-ventricular and vascular stiffening with age: implications for pressure regulation and cardiac reserve in the elderly. J Am Coll Cardiol. 1998;32:1221–7.
9. Klotz S, Hay I, Dickstein ML, Yi GH, Wang J, Maurer MS, et al. Single-beat estimation of end-diastolic pressure-volume relationship: a novel method with potential for noninvasive application. Am J Phys. 2006;291:H403–12.
10. Rain S, Handoko ML, Trip P, Gan CT, Westerhof N, Stienen GJ, et al. Right ventricular diastolic impairment in patients with pulmonary arterial hypertension. Circulation. 2013;128:2016–25.
11. Trip P, Rain S, Handoko ML, van der Bruggen C, Bogaard HJ, Marcus JT, et al. Clinical relevance of right ventricular diastolic stiffness in pulmonary hypertension. Eur Respir J. 2015;45:1603–12.
12. Sunagawa K, Yamada A, Senda Y, Kikuchi Y, Nakamura M, Shibahara T, et al. Estimation of the hydromotive source pressure from ejecting beats of the left ventricle. IEEE Trans Biomed Eng. 1980;27:299–305.
13. Kelly R, Fitchett D. Noninvasive determination of aortic input impedance and external left ventricular power output: a validation and repeatability study of a new technique. J Am Coll Cardiol. 1992;20:952–63.
14. Paulus WJ, Tschöpe C, Sanderson JE, Rusconi C, Flachskampf FA, Rademakers FE, et al. How to diagnose diastolic heart failure: a consensus statement on the diagnosis of heart failure

with normal left ventricular ejection fraction by the heart failure and echocardiography associations of the European society of cardiology. Eur Heart J. 2007;20:2539–50.

15. Schiattarella GG, Hill TM, Hill JA. Is load-induced ventricular hypertrophy ever compensatory? Circulation. 2017;136:1273–5.

16. Westerhof N. Cardio-vascular interaction determines pressure and flow. In: Jaffrin MY, Caro CG, editors. Biological flows. New York: Plenum Press; 1995.

17. Claessens TE, Georgakopoulos D, Afanasyeva M, Vermeersch SJ, Millar HD, Stergiopulos N, et al. Nonlinear isochrones in murine left ventricular pressure-volume loops: how well does the time-varying elastance concept hold? Am J Phys. 2006;290:H1474–83.

Chapter 15
The Pump Function Graph

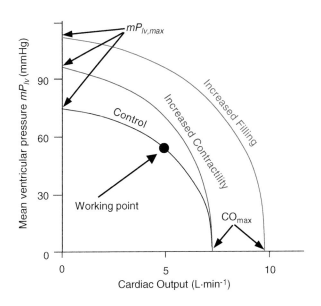

The heart as a pump can be described by the pump function graph, the relation between mean ventricular pressure, i.e., the ventricular pressure averaged over the entire cardiac cycle, and Cardiac Output. A pump function graph completely describes the heart as a pump and is similar to the characterization of industrial pumps and ventricular assist devices. When the load on the heart is increased, it will generate a higher pressure but a smaller Cardiac Output, and vice versa, as shown by the curved inverse relations. Contractility and diastolic ventricular filling modify the relation. Increased contractility 'rotates' the pump function graph around the intercept with the flow axis, as shown by the blue line. When diastolic filling is increased, the pump function graph shifts in an 'outward' manner, and $mP_{lv,max}$ and

CO_{max} both increase, as shown by the red line. Increased Heart Rate also moves the graph outward. Thus, during determination of a pump function graph contractility, diastolic filling, and Heart Rate should be constant. The working point, i.e., the pressure and flow during normal function at rest, is indicated. The maximal mean pressure, $mP_{lv,max}$, i.e., the intercept with the pressure axis, is the mean ventricular pressure when the heart beats isovolumically. The maximal cardiac output is achieved when the load is low and pressure negligible, the ventricle ejects its total volume. Stroke volume rather than CO can be used as well. The cardiac pump function graph is indirectly related to the force-velocity relation of muscle (see Chap. 13). There is a straightforward relation between the pump function graph and the end-systolic pressure-volume relation (Chap. 14).

15.1   Description

The heart is a pump that generates pressure and flow. It can be characterized in a way comparable with industrial hydraulic pumps, namely their head (pressure) – capacity (flow) curve. As an example, we consider a roller pump and make a pressure-flow relation by changing the load on the pump. In Fig. 15.1 we show the pump function graph, PFG, of a pump used in the laboratory and also known as the DeBakey roller pump used in heart-lung machines. The pump function graph of this

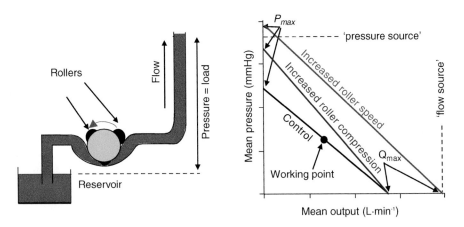

Fig. 15.1 The pump function graph of a laboratory pump. When roller speed and compression of the tube by the rollers is kept constant a pump function graph can be determined by changing the load on the pump, here obtained by changes in height of the outflow tube. An increase in pressure reduces pump output (black line). When the compression by the rollers is increased the blue line is obtained a higher maximal pressure is obtained but maximal flow against zero load remains the same. When roller speed is increased, comparable to a heart rate increase, the red pump function graph results. A pressure source is a pump that generates the same pressure for all flows obtained by the changes in load. A flow source always generates the same flow. This roller pump is neither a pressure source nor a flow source. (Adapted from Ref. [2], by permission)

roller pump can be determined by changing its load, the pressure in the outflow tube, while keeping the pump characteristics the same, i.e., roller speed, roller compression, and the inflow pressure are constant. For very high load values the pressure is maximal, $P_{lv,max}$, but the flow is negligible. Inversely, when the load is negligible flow is maximal, Q_{max}. Thus, an inverse relation between pressure and flow is obtained. The relation happens to be straight for this type of pump, and gives information about what pressures and flows the pump can generate. The pump function graph also shows that this particular roller pump is neither a pressure source, i.e., always generating the same pressure, nor a flow source, i.e., always keeping flow constant. Centrifugal Ventricular Assist Devices have a nonlinear inversed relation between pressure and flow [1] and are qualitatively similar to the cardiac pump function graph as shown below.

The pump function graph depends on the roller speed and on how much the rollers compress the tube. A higher speed results in larger pressures and flows, and both the pressure and flow intercepts, $P_{lv,max}$ and Q_{max}, increase. Better compression of the rollers, increases the pressure generating capability because less leakage is present and the $P_{lv,max}$ increases. Since at low pressures the leakage is negligible, the maximal flow, Q_{max}, is hardly affected by changes in compression of the tube. The result of the increased roller compression is a clockwise 'rotation' of the pump function graph around the intercept with the flow axis.

We can perform a similar experiment on the heart (Fig. 15.2). To avoid changes in pump function by humoral and nervous control mechanisms, these studies were

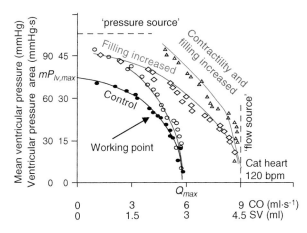

Fig. 15.2 Pump function graphs as originally measured in an isolated pumping cat heart preparation. The black line gives the control situation. An increase in contractility 'rotates' the graph around the intercept with the flow axis (Q_{max}), maximal pressure increases but mean flow is not altered (black to blue). Increased ventricular filling causes an 'outward' shift of the pump function graph (black to red). When filling and contractility are both increased the green line is found. The horizontal axis may be in terms of Stroke Volume and Cardiac Output. (Adapted from Ref. [5], by permission). Heart rate changes affect CO and mean ventricular pressure similarly so that the entire graph shifts in parallel

originally carried out in the isolated perfused and ejecting cat heart. When ventricular filling pressure, cardiac contractility and Heart Rate are kept constant, variation of the load on the heart by either changing peripheral resistance or arterial compliance, or both, results in changes of mean left ventricular pressure, mP_{lv}, and mean flow, Q_m (or Stroke Volume) [2], but leave $P_{lv,max}$ and Q_{max} unaltered. The relation between mean ventricular pressure and mean flow (Cardiac Output) results from the inverse relation between mean force and mean velocity of isolated cardiac muscle [3, 4] and thus relates to basic muscle properties. In the graph mean ventricular pressure, mP_{lv}, but not mean aortic pressure, is related with mean (aortic) flow because ventricular pressure and flow pertain to the cardiac side of heart and the effect of the very non-linear aortic valves is circumvented. Mean values of ventricular pressure and flow are used as a first order approximation, comparable with the mean aortic pressure and mean flow to determine peripheral resistance. In principle Fourier analysis (Appendix 1) of ventricular pressure and flow can be used to derive the oscillatory aspects of the pump function graph, in analogy with the derivation of arterial input impedance (Chap. 24).

From the pump function graph we can see that the heart decreases its output when a higher pressure is generated. In other words the heart does neither generate the same flow, nor the same pressure under different loading conditions. This means that the heart is neither a pressure source, i.e., pressure is independent of the load, nor a flow source, i.e., the same flow and SV for all loads. At low flows the heart starts to resemble a pressure source and at high flows a flow source is approached. The intercept of the pump function graph with the pressure axis is the mean ventricular pressure for a non-ejecting or isovolumic beat, thus mean isovolumic ventricular pressure. The intercept with the flow axis is the Cardiac Output for the 'unloaded' or 'isobarically contracting' heart, i.e., contractions without build-up of pressure.

Changes in contractility and filling are also shown in Fig. 15.2 [5]. An increase in cardiac contractility rotates the pump function graph around the flow intercept, Q_{max}. Increased filling results a 'parallel' shift of the graph. Increased Heart Rate in the physiological range results in a parallel shift of the pump function graph, which is approximately proportional to the Heart Rate increase, thus $mP_{lv,max}$ and Q_{max} are also increased proportionately. When Stroke Volume and the ventricular pressure integrated over the whole cardiac cycle are used in the pump function graph the effect of Heart Rate on the graph is negligible.

At the intercepts of the pump function graph with the pressure and flow axes, $mP_{lv,max}$ and Q_{max}, the product of pressure and flow is zero and the external power is therefore negligible as well [6]. Thus external power generation exhibits a maximum for intermediate values (Chap. 18).

The pump function graph can be approximated by a parabola of the form [7].

$$mP_{lv} = mP_{lv,max} \left(1 - Q_m^{\ 2} / Q_{max}^{\ 2}\right)$$

and maximum power output is thus found at $Q_m = \frac{1}{2}Q_{max}$ and $mP_{lv} = \frac{3}{4}mP_{lv,max}$.

15.1.1 Determination of the Pump Function Graph from Single Beats

In principle two data points are sufficient to describe the pump function graph. Estimation of the mean value of an isovolumic beat, $mP_{lv,max}$, (zero flow) together with measured mean ventricular pressure and flow, mP_{lv} and Q_m, would completely describe the graph. However, using the method discussed in Chap. 14 to derive an isovolumic beat has not been shown to result in acceptable estimates of $mP_{lv,max}$.

15.1.2 Relation Between the Pump Function Graph and the End-Systolic Pressure-Volume Relation

Figure 15.3 shows a comparison between the pressure-volume relation and the pump function graph. We see a 'mirrored' relation between the two characterizations of the heart. This follows from the fact that Stroke Volume implies a decrease in ventricular volume during ejection. The main difference between the relations is that in the pressure-volume relation the end-systolic ventricular pressure is used, while in the pump function graph the mean ventricular pressure is used.

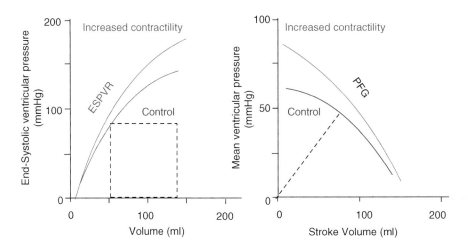

Fig. 15.3 The end-systolic pressure-volume relation (ESPVR, left) and the pump function graph (right) show a 'mirrored' relationship. Increased contractility rotates the relations (red). Diastolic filling does not affect the ESPVR but shifts the pump function graph. The ESPVR is obtained by preload changes, i.e., changes in cardiac filling and the Pump Function Graph by afterload changes, i.e., changes in arterial resistance or compliance. (Note the scale difference in the pressure axes)

15.2   Physiological and Clinical Relevance

The pump function graph describes the pump function of the heart for constant filling, Heart Rate and contractility. The graph is a relation between mean ventricular pressure, not mean aortic pressure, and Cardiac Output. The pump function graph teaches us that the heart is neither a flow source nor a pressure source. The flow source or in German the 'Harte Brunne' was the assumed heart model used until the 1960s. We see (Fig. 15.2) that contractility at constant loading pressure has only a small effect on Cardiac Output. Heart Rate and diastolic filling contribute more importantly to CO.

15.2.1   The Frank-Starling Law

Figure 15.4 shows the effect of filling on the pump function graph and its meaning with respect to the Frank-Starling mechanism. Frank studied the effect of filling on both ejecting and isovolumic contractions, but here the effect of filling on isovolumic beats are shown. The effect of an increase in ventricular filling on non-ejecting, i.e., isovolumic contractions is given by the intercepts of the pump function graphs with the pressure axis, $mP_{lv,max}$, and identified here as Frank. Starling studied the effect of filling on Cardiac Output in the heart-lung preparation where aortic pressure and thus ventricular pressure was kept constant: Cardiac Output (and Stroke Volume) increases with cardiac filling.

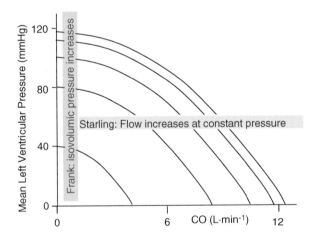

Fig. 15.4 The cardiac pump function graph is a generalized description of the Frank-Starling mechanism. With increased cardiac filling the graph moves outwardly. One of Frank's experiments pertains to isovolumic conditions where pressure increases with filling. Starling's experiment is one that keeps aortic pressure, and thus also ventricular pressure, constant so that cardiac output increases with filling at constant arterial pressure

15.2.2   Concentric Hypertrophy and Heart Failure

Figure 15.5 shows the pump function graph in hypertension and failure. In hypertrophy a flow source is approached while in failure the heart acts more like a pressure source [8].

These changes in pump function have an effect on reflected waves (Chap. 22). In ventricular hypertrophy the reflected pressure wave is reflected positively at the heart (flow source) and is added to the forward pressure wave resulting in augmentation of the measured pressure wave. This increased augmentation of pressure in hypertrophy shows the contribution of the hypertrophied heart to hypertension. In failure, when the heart approaches a pressure source the reflected flow wave affects the forward flow wave negatively resulting in a decrease in Cardiac Output (Chaps. 12 and 22). Understanding of the contribution of the heart to reflected pressure and flow waves may assist in giving suggestions for possible therapy in heart failure [9].

From Fig. 15.6 illustrates the way the pump function graph approaches a pressure source in chronic heart failure. Beta-blockers may be beneficial even though blood pressure may be low already. A decrease in contractility combined with blockade of sympathetic and adrenergic stimulation allows improved survival. Peripheral vasodilation, by Renin-angiotensin inhibition or calcium antagonism affects pressure little but increases Cardiac Output, because of the 'pressure-source' behavior of the heart. Improved survival by beta-blockade was indeed shown in patients with severe chronic heart failure [10].

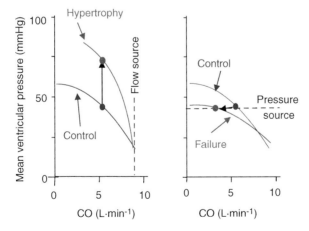

Fig. 15.5 The pump function graph in hypertrophy and failure. The graph in hypertrophy has a greater slope in the working point, indicating that the heart approaches a flow source. In failure a pressure source is approached. The filled circles show the working points. Pressure wave reflections against a flow source augment the pressure without affecting the flow; thus reflection against the heart increases the pressure. Reflection against a pressure source, as in failure, decreases flow but does not affect the pressure. Thus in failure cardiac output is diminished by reflections

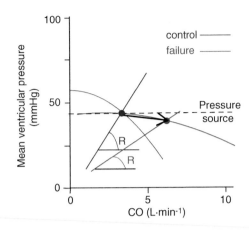

Fig. 15.6 The pump function graph shows that in chronic failure a pressure source is approached (red), and that vasodilation affects pressure only little but increases cardiac output

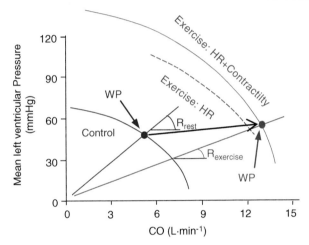

Fig. 15.7 During exercise vascular resistance decreases (red line) and the pump function graph 'shifts' due to the heart rate increase (dashed) and also 'rotates' since contractility and filling increase (fully drawn). As a result cardiac output increases strongly with a limited increase in pressure

15.2.3   Exercise

Figure 15.7 shows what happens in (moderate, supine) exercise. The major effect is the increase in Heart Rate: the pump function graphs shifts outwardly. The increase in contractility causes a small rotation as well, but filling changes are negligible [11]. The systemic peripheral resistance is decreased. The overall result is an increase in Cardiac Output with only a small increase in pressure.

15.2.4   Limitations

The pump function graph is a global description of the heart as a pump. Changes in muscle contractility, in synchronicity or effects of local ischemia or infarction, all affect this global description. The pump function graph determined on the basis of a single beat has not been shown to be accurate.

Since the heart is under the influence of nervous and humoral control and the fact that diastolic filling shifts the pump function graph, the determination of the pump function graph *in situ* is difficult. During arterial load changes filling, Heart Rate and contractility may change due to control mechanisms so that the operating points move over a family of pump function graphs.

References

1. Moazami N, Fukamachi K, Kobayashi M, Smedira NG, Hoercher KJ, Massiello A, et al. Axial and centrifugal continuous-flow rotary pumps: a translation from pump mechanics to clinical practice. J Heart Lung Transplant. 2013;32:1–11.
2. Elzinga G, Westerhof N. How to quantify pump function of the heart. Circ Res. 1979;44:303–8.
3. Elzinga G, Westerhof N. Isolated cat trabeculae in a simulated feline heart and arterial system. Circ Res. 1982;51:430–8.
4. Noble MIM. The cardiac cycle. Oxford/London: Blackwell Scientific Publications; 1979.
5. Elzinga G, Westerhof N. The effect of an increase in inotropic state and end-diastolic volume on the pumping ability of the feline left heart. Circ Res. 1978;42:620–8.
6. Elzinga G, Westerhof N. Pump function of the feline left heart: changes with heart rate and its bearing on the energy balance. Cardiovasc Res. 1980;14:81–92.
7. Van den Horn GJ, Westerhof N, Elzinga G. Optimal power generation by the left ventricle. A study in the anesthetized open thorax cat. Circ Res. 1985;56:252–61.
8. Elzinga G, Westerhof N. Workload as a determinant of ventricular hypertrophy. Cardiovasc Res. 1985;19:524.
9. Westerhof N, O'Rourke MG. Haemodynamic basis for the development of left ventricular failure in systolic hypertension and for its logical therapy. J Hypertension. 1995;13:943–52.
10. Rouleau JL, Roecker EB, Tendera M, Mohacsi P, Krum H, Katus HA, et al. Influence of pretreatment systolic blood pressure on the effect of carvedilol in patients with severe chronic heart failure (Copernicus study). J Am Coll Cardiol. 2004;43:1423–9.
11. Roest AA, Kunz P, Lamb HJ, Helbing WA, van der Wall EE, de Roos A. Biventricular response to supine physical exercise in young adults assessed with ultrafast magnetic resonance imaging. Am J Cardiol. 2001;87:601–5.

Chapter 16
Cardiac Work, Energy and Power

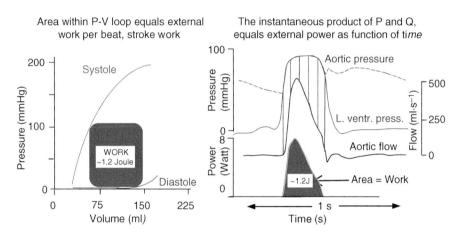

Left: External work per beat, stroke work, can be determined from the area contained in the pressure-volume loop, mmHg·ml or Joule, as first suggested by Frank [1]. Multiplication of stroke work by Heart Rate gives cardiac power (mmHg.ml/s or Watt). Right: External power (work per unit time) can be calculated from the instantaneous product of ventricular (or aortic) pressure, $P(t)$, and flow, $Q(t)$: Power = $P(t)\cdot Q(t)$, mmHg·ml·s^{-1} or Watt. The area under the power curve is stroke work mmHg·ml or Joule. The calculation of energy and power does not require a linear system, as, for example, in the calculation of resistance and impedance. This makes the use of energy and power very broadly applicable in hemodynamics. Power and work are a characterization of heart and load together, while the End-Systolic Pressure-Volume Relation and Pump Function Graph characterize the heart; resistance and impedance characterize the arterial system.

© Springer International Publishing AG, part of Springer Nature 2019
N. Westerhof et al., *Snapshots of Hemodynamics*,
https://doi.org/10.1007/978-3-319-91932-4_16

16.1   Description

Work and the potential to do work, energy, are based on the product of force times displacement, the units being Newton times meter (Nm or Joule). When work is expressed per unit time it is power (Nm/s or Watt). In hemodynamics this translates to pressure times volume (Joule or mmHg·ml) and pressure times flow (watt or Joule or mmHg·ml/s), respectively. Linearity of the relations between pressure and volume or flow is not required in the calculation of work and power, while linearity is required in the calculation of resistance and input impedance. However, work and power depend on heart and load, while the ventricular pressure volume relation and the pump function graph describe the heart and vascular resistance describes the vascular system.

In the heart, external work can be derived from pressure and volume through the pressure-volume loop, as first suggested by Otto Frank in 1898 [1], it is the area contained within that loop. The so calculated work is, of course, the external work produced by the heart during that heartbeat and called work per beat or stroke work.

Power delivered by the heart to the arterial load equals the instantaneous pressure times flow (Figure in Box). Both pressure, P, and flow, Q, vary with time, and the instantaneous power, calculated as $P(t)·Q(t)$ also varies with time. This means that instantaneous power varies over the heartbeat and is zero in diastole because aortic flow is zero. Thus, external work and power are only generated during ejection. Total energy is the integral of power, in mathematical form $\int P(t)·Q(t)\,dt$, the integral sign, $\int$, together with dt implies that at all moments in time pressure and flow values are multiplied and the products added. The integration is carried out over the heart period T, but since flow is zero in diastole (assuming patent valves) integration over the ejection period is adequate. The average power over the heart beat is $(1/T)·\int P(t)·Q(t)·dt$. Since aortic pressure and left ventricular pressure are practically equal during ejection, both ventricular pressure and aortic pressure may be used in the calculation.

Sometimes mean power is calculated as the product of mean pressure and mean flow (Cardiac Output). Here aortic pressure is to be used because it is the mean power delivered to the arterial system that we want to calculate. Since mean aortic pressure is about 2–3 times higher than mean left ventricular pressure, using ventricular pressure would lead to considerable errors [2]. The difference between total power and mean power $(1/T)·\int P(t)·Q(t)·dt - mP_{aorta}$ is pulsatile power (also called oscillatory power). Pulsatile power is about 15% of total power in the systemic circulation and increases in hypertension. The oscillatory power fraction is about 23% in the pulmonary circulation and the same in health and pulmonary hypertension [3] (see Chap. 28).

16.2 Physiological and Clinical Relevance

It has sometimes been reasoned that it is the mean power that is related to useful power while pulsatile power is related to moving blood forward and reflected only. In other words it was thought that only mean power and work were useful quantities. The logical consequence was then to assume that pulsatile power should be minimal in physiological conditions. This in turn, was used to argue that if the Heart Rate is related to the frequency of the minimum in the input impedance modulus (Chap. 24), pulsatile power would be minimal. However, this is not correct since it is the real part of the impedance that is related to power, not the impedance modulus. Thus, the separation of mean and pulsatile power is not very useful as a measure of ventriculo-arterial coupling. Under physiological conditions the heart pumps at optimal external power (Chap. 18) [4]. Total power is most important.

Work and energy find their main importance in relation to cardiac oxygen consumption, metabolism, and optimal efficiency in ventriculo-arterial coupling.

References

1. Frank O. Die Arbeit des Herzens und ihre Bestimmung durch den Herzindicator. Sitzungsbericht Gesell Morphol Physiol. 1898;14:147–56.
2. Williams SG, Jackson M, Cooke GA, Barker D, Patwala A, Wright DJ, et al. How do different indicators of cardiac pump function impact upon the long-term prognosis of patients with chronic heart failure? Am Heart J. 2005;150:983.e1–6.
3. Saouti N, Westerhof N, Helderman F, Marcus JT, Boonstra A, Postmus PE, et al. Right ventricular oscillatory power is a constant fraction of total power irrespective of pulmonary artery pressure. Am J Respir Crit Care Med. 2010;182:1315–20.
4. Toorop GP, Van den Horn GJ, Elzinga G, Westerhof N. Matching between feline left ventricle and arterial load: optimal external power or efficiency. Am J Phys. 1988;254:H279–85.

Chapter 17
Cardiac Oxygen Consumption and Hemodynamics

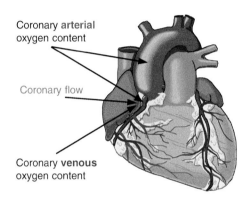

Coronary arterial oxygen content

Coronary flow

Coronary venous oxygen content

Cardiac oxygen consumption can be determined from the product of coronary flow, Q_{coron}, and arterio-venous oxygen content difference, ΔAVO_2. Coronary arterial oxygen content can be obtained from any arterial blood sample. Coronary venous or great cardiac vein oxygen content requires blood sampling at that location. Total coronary flow can be determined in the main stem coronary artery (ultrasound, catheter-tipped) flow meter, MRI (non-invasive), with microspheres, or at the venous side with thermodilution. To circumvent these preferentially simultaneous but difficult determinations, many indices for estimating cardiac oxygen consumption from hemodynamic variables have been proposed. It has been shown that heart rate is a primary determinant of oxygen consumption. The second major determinant is tension (stress) generation of the cardiac muscle, mostly measured as ventricular pressure. Muscle stress (pressure) generation costs more oxygen than muscle shortening (flow). Therefore many methods to derive oxygen consumption from hemodynamics are based on heart rate and pressure. The most used methods are the Rate Pressure Product (RPP, systolic pressure times Heart Rate), often used in biochemical studies, and the Tension Time Index (TTI, mean pressure during ejection). Total oxygen consumption depends two terms each consisting of two

© Springer International Publishing AG, part of Springer Nature 2019
N. Westerhof et al., *Snapshots of Hemodynamics*,
https://doi.org/10.1007/978-3-319-91932-4_17

sub-terms. The first is the 'unloaded' contraction, consisting of 'cell maintenance' plus excitation-contraction coupling (E_{es}, the slope of the End-Systolic Pressure-Volume relation). The second is the hemodynamic part namely the Pressure-Volume Area (PVA) that is the sum of external work plus potential energy measurable from the Pressure-Volume Relation.

17.1   Description

It was shown by Sarnoff et al. [1] that the production of pressure costs much more oxygen than the production of flow or Cardiac Output (see Fig. 17.1). Also, it has been shown that oxygen consumption, VO_2, is almost proportional to Heart Rate. These findings imply that the main mechanical variables determining cardiac oxygen consumption are pressure and Heart Rate. If oxygen consumption is expressed per beat, pressure remains as major determinant.

17.1.1   Rate Pressure Product and Tension Time Index

In approximation, the product of the systolic ventricular pressure and Heart Rate can be used to estimate oxygen consumption. This so-called Rate Pressure Product, RPP, is simple to use. The triple product, defined as $HR \cdot P_{syst} \cdot dP_{lv}/dt$, with dP_{lv}/dt the

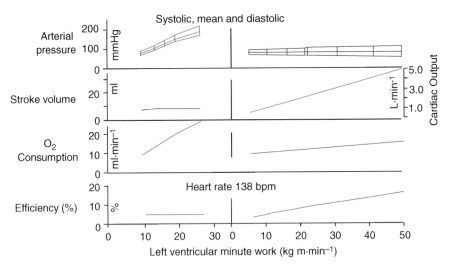

Fig. 17.1 Oxygen consumption as a function of minute work (power) was studied in experiments where Heart Rate was kept constant and cardiac filling and load were manipulated. Left panels: Arterial pressure was increased by diastolic cardiac filling while stroke volume was kept the same by a load increase. Right panels: stroke volume is increased by increased filling and decreased load while keeping pressure constant. Efficiency is the ratio of Stroke Work and oxygen consumption. Oxygen consumption changes much less with minute work during a stroke volume increases than with a pressure increase. (Adapted from Ref. [1], used by permission)

Fig. 17.2 TENSION TIME INDEX equals the
area under the pressure curve during ejection (red),
and is a simple method to estimate cardiac oxygen
consumption per beat

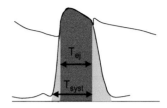

maximal rate of rise of ventricular pressure, has also been suggested as a measure
of cardiac oxygen consumption.

Sarnoff introduced the Tension Time Index, TTI, based on the results presented
in Fig. 17.1 [1]. The oxygen consumption per beat is assumed to be proportional to
the area under the ventricular (or aortic pressure when no stenosis is present) during
the ejection period (red area Fig. 17.2). Often the whole contraction period is used
instead, thus the green plus red area (Fig. 17.2). When we can neglect the contribution in diastole this area equals mean ventricular pressure, $P_{lv,mean}$ times heart period,
T, i.e., TTI $\approx P_{lv,mean} \cdot T$. In isolated heart studies where isovolumic contractions are
studied, and the ejection period is negligible, the total area under the *ventricular*
pressure curve, thus $P_{lv,mean} \cdot T$ can be used as a measure of cardiac oxygen consumption. The TTI is a global measure of cardiac oxygen consumption, and the term
tension is not meant to be local stress, but is pressure. The TTI is more difficult to
measure than the RPP.

17.1.2 Cardiac Oxygen Consumption and the Pressure Volume Area

Another way to estimate oxygen consumption per beat is the Pressure Volume Area
(PVA, the red area in the top part of Fig. 17.3) is the sum of external work (EW,
Chap. 16) and Potential Energy, PE [2]. This method requires measurement of ventricular pressure and volume for at least two, and preferably more cardiac filling
conditions to obtain the End-Systolic Pressure-Volume Relation (Chap. 14). The
relation between oxygen consumption, VO_2 per beat and 100 ml muscle, and PVA
is shown in the bottom part of Fig. 17.3, and can be written as:

$$VO_2 = a_1 \cdot PVA + a_2 \cdot E_{es} + a_3$$

where E_{es}, is the slope of the End-Systolic Pressure-Volume Relation (ESPVR),
giving a measure of contractile state. The first term is the relation between mechanics and oxygen consumption. The two other terms together give the oxygen consumption for the unloaded contraction or isobaric contraction, i.e., a contraction
without buildup of pressure. The second term, $a_2 \cdot E_{es}$, is the energy cost of excitation-
contraction coupling, mainly Calcium handling, and depends on the contractile state
of the cardiac muscle, expressed as *Ees*. The last term is the basal oxygen consumption, used for the maintenance of cell structure, etc. For details see Suga [2].

Fig. 17.3 The pressure-volume area (PVA) is the sum of external work (EW) and Potential Energy (PE). PVA relates to cardiac oxygen consumption. Oxygen consumption is also determined by basal (non-contractile) processes such as cell integrity and ion pumps, and by excitation-contraction coupling (activation energy, Calcium handling). Increased contractility increases activation energy. The PVA determines the third part of the energy. The inverse slope of the relation between PVA and VO_2 (red line) is the contractile efficiency. Overall efficiency equals EW/VO_2. (Adapted from Ref. [2], used by permission)

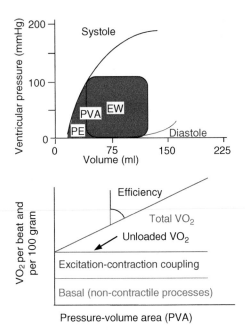

Ventricular efficiency is EW/VO_2. The PVA – VO_2 relation shows that pressure contributes more to VO_2 than flow for similar changes in EW, but the difference is smaller than suggested by Sarnoff et al. [3]. Increased contractility does not change the a_1 and a_3 but increases *Ees* implying that with similar PVA and similar External Work more oxygen is used due to increased energy utilization associated with excitation-contraction coupling and efficiency is lowered [4]. This may be called oxygen wasting by enhanced contractility.

In hypertrophy, with increased *Ees* due to wall thickening, the intercept and the slope of the VO_2-PVA relation is not affected [2]. Comparing a shortening contraction where PVA = PE + EW and an isovolumic contraction with the same systolic pressure where PVA = PE shows that the shortening contraction costs more oxygen in agreement with the Fenn-effect shown in muscle studies.

Local measures of oxygen consumption have been suggested as well. The Stress Time Index, i.e., mean wall stress, derived from left ventricular pressure, times heart period, is the local formulation of the TTI. In analogy with the PVA the local Force (Tension or Stress) Length Area (FLA) has been suggested in analogy with Fig. 17.3.

Most hemodynamic indices predict oxygen consumption per beat, oxygen consumption per second or minute is found by multiplication with Heart Rate. If we assume the TTI to be equal to the mean ventricular pressure times heart period, multiplying with Heart Rate results in mean pressure as a measure of oxygen consumption.

An overview of other, more complex hemodynamic indicators of cardiac oxygen consumption can be found in Rooke and Feigl's report [5].

17.1.3   Heterogeneity of Metabolism

Not only local perfusion (Chap. 19), but also local myocardial oxygen consumption is heterogeneously distributed in the myocardium [6]. Thus perfusion and metabolism seem related [7] but the reason for the heterogeneity is still disputed.

17.2   Physiological and Clinical Relevance

Cardiac oxygen consumption, or oxygen demand, and cardiac oxygen supply, are in equilibrium in the normal healthy heart. The above indices give hemodynamic measures of oxygen demand. Oxygen supply depends on coronary perfusion. Perfusion, especially to the subendocardial layers, mainly takes place in diastole when the cardiac muscle is relaxed. Thus, aortic pressure in diastole and the duration of diastole, together, quantified by the area under the diastolic aortic pressure curve, and called the diastolic pressure-time index, gives a measure of oxygen supply. The Tension Time Index, the area under the systolic pressure, is a simple measure of oxygen demand. It has therefore been proposed that the ratio of areas under the diastolic aortic pressure curve and the area under the systolic pressure curve, gives an estimate of the supply-demand ratio of the subendocardial layers of the heart [8].

With increasing age systolic pressure increases and diastolic pressure decreases a little (Chap. 25), resulting in an increase in mean systolic pressure see Fig. 17.4. This means that with age the supply-demand ratio decreases, which may result in ischemia in subendocardial layers. A similar reasoning can be applied to aortic valvular disease and tachycardia.

17.2.1   Limitations

The hemodynamic determinants of oxygen consumption, discussed above, can be used in individual hearts in situ and isolated hearts during acute experiments, such a pharmacological or loading interventions. The use of the hemodynamic parameters in different hearts, animals or in disease, should be done with care. When a dilated heart is compared with a normal heart, pressures and Heart Rates may be

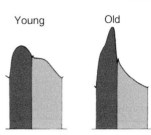

Young   Old

Fig. 17.4 The oxygen demand and supply relate to the areas under the systolic (red) and diastolic part (blue) of the pressure curve, respectively. The supply-demand ratio may be unfavorably influenced with increasing age

similar, but with more muscle mass, and different wall stress, oxygen consumption is not. In compensated concentric hypertrophy ventricular pressure is increased and wall thickness is increased in proportion while lumen radius is hardly changed, thereby keeping wall stress the same (Chap. 9). The Pressure Volume Area, PVA, as measure of oxygen per beat and per 100 g muscle allows for comparison of normal and hypertrophied hearts [2]. In the formula for the Pressure Volume Area the coefficients in the equation depend on animal size.

By applying the Rate Pressure Product to mouse and man, where systolic ventricular pressure and wall stress are similar but Heart Rate differs by a factor ten, it cannot be concluded that cardiac metabolism in the mouse heart is ten times that of the human heart (Chap. 32).

References

1. Sarnoff SJ, Braunwald E, Welch GH, Case RB, Stainsby WN, Macruz R. Hemodynamic determinants of oxygen consumption of the heart with special relevance to the tension-time index. Am J Phys. 1958;192:148–56.
2. Suga H. Ventricular energetics. Physiol Rev. 1990;70:247–77.
3. Suga H, Hisano R, Hirata S, Hayashi T, Ninomiya I. Mechanism of higher oxygen consumption rate: pressure-loaded vs. volume-loaded heart. Am J Phys. 1982;242:H942–8.
4. Suga H, Hisano R, Goto Y, Yamada O, Igarashi Y. Effect of positive inotropic agents on the relation between oxygen consumption and systolic pressure volume area in canine left ventricle. Circ Res. 1983;53:306–18.
5. Rooke GA, Feigl EO. Work as a correlate of canine left ventricular oxygen consumption, and the problem of catecholamine oxygen wasting. Circ Res. 1982;50:273–86.
6. van Beek JH, van Mil HG, King RB, de Kanter FJ, Alders DJ, Bussemaker J. A (13)C NMR double-labeling method to quantitate local myocardial O(2) consumption using frozen tissue samples. Am J Phys. 1999;277:H1630–40.
7. Alders DJ, Groeneveld AB, de Kanter FJ, van Beek JH. Myocardial O2 consumption in porcine left ventricle is heterogeneously distributed in parallel to heterogeneous O2 delivery. Am J Phys. 2004;287:H1353–61.
8. Hoffman JI, Buckberg GD. The myocardial oxygen supply: demand index revisited. J Am Heart Assoc. 2014;3:e000285.

Chapter 18
Cardiac Power and Ventriculo-Arterial Coupling

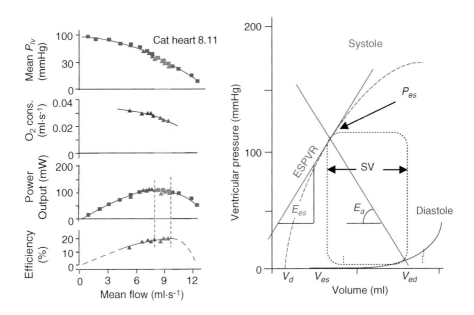

In health the heart pumps close to maximal external power and efficiency. The left panel shows in the isolated pumping heart. From top to bottom the Pump Function Graph, Oxygen Consumption, Mean Power Output (pressure times flow) and Cardiac Efficiency (ratio of Power Output and O_2 consumption). In this example the cardiac load was changed but filling, contractility and heart rate kept constant. Both power and efficiency exhibit shallow relations with flow, without sharply defined maximum implying that under normal conditions the heart pumps close to maximal efficiency and maximal power, with an efficiency of about 25%. Whether the heart is pumping at optimal efficiency or optimal power (ventriculo-arterial

© Springer International Publishing AG, part of Springer Nature 2019
N. Westerhof et al., *Snapshots of Hemodynamics*,
https://doi.org/10.1007/978-3-319-91932-4_18

coupling), or neither, depends on both the cardiac and the arterial state. To test if efficiency is maintained in disease ventriculo-arterial coupling analysis can be used (right panel). The slope of the ESPVR (E_{es}, see Chap. 14) characterizes the ventricle and the effective arterial elastance (E_a), which approximately equals total peripheral resistance over heart period, R/T, characterizes the arterial system. When $E_{es}/E_a \approx 1$, external work is maximized, and when $E_{es}/E_a \approx 2$ cardiac efficiency is maximal.

18.1 Description

18.1.1 Power and Efficiency

Cardiac efficiency is defined in analogy to that of a hydraulic pump. The produced power by the heart is pressure times flow (Chap. 16) and the 'input power' is calculated from cardiac oxygen consumption (Chap. 17). The ratio of produced or external power and input power is defined as efficiency. Therefore, both external power and input power need to be expressed in the same units. When glucose or free fatty acids are consumed oxygen consumption can be expressed in Joules and oxygen consumption per time in Watts, through the so-called oxygen caloric equivalent. For carbohydrate and fat metabolism it holds that 1 ml $O_2 \approx 20$ J and 1 ml O_2/min ≈ 0.33 Watt. A review on cardiac energetics has been published by Suga [1].

18.1.2 Maximum Cardiac Efficiency and Maximum Power in the Intact Animal

The pressure and flow generated by the heart and the arterial load can be studied while keeping the Heart Rate, diastolic filling and contractility unaltered [2]. Power can be calculated from the pressure and flow. The Figure in the Box, on the left, shows that, when power is plotted as a function of Cardiac Output it exhibits an optimal value. This can be understood with the cardiac pump function graph in mind, (top panel of Box Figure, and Chap. 15). At a high load (isovolumic contraction) flow is negligible and for a very low load pressure negligible, and at both extremes power, the product of pressure and flow, is negligible. Thus, power, at some intermediate value of Cardiac Output, must be maximal. This power maximum was found, in the intact cat [3], to coincide with the working point, i.e., when a physiologic arterial load is present (see Fig. 18.1). It has also been reported that the left ventricle works at maximal efficiency [4]. The shallow relation between power and efficiency allows to state that the heart pumps at about maximal power output and efficiency.

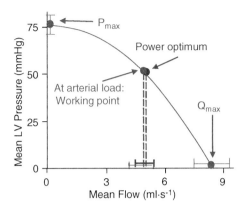

Fig. 18.1 In health the heart pumps at optimal power output. Power output of the heart as studied in the intact animal for different arterial loads. Other determinants of pressure and flow, heart rate, diastolic filling and contractility, are kept constant. When the physiological arterial load is present, called working point, power transfer is maximal. (Adapted from Ref. [3], used by permission)

18.1.3   Local Work and Power

It is of great interest if local power and efficiency could be derived. However, this is difficult since local work, and local oxygen consumption are hard to measure accurately. Local PET based O2 consumption is feasible but complex. Local work can be derived by local shortening times local stress. The first, local shortening, can be obtained from (surface) markers attached to the muscle or by MRI-tagging (magnetically induced 'markers' in the myocardium). Local forces are only possible to derive indirectly from pressure and anatomy (sophisticated forms of Laplace's law, Chap. 9). This technique was used by Prinzen et al., to study effect of pacing site on local work [5]. When local oxygen consumption is also determined [6–8] local efficiency can be derived. However, local stresses derived from pressure are difficult to verify.

18.1.4   Heat Production and Transport

Oxygen is used for cell maintenance, excitation-contraction and mechanics (Chap. 17), all metabolic processes producing heat. Heat is transported by convection by coronary flow, and diffusion to thorax and cardiac lumen (Fig. 18.2). In the mid-wall of the myocardium the temperature is a few tenths of a degree Celsius higher than in subepicardial and subendocardial layers allowing for diffusion of heat [9]. All in all the heart is about 25% efficient.

18.1.5   Assessment of Ventriculo-Arterial Coupling

Optimum power and efficiency are assumed measures of ventriculo-arterial coupling. Whether the heart functions on optimum power-efficiency can be derived from hemodynamic principles [10]. The Pressure-Volume relations (Chap. 14)

Fig. 18.2 Oxygen is used for cell maintenance, excitation-contraction processes and mechanics, all producing heat, with overall mechanical efficiency ~ 25%. Heat is transported by convection, i.e., coronary flow, and diffusion to thorax and cardiac lumen. Convection and diffusion contribute about equally depending on the magnitude of the coronary flow

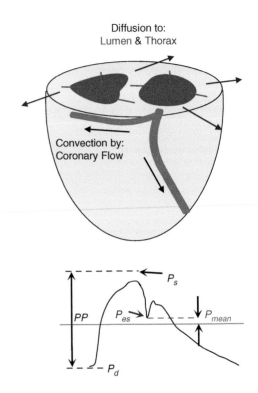

Diffusion to:
Lumen & Thorax

Convection by:
Coronary Flow

Fig. 18.3 End-systolic pressure is close to mean aortic pressure, allowing for non-invasive determination of P_{es}

stand at the basis of determination of ventriculo-arterial coupling. The two parameters to quantify coupling are the slope of the left ventricular End-Systolic Pressure-Volume Relation, E_{es}, (Chap. 14) and the effective arterial elastance, E_a, see the Figure in the Box, right panel. The effective arterial elastance is defined as $E_a = P_{es}/SV$, i.e., end-systolic (ventricular or aortic) pressure over Stroke Volume. The ratio E_{es}/E_a is considered a ventriculo-arterial coupling parameter and when $E_{es}/E_a \approx 1$, external work is maximized, while for $E_{es}/E_a \approx 2$ cardiac efficiency is maximal [10].

To determine these two parameters in practice several simplifications have been used. The E_a can be approximated as follows. End-systolic pressure is assumed equal to mean arterial pressure, P_{mean}, as shown in Fig. 18.3 [11]. Others have assumed a P_{es} 90% of systolic pressure. With Stroke Volume being Cardiac Output, $CO/HR = CO \cdot T$ and T heart period we find that

$$E_a = P_{es} / SV \approx P_{mean} / CO \times T = R_p / T$$

Thus the effective arterial elastance, E_a, is primarily a measure of vascular or peripheral resistance, R_p, and hardly reflects the compliant properties of the large conduit arteries [10], and the term 'elastance' is therefore misleading. Note that E_a depends both on vascular resistance, which is a purely arterial variable, and on heart period, T, which is a purely cardiac variable. Therefore, E_a is a coupling parameter by itself. The E_a can be derived from noninvasive measurements: mean pressure (by sphygmomanometer), Cardiac Output (US or MRI), and Heart Rate.

The End-Systolic elastance, E_{es} is calculated from $E_{es} = P_{es}/(V_{es} - V_d)$. End-Systolic volume can be obtained by MRI of US Echo. End-systolic pressure can be estimated noninvasively (see above), but V_d requires at least one other point on the ESPVR. This would require changes in diastolic filling that are often not feasible in patients and in epidemiological studies. When ventricular pressure wave shape and ventricular volume can be measured the single beat method explained in Chap. 14 can be applied to derive E_{es} and V_d. Other methods to derive E_{es} noninvasively have been published using the standard $E(t)$ curve discussed [12] see also in Chap. 14. However, assuming a linear ESPVR may result in an erroneous estimate of V_d and single beat methods have been seriously criticized [13]. The coupling parameter E_{es}/E_a can be written as $E_{es}/E_a = SV/(V_{es} - V_d) = EF/[1 - EF - (V_d/V_{ed})]$.

In a number of studies it has simply been assumed that $V_d = 0$ [14, 15]. This assumption disregards the principle of optimal coupling and calculates an $E_{es}*$ by assuming the intercept volume $V_d = 0$. The so-calculated $E_{es}* = P_{es}/V_{es} = P_{es}/(V_{ed} - SV)$, is not equal to E_{es} and thus not a load-independent cardiac parameter, and the ratio $E_{es}*/E_a$ is not based on energetic coupling.

$$E_{es}*/E_a = (P_{es}/V_{es})/(P_{es}/SV) = SV/V_{es} = SV/(V_{ed} - SV) = EF/(1 - EF)$$

with EF, the Ejection Fraction. We see that the P_{es} disappears altogether only leaving the Ejection Fraction in this ratio. The $E_{es}*/E_a$ and EF both are coupling parameters since they depend on heart and load, but EF is not based on efficiency. The V_d is in general not equal zero, especially in the dilated ventricle.

Under the same assumption that $V_d = 0$ the ratio $SV/V_{es} = E_{es}*/E_a$ has been suggested as coupling parameter. However, as mentioned this ratio is not based on efficiency.

Using the pump function graph (Chap. 15) a mean ventricular power can be calculated (Fig. 18.1) $Q_m \cdot P_{v,m} = Q_m \cdot P_{lv,max}(1 - Q_m^2/Q_{max}^2)$ and its maximum is found at $Q_m = Q_{max}/2$ or at $P_{v,m} = \frac{3}{4}P_{v,max}$. In other words when Q_m is unequal $Q_{max}/2$ or $P_{v,m}$ unequal $\frac{3}{4}P_{v,max}$ the heart does not work on optimal power and is not maximally efficient [3].

18.2 Physiological and Clinical Relevance

Cardiac oxygen consumption and efficiency can now be obtained in the patient [7, 8]. Modern techniques, such as Positron Emission Tomography (PET) and Magnetic Resonance Spectroscopy (MRS) are presently available. Assessment of glucose metabolism with ^{18}F-fluorodeoxyglucose measures glucose uptake into myocardial cells, but not its conversion by glycolysis. Myocardial oxidative metabolism can be measured by ^{11}C-labeled acetate PET. For lipid metabolism, tracer examples are ^{123}I-beta-methyl-p-iodophenyl pentadecanoic acid and

[15]-(Ortho-^{123}I-phenyl)-pentadecanoic acid. These tracers can be detected by planar scintigraphy and single-photon emission computed tomography (SPECT), which are more economical and more widely available than PET. With current MRS techniques, ^{31}P-labeled magnetic resonance spectroscopy, Phosphate/Creatine and/or pH can be obtained in humans but this is not common yet.

The hemodynamic determinants for oxygen consumption, as discussed in Chaps. 16 and 17 and the hemodynamic parameters determining coupling as discussed here, are a good surrogate.

18.2.1   Theory of Optimal Heart Size

Why does the left ventricle pump at maximum power, while a feedback control for power is not known to exist? A simple answer to this question can be given based on the following reasoning [16]. Consider the pump function graph (Fig. 18.4). The working point, i.e., the point where maximum power is found, is for a flow which is about 50% maximal flow, Q_{max}. Mean ventricular pressure and Cardiac Output together determine the working point. Pressure is similar in mammals and Cardiac Output is determined by body size (Chap. 30). Several pump function graphs can be drawn through this working point. We begin by assuming that muscle stress is a given quantity, and that the ventricle is a sphere. On the one hand, a larger intercept of the pump function graph with the flow axis, i.e., a larger Q_{max}, implies a larger ventricular lumen requiring a thicker wall (Law of Laplace), to

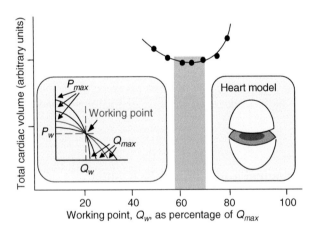

Fig. 18.4 Total ventricular volume, i.e., wall plus lumen volume, can be calculated assuming a spherical shape, right, and a fixed, maximal, wall stress for isovolumic contractions, σ_m / P_m. Many pump function graphs through the working point are possible, left, but the pump function graph where the working point is about 60% of Q_{max}, i.e., where maximal power and efficiency are found, corresponds with the smallest total ventricular volume. (Adapted from Ref. [16], used by permission)

maintain muscle, or wall stress. On the other hand, with a larger Q_{max} a smaller $P_{lv,max}$ results so that the wall may be less thick. In this way it is possible to calculate ventricular volume for the different pump function graphs through the working point, each with its own Q_{max}. Plotting ventricular volume as a function of Q_{max}, results in the graph given in Fig. 18.4. The minimum volume is found when the working point is at about 50–60% of Q_{max}, and this is the same value as where maximum power and efficiency are found. The minimum in heart volume thus corresponds to a working point where power and efficiency are about maximal. In other words, the size of the heart is minimized, and, for this minimal heart volume the heart pumps at maximal power.

18.2.2   Related issues

Contractile efficiency   On the basis of the Pressure Volume Area concept (Chap. 17) the contractile efficiency has been defined as the inverse of the slope of the Pressure Volume Area-VO$_2$ relation [17]. This definition of efficiency only accounts for the mechanical aspects of oxygen consumption and does not take into account the oxygen expenditure related to activation and basic metabolism. Therefore this contractile efficiency is about twice the actual cardiac efficiency.

Power in cardiogenic shock   Although power is a rather abstract measure, it has been shown that it is the strongest hemodynamic correlate of mortality in cardiogenic shock [18].

Economy   At the extremes of the pump function graph, the heart generates neither pressure nor flow. External power and then efficiency is zero. In isolated heart studies (Langendorff preparations) where the heart is contracting isovolumically or in isolated cardiac muscle studies, when the muscle contracts isometrically, contraction economy can be used instead. Economy of contraction is defined as oxygen consumption used for isovolumic contraction.

References

1. Suga H. Ventricular energetics. Physiol Rev. 1990;70:247–77.
2. Elzinga G, Westerhof N. Pump function of the feline left heart: changes with heart rate and its bearing on the energy balance. Cardiovasc Res. 1980;14:81–92.
3. Toorop GP, Van den Horn GJ, Elzinga G, Westerhof N. Matching between feline left ventricle and arterial load: optimal external power or efficiency. Am J Phys. 1988;254:H279–85.
4. Burkhoff S, Sagawa K. Ventricular efficiency predicted by an analytical model. Am J Phys. 1986;250:R1021–7.
5. Prinzen FW, Hunter WC, Wyman BT, Mcveigh ER. Mapping of regional myocardial strain and work during ventricular pacing: experimental study using magnetic resonance imaging tagging. J Am Coll Cardiol. 1999;33:1735–42.

6. van Beek JH, van Mil HG, King RB, de Kanter FJ, Alders DJ, Bussemaker J. A (13)C NMR double-labeling method to quantitate local myocardial O(2) consumption using frozen tissue samples. Am J Phys. 1999;277:H1630–40.
7. Wong YY, Westerhof N, Ruiter G, Lubberink M, Raijmakers P, Knaapen P, et al. Systolic pulmonary artery pressure and Heart Rate are main determinants of oxygen consumption in the right ventricular myocardium of patients with idiopathic pulmonary arterial hypertension. Eur J Heart Fail. 2011;13:1290–5. Erratum in: Eur J Heart Fail 2012;14:1190.
8. Güçlü A, Knaapen P, Harms HJ, Vonk AB, Stooker W, Groepenhoff H, et al. Myocardial efficiency is an important determinant of unctional improvement after aortic valve replacement in aortic valve stenosis patients: a combined PET and CMR study. Eur Heart J Cardiovasc Imaging. 2015;16:882–9.
9. ten Velden GH, Elzinga G, Westerhof N. Left ventricular energetics. Heat loss and temperature distribution of canine myocardium. Circ Res. 1982;50:63–73.
10. Sunagawa K, Maughan WL, Sagawa K. Optimal arterial resistance for the maximal stroke work studied in the isolated canine left ventricle. Circ Res. 1985;56:586–95.
11. Kelly RP, Ting CT, Yang TM, Liu CP, Maughan WL, Chang MS, et al. Effective arterial elastance as index of arterial vascular load in humans. Circulation. 1992;862:513–21.
12. Chen CH, Fetics B, Nevo E, Rochitte CE, Chiou KR, Ding PA, et al. Noninvasive single-beat determination of left ventricular end-systolic elastance in humans. J Am Coll Cardiol. 2001;38:2028–34.
13. Kjorstad KE, Korvald C, Myrmel T. Pressure-volume-based single beat estimations cannot predict left ventricular contractility in vivo. Am J Phys. 2002;282:H1739–50.
14. Grosu A, Bomgrosu A, Bombardini T, Senni M, Duino V, Gori M, et al. End-systolic pressure/volume relationship during dobutamine stress echo: a prognostically useful non-invasive index of left ventricular contractility. Eur Heart J. 2005;26:2404–12.
15. Sanz J, García-Alvarez A, Fernández-Friera L, Nair A, Mirelis JG, Sawit ST, et al. Right ventriculo-arterial coupling in pulmonary hypertension: a magnetic resonance study. Heart. 2012;98:238–43.
16. Elzinga G, Westerhof N. Matching between ventricle and arterial load. An evolutionary process. Circ Res. 1991;68:1495–500.
17. Senzaki H, Iwamoto Y, Ishido H, Masutani S, Taketazu S, Kobayashi T, et al. Ventricular–Vascular stiffening in patients with repaired coarctation of aorta. Circulation. 2008;118:191–8.
18. Fincke R, Hochman JS, Lowe AM, Menon V, Slater JN, Webb JG, et al. Cardiac power is the strongest hemodynamic correlate of mortality in cardiogenic shock: a report from the SHOCK trial registry. J Am Coll Cardiol. 2004;44:340–8.

Chapter 19
Coronary Hemodynamics

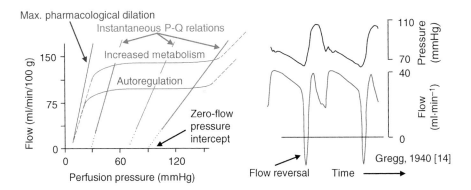

The relation between mean coronary flow and mean perfusion pressure (red & purple lines, left panel) is under the influence of autonomic, neural and hormonal control. Autoregulation is seen in two ways. It is the rather constant flow for the physiological range of pressures, and the change in flow with cardiac metabolism. Autonomic coronary flow regulation consists of three mechanisms: metabolic, myogenic and endothelium mediated vasoactivity. The so-called instantaneous pressure-flow relations (green) are obtained in diastole to avoid the effect of cardiac muscle contraction, and so rapid that vasomotor tone does not change. The relations describe the state of the coronary bed. For a low steady state perfusion pressure the relation has a small resistance (steep line) and a small intercept with the pressure axis: the zero flow pressure intercept. For larger perfusion pressure the resistance and intercept increase. Maximal pharmacological dilation results in smaller resistance and intercept than can be obtained by lowering pressure and gives "functional the anatomy" of the coronary bed. Cardiac contraction reduces coronary arterial inflow (right side) and augments venous outflow in systole. This effect results from three mechanisms: The direct effect of increased muscle stiffening (varying elastance), the indirect effect of increased ventricular pressure producing an

N. Westerhof et al., *Snapshots of Hemodynamics*,
https://doi.org/10.1007/978-3-319-91932-4_19

intramyocardial (interstitial, wall) pressure, and the thickening of the muscle during shortening contractions at the expense of vascular lumen. All three mechanisms decrease coronary vascular diameters, and together can be called the 'intramyocardial pump'. The decrease in vessel diameters during muscle contraction implies an increase in resistance and the rate of change of the volume decrease causes a blood flow, reducing arterial inflow and increasing venous outflow. Cardiac contraction is the main reason why the subendocardial layers are most prone to ischemia.

19.1   Description

The relations between arterial pressure and flow in the coronary bed are under the influence of the humoral-nervous systems, subject to cardiac contraction, and under local control, i.e. autoregulation. Several mutual interactions of smaller magnitude between the coronary vasculature and the cardiac muscle exist, which will be discussed below. The quantitative contribution of humoral and nervous control will not be discussed here. For a comprehensive description of coronary hemodynamics see Refs. [1–3].

19.1.1   Autoregulation of Coronary Flow

In the beating heart and in the physiological pressure range (40–140 mmHg) the relation between mean coronary flow and mean perfusion pressure shows a rather constant mean coronary flow (left part of Figure in the Box). With increased and decreased cardiac metabolism the plateau of the relationship is higher or lower, respectively. This dependence on cardiac metabolism suggests that metabolic autoregulation is a primary control of resistance vessels that are in close contact with the cardiac muscle. There is a fundamental difference in the equations required to express the effects of vasodilating metabolic products such as adenosine, carbon dioxide, pH, and ions and those for low oxygen content, releasing oxygen mediated vasoconstriction. Mathematical modeling [4] and the proven relation between coronary vascular resistance and tissue and venous oxygen tension [5] suggest an important role of oxygen, and provides a statistically better fit to observed data than models based on vasodilating metabolic products.

Whereas metabolic autoregulation provides flow adaptation to myocardial oxygen consumption (MVO2), an increase in pressure induces myogenic autoregulation by vascular smooth muscle (Fig. 19.1).

The response time of metabolic and myogenic regulation is in the order of seconds. It is of interest to remark that almost the same relationship was found between coronary conductance (inverse of resistance) and coronary venous PO_2 (reflecting tissue PO_2), for perfusion pressure changes and for pacing-induced changes in MVO_2 [6]. This suggests that tissue PO_2 may also play a part in pressure adaptation, in this case increases of pressure causing increasing PO_2 which causes vasoconstriction.

Fig. 19.1 The myogenic response. An increase in pressure increases vessel diameter and wall stress. Subsequent smooth muscle contraction reduces the diameter, to smaller than initial values, and restores wall stress

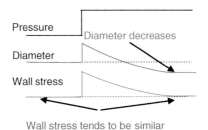

Fig. 19.2 Autoregulation gain, G, is defined as one minus the ratio of the local slope ($\Delta Q/\Delta P$) and the slope of the line through the origin (Q/P), i.e., 1/Resistance. Thus $G = 1 - (\Delta Q/\Delta P)/(Q/P)$. Gain depends on perfusion pressure

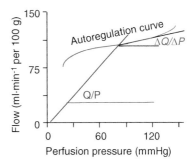

Endothelium mediated vasoactivity results from the fact that perfusion flow determines shear stress on the endothelial cells, which liberate vasodilators such as NO and prostaglandins. The main effect is in the larger vessels, rather than in the resistance vessels [7]. Especially during strong vasodilation and thus large flow, increased diameters keep the pressure drop over the conduit system minimal.

19.1.2   Autoregulation Gain

Autoregulation gain (Fig. 19.2), G, is a measure of the strength of autoregulation, and can be calculated as:

$$G = 1 - \left(\Delta Q / \Delta P\right)/\left(Q / P\right) = 1 - \left(\Delta Q / Q\right)/\left(\Delta P / P\right)$$

with $\Delta Q/\Delta P$ the slope of the mean pressure-mean flow relation and Q/P the slope of the line through the point of determination, the working point, and the origin of the graph, the inverse of resistance. It can be seen that for perfect autoregulation the gain equals 1 and for no autoregulation, assuming the pressure-flow relation would go through the origin, the gain equals zero. Since the pressure-flow relation does, in general, not go through the origin, it has been suggested to use the slope of the instantaneous pressure-flow relation (see below) instead of Q/P. Autoregulation gain can be plotted as a function of pressure to obtain the range of regulation.

19.1.3 Reactive Hyperemia and Maximal Vasodilation

When cardiac oxygen demand increases, as in exercise, coronary flow will increase and the increase is called exercise hyperemia. During a (short) coronary occlusion the coronary vessels dilate and after the release of the occlusion the flow is temporarily enhanced, a phenomenon called reactive hyperemia. In the normal coronary bed the maximal increase in flow is about fourfold.

Even during maximal exercise a brief coronary occlusion still results in reactive hyperemia [8]. It is possible to increase coronary flow pharmacologically (e.g., adenosine) and maximal pharmacologic vasodilation can lead to a smaller resistance than physiologic dilation (see left part of Figure in the Box). When a coronary stenosis is present the magnitude of the reactive hyperemia is reduced. Quantification is then usually presented as Flow Reserve or Fractional Flow Reserve (see Chap. 5).

19.1.4 Instantaneous Pressure-Flow Relations

A complicating factor with the coronary circulation is the effect of the cardiac contraction on the vessels. Bellamy [9] studied pressure-flow relations of long diastoles, obtained by vagal stimulation, thereby minimizing the effect of cardiac muscle contraction (Fig. 19.3). It was also assumed that over a single long diastole, about 1–2 s, vascular tone does not change. The instantaneous pressure-flow relations (see Figure in the Box, left panel) show an intercept, P_{zf}, with the pressure axis, the so-called zero-flow pressure. The zero-flow pressure and the inverse slope of the Q/P (green lines) increase with vasomotor tone. Since the intercept pressure also is present with crystalloid perfusion, it is not the effect of plugging by blood cells [10]. Surface tension [11] has been proposed as a mechanism as well, but the changes in intercept with tone are hard to explain with this theory. The most likely explanation is that the intercept (zero flow) pressure results from (micro)vascular compliance which increases with the lowering of pressure [12, 13], but would decrease with increased tone (stiffer vascular walls). See also Chap. 7, nonlinear pressure-flow relation.

Fig. 19.3 The instantaneous pressure-flow relation can be determined from a long diastole. It gives the 'state' of the bed, without the mechanical effect of cardiac muscle contraction, and during assumed constant vasomotor tone. (Adapted from Ref. [9], by permission)

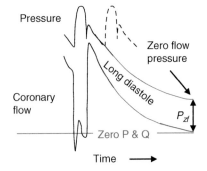

19.1.5   Cardiac Contraction and Coronary Flow

Coronary arterial inflow is impeded and venous outflow is augmented during cardiac contraction. When the coronary bed is vasodilated and cardiac muscle contractility is high, arterial flow may even reverse in early systole (see right part of the Figure in the Box [14]).

The contracting cardiac muscle exerts its effect on the vasculature in three ways [3]. The increasing stiffness of the muscle in systole (see $E(t)$, Chap. 14) has a similar effect on the interstitial volume and the blood vessels as it has on the lumen of the ventricle (Fig. 19.4). This pumping action causes the vascular diameters and thus, vascular volume to decrease in systole, and as there are no valves, blood is pumped to the arterial and to the venous side, with the amount depending on aortic and venous pressures. Figure 19.5 shows that compression of the vasculature occurs even when there is no increase in cavity pressure, indicating a direct effect of the contracting cardiac muscle (via stiffness changes) upon the vasculature [15].

In the vascular waterfall theory (Fig. 19.6 and Chap. 6), intramyocardial pressure is assumed to be equal to ventricular pressure at the subendocardium and negligible

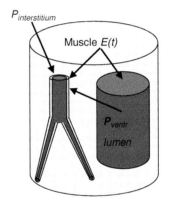

Fig. 19.4 Cardiac muscle contraction and shortening stand at the basis the cardiac pump. Contraction implies increased stiffness of the muscle. For the ventricular interstitium the increase in muscle stiffness affects the intramyocardial blood vessels. Ventricular pressure is also transmitted to interstitium, thus producing an intramyocardial pressure. Muscle thickening during shortening also affects the vessels. The result of these three mechanisms is that cardiac contraction decreases vascular volume (the 'intramyocardial pump') and increases coronary vascular resistance

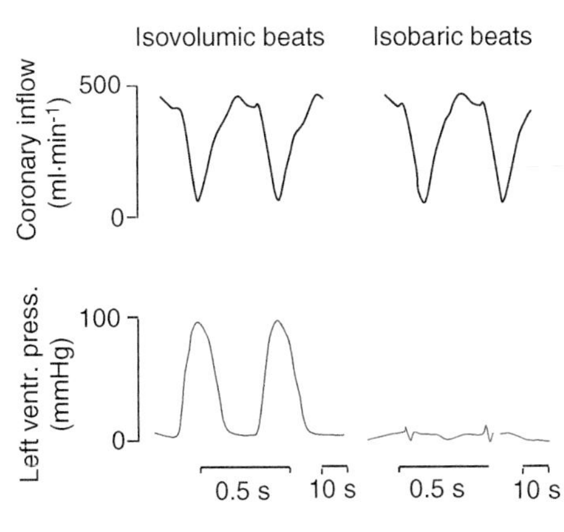

Fig. 19.5 Coronary flow during isovolumic beats, left, and isobaric contractions, right, of the isolated blood perfused cat heart. (From Ref. [15], by permission)

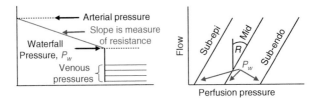

Fig. 19.6 The waterfall model is used to explain the effect of cardiac contraction on coronary arterial inflow. The waterfall pressure, P_w, is assumed to be proportional to left ventricular pressure with $P_w = P_{lv}$ sub-endocardially, and negligible sub-epicardially. Resistance = $(P_{arterial} - P_{waterfall})/$ mean flow. See also Chap. 6

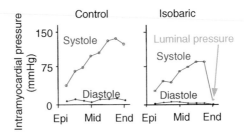

Fig. 19.7 Intramyocardial pressures measured in the beating heart using the servo-null technique. The intramyocardial pressure is high in isobaric beats where ventricular luminal pressure is negligible. (Adapted from Ref. [20], used by permission)

at the subepicardium [16]. However, there is some doubt regarding this assumption, since intramyocardial pressure is still considerable even when ventricular luminal pressure is negligible as in isobaric contraction (Fig. 19.7). Also the waterfall model does not explain the increase in venous outflow during cardiac contraction [17].

Finally muscle shortening and thickening affects the vasculature since by shortening the muscles increase in diameter. The increase in muscle diameter takes place at the expense of the vessels, thereby decreasing their diameters [3, 18]. When one considers the interplay of the effect on vessels of shortening, inversely related to pressure and wall force, there is plenty of material for vibrant debate rather than firm conclusions, including the mechanism of mean flow decrease in systolic arrest [19].

Detailed calculations have shown that the varying stiffness of the cardiac muscle, the thickening of the shortening muscle, and the increased intramyocardial pressure resulting from left ventricular pressure during contraction all contribute to decreased vessel size and therefore the increased resistance and the intramyocardial pumping. The contribution of these effects depends on the layer, mode of contraction and the contractility [18].

The summary of the effects of cardiac contraction on the coronary vessels is given in Fig. 19.8. The pressure-flow relations show an intercept that depends on the layer, on contractility, left ventricular pressure, and muscle shortening.

When it is assumed that coronary perfusion only takes place in diastole we can approximate the coronary fractional perfusion time, i.e., the perfusion time relative

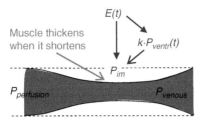

Fig. 19.8 Summary of effects of cardiac contraction on coronary flow. Muscle contraction results in stiffer environment and in ventricular pressure, both leading to P_{im}. When the muscle shortens it thickens at the expense of the vasculature. These three mechanisms all play a role depending on the layer in the heart wall. The variations in vascular diameters result in 'pumping' of blood retrograde to aorta and antegrade to the veins, the amounts depending on aorta and venous pressures

to the heart period T, as $T_d/T = 1 - T_s/T$, with T_d and T_s the duration of diastole and systole, respectively. Thus with a Heart Rate of 60 bpm, and the duration of systole being 0.35 s, the coronary fractional perfusion time is $1-0.35/1 = 0.65$. When Heart Rate is increased as in exercise to 120 bpm, i.e., $T = 0.5$ s, and the ejection period decreases to 0.3 s the coronary fractional perfusion time is $1-0.3/0.5 = 0.4$ s/s, thus decreasing the time for coronary perfusion.

19.1.6 Microvascular Aspects

Intramyocardial pressure and micro vessel diameters have been measured with different techniques [3, 20–22]. One method is the measurement of intramyocardial pressure with the servo-null technique, using micropipettes (diameter in the micron range) so as to cause minimal damage [20], see Fig. 19.7. The varying elastance hypothesis was applied to explain why intramyocardial pressure is present and similar in isobaric and isovolumic beats [3]. Both arteriolar and venular diameters decrease in systole [22] but the lower venous pressure results in a larger decrease in venous diameters thereby protecting arterioles from large changes in diameter [23].

So-called bridging occurs when an epicardial vessel, instead of running on the surface of the myocardium, is located in the heart wall, the vessel is greatly affected by cardiac contraction and may limit perfusion.

Microvascular perfusion pressure, expressed as arteriolar minus venular pressure (see Fig. 19.9) is considerably lower in subendocardial layers than in subepicardial layers [24]. This is caused by the pressure drop over the transmural arteries and transmural veins and may, in part, explain why the subendocardium is more vulnerable to ischemia than the subepicardial layers.

Coronary flow heterogeneity is shown by different local flows between locations, and may vary from less than 50% to more than twice the mean overall perfusion flow. A partial explanation is based on the fractal rules of coronary geometry [25], but a complete explanation has not yet been given. Another explanation may be that cardiac myocytes are quite different in length and cross-section and larger

Fig. 19.9 The net perfusion pressure, expressed as microvascular pressure gradient, is significantly smaller in the sub-endocardium than in the sub-epicardium. (Adapted from Ref. [24], by permission)

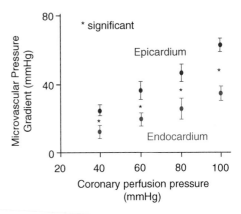

cells require more oxygen. In studies on local coronary flow by Positron Emission Tomography (PET) it was observed that heterogeneity is present in patients with different degrees of stenosis [26]. Some authors report on the so-called Gregg effect, a sort of garden-hose action where the coronary arteries are pumped up by perfusion and muscle Ca-handling appears increased [27], but there is doubt about its role as it is not seen in the intact animal when aortic pressure is increased.

Both the endocardial and the vascular endothelium generate nitric oxide and experimental removal or damage of the endocardial endothelium results in a lower and shortened myocardial force generation [28], and plays a role in Heart Failure with Preserved Ejection Fraction [29].

Cardiac efficiency is about 20–25% (Chap. 18), implying that about 75% of the oxygen consumed is converted into heat. At the normal level of coronary flow, i.e., ~90 ml/min/100 g, about 70% of the heat is carried away by the coronary flow and 30% by diffusion to thorax and ventricular lumen [30].

19.2 Physiological and Clinical Relevance

19.2.1 Coronary Flow in Layers

Coronary heart disease is a major problem in the western world and understanding of the factors that determine the pathology of coronary function is therefore of utmost clinical importance.

The coronary flow has to be matched to cardiac metabolism and should thus vary with activity and exercise (Fig. 19.10). The explanation that cardiac ischemia is earlier apparent in subendocardial layers than in subepicardial layers is partly due to cardiac contraction and partly the due to the pressure drop over the transmural vessels (Fig. 19.9).

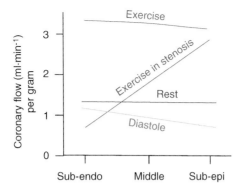

Fig. 19.10 Blood flow distribution in cardiac layers. In diastole mean flow is about 20% larger in subendocardial than in subepicardial layers (green). During rest mean flow is equally distributed over the different layers (blue). During exercise flow in the sub-endocardium tends to be smaller than in the sub-epicardium (purple). During exercise in the presence of a mild stenosis, coronary sub-endocardial flow will fall short (red)

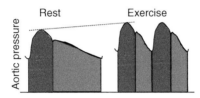

Fig. 19.11 The systolic (red) and diastolic (green) pressure-time areas. Their ratio is considered to be a measure of the myocardial, sub-endocardial, supply-demand ratio. During exercise the diastolic area decreases and the systolic area increases

19.2.2 Supply-Demand

Although the anatomy is such that coronary vascular resistance in diastole is the smallest in the subendocardial layers, contraction still reduces flow so much in this layer that perfusion only takes place during diastole. Thus the perfusion pressure and the duration of diastole are the main determinants of flow when the vasculature is dilated to its physiological maximum. This has led to the supply-demand ratio. The area under the systolic part of aortic or left ventricular pressure curve is an index of oxygen consumption, see the Tension Time Index (Chap. 17). The area under the diastolic pressure curve is a measure of supply. The supply-demand ratio appears an acceptable indication for subendocardial ischemia [31]. In exercise the supply-demand ratio is strongly decreased (Fig. 19.11).

The effect of a coronary stenosis, in terms of perfusion, is quantified by coronary flow reserve, CFR, and by fractional flow reserve, FFR. The hemodynamic effect of the stenosis is discussed Chap. 5. Wave Intensity Analysis has been extensively used in the analysis of coronary hemodynamics (Chap. 23).

Aortic balloon pumping reduces the aortic pressure in systole (reduced load, thus reduced demand) and increases aortic pressure in diastole (increased supply) and helps patients with cardiogenic shock.

References

1. Hoffman JIE, Spaan JAE. Pressure-flow relations in the coronary circulation. Physiol Rev. 1990;70:331–90.
2. Spaan JA. Coronary blood flow. Dordrecht: Kluwer; 1991.
3. Westerhof N, Boer C, Lamberts RR, Sipkema P. Cross-talk between cardiac muscle and coronary vasculature. Physiol Rev. 2006;86:1263–308.
4. Dankelman J, Spaan JAE, van der Ploeg CPB, Vergroesen I. Dynamic response of the coronary circulation to a rapid change in perfusion in the anaesthetised goat. J Physiol Lond. 1989;419:703–15.
5. Vergroesen I, Noble MIM, Wieringa PA, Spaan JAE. Quantification of O_2 consumption and arterial pressure as independent determinants of coronary flow. Am J Phys. 1987;252:H545–53.
6. Drake-Holland AJ, Laird JD, Noble MIM, Spaan JAE, Vergroesen I. Oxygen and coronary vascular resistance during autoregulation and metabolic vasodilation in the dog. J Physiol. 1984;348:285–300.
7. Kuo L, Davis MJ, Chilian WM. Longitudinal gradients for endothelium-dependent and -independent vascular responses in the coronary microcirculation. Circulation. 1995;92:518–25.
8. Duncker DJ, Bache RJ. Regulation of coronary blood flow during exercise. Physiol Rev. 2008;88:1009–86.
9. Bellamy RF. Diastolic coronary artery pressure-flow relations in the dog. Circ Res. 1978;43:92–101.
10. Van Dijk LC, Krams R, Sipkema P, Westerhof N. Changes in coronary pressure-flow relation after transition from blood to Tyrode. Am J Phys. 1988;255:H476–82.
11. Sherman IA. Interfacial tension effects in the microvasculature. Microvasc Res. 1981;22:296–307.
12. Sipkema P, Westerhof N. Mechanics of a thin walled collapsible microtube. Ann Biomed Eng. 1989;17:203–17.
13. Spaan JA. Coronary diastolic pressure-flow relation and zero flow pressure explained on the basis of intramyocardial compliance. Circ Res. 1985;56:293–309.
14. Gregg DE, Green HD. Registration and interpretation of normal phasic inflow into the left coronary artery by an improved differential manometric method. Am J Phys. 1940;130:114–25.
15. Krams R, van Haelst ACTA, Sipkema P, Westerhof N. Can coronary systolic-diastolic flow differences be predicted by left ventricular pressure of by time-varying intramyocardial elastance? Basic Res Cardiol. 1989;84:149–59.
16. Downey JM, Kirk ES. Inhibition of coronary blood flow by a vascular waterfall mechanism. Circ Res. 1975;36:753–60.
17. Spaan JA, Breuls NPW, Laird JD. Diastolic-systolic coronary flow differences are caused by intramyocardial pump action in the anesthetized dog. Circ Res. 1981;49:584–93.
18. Vis MA, Bovendeerd PH, Sipkema P, Westerhof N. Effect of ventricular contraction, pressure, and wall stretch on vessels at different locations in the wall. Am J Phys. 1997;272:H2963–75.
19. Sipkema P, Takkenberg JJM, Zeeuwe PEM, Westerhof N. Left coronary pressure-flow relations of the beating and arrested rabbit heart at different ventricular volumes. Cardiovasc Res. 1998;40:88–95.
20. Mihailescu LS, Abel FL. Intramyocardial pressure gradients in working and nonworking isolated cat hearts. Am J Phys. 1994;266:H1233–41.

21. Westerhof N. Physiological hypothesis. Intramyocardial pressure. Basic Res Cardiol. 1990;85:105–19.
22. Yada T, Hiramatsu O, Kimura A, Goto M, Ogasawara Y, Tsujioka K, et al. In vivo observation of subendocardial microvessels in the beating porcine heart using a needle-probe videomicroscope with a CCD camera. Circ Res. 1993;72:939–46.
23. Vis MA, Sipkema P, Westerhof N. Compression of intramyocardial arterioles during cardiac contraction is attenuated by accompanying venules. Am J Phys. 1997;273:H1002–11.
24. Chilian WM. Microvascular pressures and resistances in the left ventricular subendocardium and subepicardium. Circ Res. 1991;69:561–70.
25. Bassingthwaightc JB, King RB, Roger SA. Fractal nature of regional myocardial blood flow heterogeneity. Circ Res. 1989;65:578–90.
26. Danad I, Raijmakers PG, Harms HJ, Heymans MW, van Royen N, Lubberink M, et al. Impact of anatomical and functional severity of coronary atherosclerotic plaques on the transmural perfusion gradient: a [15O]H2O PET study. Eur Heart. 2014;35:2094–105.
27. Lamberts RR, Van Rijen MH, Sipkema P, Fransen P, Sys SU, Westerhof N. Coronary perfusion and muscle lengthening increase cardiac contraction: different stretch-triggered mechanisms. Am J Physiol Heart Circ Physiol. 2002;283:H1515–22.
28. Brutsaert DL. Cardiac endothelial-myocardial signaling: its role in cardiac growth, contractile performance, and rhythmicity. Physiol Rev. 2003;83:59–115.
29. Paulus WJ, Tschöpe C. A novel paradigm for heart failure with preserved ejection fraction: comorbidities drive myocardial dysfunction and remodeling through coronary microvascular endothelial inflammation. J Am Coll Cardiol. 2013;62:263–71. Review.
30. Ten Velden GHM, Westerhof N, Elzinga G. Left ventricular energetics: heat loss and temperature distribution in the canine myocardium. Circ Res. 1982;50:63–73.
31. Hoffman JIE, Buckberg JD. Myocardial supply:demand ratio – a critical review. Am J Cardiol. 1978;41:327–32.

Chapter 20
Assessing Ventricular Function

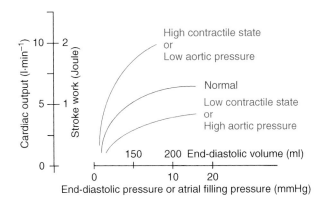

The ventricular function curve relates cardiac output or stroke work with end-diastolic ventricular volume, end-diastolic ventricular pressure, or atrial filling pressure. End-diastolic volume is a measure of end-diastolic muscle length and therefore the preferred variable. However, in practice filling is often expressed in terms of filling pressure, because pressure is an easier measure than end-diastolic volume (e.g., pulmonary arterial wedge pressure as measure of atrial filling pressure). Both Cardiac Output and Stroke Work are used as dependent variables. The Ventricular Function Curve is often obtained under conditions where the arterial load changes together with the ventricular filling. This means that a changed Ventricular Function Curve includes cardiac and arterial changes. Thus while the Ventricular Function Curve can explain in vivo adjustments of the heart and the circulation, it is not a characterization of the heart alone. The above figure makes this clear.

Starling studied the heart-lung preparation of the dog and the left ventricle was loaded with a Starling resistor. This device kept the aortic pressure constant during ejection and under this condition the Ventricular Function Curve describes the

© Springer International Publishing AG, part of Springer Nature 2019
N. Westerhof et al., *Snapshots of Hemodynamics*,
https://doi.org/10.1007/978-3-319-91932-4_20

heart alone. For isovolumic contractions as studied by Frank no equivalent Ventricular Function Curve is possible because no ejection takes place. We can explain the ventricular function curve on the basis of the Pressure-Volume relations and the Cardiac Pump Function graph. Thus, while the Frank-Starling mechanism relates end-diastolic ventricular volume with cardiac output at constant heart rate and contractility, and thus characterizes the heart, the Ventricular Function Curve also depends on the arterial load.

20.1   Description

In the intact organism the Ventricular Function Curve is usually presented as the relation between Stroke Volume (or Cardiac Output or Stroke Work) and ventricular filling. The idea arose from the fact that increased muscle length produces stronger contraction (Chap. 13). Frank showed that a similar relationship held true in the intact heart where he reported that when the isovolumic frog heart beats from an increased starting volume the pressure developed by contraction is increased. Starling kept the pressure development constant, using a 'Starling Resistor' and found that increased starting volume (and end-diastolic ventricular pressure) increased the cardiac output. This led to the popular "Ventricular Function Curve" relating cardiac output or stroke volume or Stroke Work to indices of filling, the end-diastolic ventricular pressure or volume. In the intact organism Cardiac Output is indeed increased by increased end-diastolic volume but the increased blood flow causes an increase in pressure, so that the Starling data does not adequately apply *in vivo* (see Fig. 14.1). Indeed, there also is a complicated adjustment of the circulation which depends on neural and humoral regulatory mechanisms. Thus, an increase in filling volume results in a smaller increase in Cardiac Output than under the assumption of a constant arterial pressure, as in Starling's experiment (Fig. 20.1). We thus see that the Ventricular Function Curve as measured in an intact organism depends on the heart in combination with the arterial load, and therefore characterizes ventriculo-arterial coupling and not the heart alone. The relation between diastolic filling and Cardiac Output is therefore more difficult to interpret than the original experiments by Frank and Starling.

Before the cardiac Echo technique became available, ventricular filling pressure or diastolic ventricular pressure was easier to determine than end-diastolic volume and the Ventricular Function Graph was therefore often presented as the relation between diastolic ventricular pressure with Stroke Work (SW). The graph is, in general, more linear when ventricular volume is used as independent variable than when filling pressure is used, because of the nonlinear diastolic pressure-volume relation. The relation between Stroke Work and ventricular diastolic volume is the so-called Preload Recruitable Stroke Work with slope M_w [1].

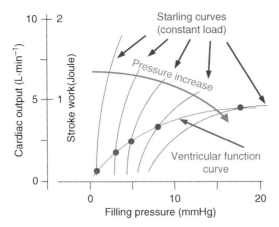

Fig. 20.1 The ventricular function curve is the relation between left ventricular filling pressure and cardiac output. The function curve depends on the pressure in systole, or more simply, aortic pressure, and is therefore load dependent. The family of curves, blue lines, can be derived from Starling's experiments each at constant aortic pressure. When the actual arterial load is present increased filling results in increased output and increased pressure, thus a lower Cardiac Output than the Starling curve predicts ventricular function curve (red line)

20.1.1 Global Left Ventricular Contractile Function Compared Between Patients

Indices of contractile function or contractility are dominated by the contribution of left ventricular (LV) cavity volume because arterial pressures are usually similar between patients. Nowadays clinical assessment of contractile function is made using ejection fraction (EF): the ratio of stroke volume (SV, the amount of blood ejected each beat) to end-diastolic volume (EDV, the starting volume for contraction at the end of diastole), EF = SV/EDV. When end-systolic volume (ESV) and end-diastolic volume (EDV) are increased, while Stroke Volume, is not changed, Ejection Fraction (EF) is decreased. At its simplest, if one can detect an increase in EDV in a patient free of valvular disease, it is almost as good as measuring EF. Sometimes one can do this by physical examination of the patient's chest. More sophisticated methods are (a) echocardiography in which one relies on ultrasound echoes to measure the end-systolic and end-diastolic diameters, (b) left ventriculography, when a patient is undergoing cardiac cauterization and X-ray contrast medium is injected into the LV cavity, (c) MUGA, Multiple Gated Acquisitions, is a better method of assessment, at least in theory, because a radioisotope can simply be injected intravenously and the radioactive counts from the LV cavity, when the blood is labeled, are proportional to volume, (d) imaging the heart by Magnetic Resonance Imaging (MRI). (e) in patients undergoing cardiac catheterization, a can be inserted into the LV, to measure volume continuously, that has a pressure transducer also mounted. The PV loops (giving values of EF) displayed from these transducers are more reliable for small hearts of animals than for humans, but it was possible with this approach in patients to show that with a strong post-ectopic beat, the ESV at similar pressure was smaller than in the normal beats, i.e., the strength of the post-ectopic beat not only depends on more filling, but also on increased contractility.

20.1.2   Invasive Assessment of Local Ventricular Function in the Patient

The maximum rate of rise of left ventricular pressure, dP_{lv}/dt_{max}, can be determined by measuring left ventricular pressure (LVP) with a catheter-tip manometer and passing the signal through an electronic differentiator. If the signal has a prominent positive maximum before valve opening, dP_{lv}/dt_{max} is an index of global LV contractile function and contractility. An argument in favor of the use of dP_{lv}/dt_{max} can be based on the Pressure Volume loop. It was shown (Chap. 14) that the $E(t)$-curve has a 'universal' shape and before valve opening ventricular pressure is proportional to $E(t)$ and thus dP_{lv}/dt_{max} then is a measure of global contractility.

To be a measure of muscle function dP_{lv}/dt should be related to wall stress σ. This can be done using Laplace's law (Chap. 9).

$$\sigma = P_{lv} \cdot g_f$$

with g_f a geometry factor accounting for the (local) radius of curvature and myocardial wall thickness. By the chain rule, differentiating with respect to time, we obtain:

$$d\sigma / dt = g_f \cdot dP_{lv} / dt + P_{lv} \cdot dg_f / dt$$

This shows that it is important to determine dP_{lv}/dt_{max} during isovolumic conditions so that g_f may be assumed constant, i.e., $dg_f/dt = 0$, and

$$dP_{lv} / dt = \left(1 / g_f\right) \cdot d\sigma / dt$$

With changes in filling the geometric factor g_f will change limiting its use as contractility index. At low volumes, such as during cardiac surgery with open chest, a change in dP_{lv}/dt_{max}, may result both from changes in muscle function and filling. In the closed chest, and in the catheter laboratory the geometric factor does, in general, not change so that dP_{lv}/dt_{max} gives useful information on averaged global muscle function. At very large ventricular volumes an increase in the factor g_f may even result in a decrease in dP_{lv}/dt_{max}. Thus dP_{lv}/dt_{max} can be used only as a convenient volume independent index for changes in cardiac contractility in the catheter

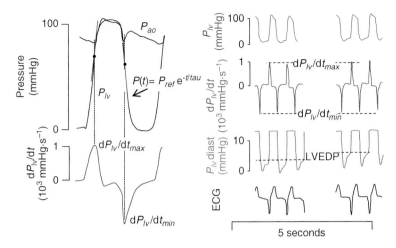

Fig. 20.2 Time derivative of left ventricular pressure, dP_{lv}/dt_{max}, when falling before valve opening (left panel) is used as a measure of contractility. The right panel shows that increased filling, resulting in an increase in end-diastolic pressure (LVEDP, dashed line) does not affect dP_{lv}/dt_{max} since this index is sensitive to inotropic interventions and not, in this range, depending on filling pressure. The rate of ventricular relaxation is defined by the time constant tau, and relates with left ventricular end-diastolic pressure. The dP_{lv}/dt_{min} is a measure of ventricular relaxation. (Right panel adapted from Ref. [2], by permission)

laboratory. In Fig. 20.2 the record on the left was obtained with the patient in head-up tilt and the record on the right with the patient in head-down tilt. It can be seen that the left ventricular end-diastolic pressure is higher in the right hand record due to the increase in ventricular volume, but dP_{lv}/dt_{max} is unchanged [2].

The isovolumic ventricular relaxation phase can be characterized by the exponential decay constant tau. In patients with diastolic heart failure with preserved ejection fraction (HFpEF) the time constant is prolonged and filling pressure is increased [3], leading to lower filling volume. There is also a prominent negative maximum, dP_{lv}/dt_{min}, which is used as a measure of ventricular relaxation (lusitropy).

20.1.3 Merits and Drawbacks of dP_{lv}/dt_{max}, ESPVR and E_{es} as Assessments of Global Contractility

The dP_{lv}/dt_{max} has limited value for comparing the contractility of patients [4] because it is also an index of the synchronicity of contraction and muscle mass. Figure 20.3 shows, as an example, that during conduction defects, e.g., bundle branch block or inappropriate pacing sites, dP_{lv}/dt_{max} is different [5]. In general, the dP_{lv}/dt_{max} is highest during sinus rhythm (extreme right hand point in Fig. 20.3). The End-Systolic Pressure-Volume Relation, ESPVR, has the same shortcoming. In

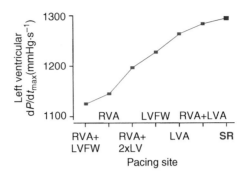

Fig. 20.3 LVdP/dt$_{max}$ depends on pacing site. During ventricular pacing from various sites LVdP/dt$_{max}$ is compared with its value during sinus rhythm (SR, blue). RVA Right Ventricular Apex, LVFW Left Ventricular Free Wall, LVA Left Ventricular Apex, 2xLV LV free wall and apex. (Redrawn from Ref. [5], used by permission)

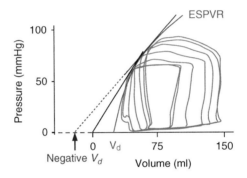

Fig. 20.4 End-Systolic Pressure-Volume relation, ESPVR, as a measure of global ventricular function. Several pressure-volume loops, preferably obtained with changes in cardiac filling, are required to determine this relation (red line). Approximations by assuming a straight relation (blue line, with negative intercept), or using a single loop and assuming linearity and zero intercept volume (black line) may lead to unacceptable errors

other words, the two quantities do not quantify muscle contractility alone but depend on muscle mass and synchronicity of muscle contraction and pacing site as well.

The theoretical gold standard for assessment of cardiac contractility is the slope of the End-Systolic Pressure-Volume Relation (ESPVR, Fig. 20.4), but in practice this ESPVR is usually only obtainable invasively, as during cardiac surgery. Volume changes are required and they can be obtained by, partial, occlusion and release of the vena cavae. An increase in contractility corresponds to a 'rotation' around V_d of the ESPVR (Chap. 14). The slope of the relation, E_{es}, is only an acceptable index of contractility if the relation is straight. For a curved relation the slope depends on the chosen pressure. The straight-line extrapolation often suggests a negative, physically impossible, and thus virtual, intercept with the volume axis. Thus when volume and pressure can be measured, the ESPVR-curve should be reported because it gives much more accurate information than its (locally dependent) slope, the E_{es}.

20.1.4   Noninvasive Assessment of Global Ventricular Function in the Patient

By definition, noninvasive assessment rules out methods such as catheter-tip manometry and conductance catheter volume measurement. One approach that gained some popularity is calculating E_{es} by dividing peak aortic pressure, as an index of end-systolic left ventricular pressure, by end-systolic volume, obtained by Echo or MRI. In addition to the assumption of linearity of the ESPVR, the intercept volume is assumed to be negligible. These noninvasive approaches are subject to errors (see Chaps. 14 and 18).

The assessment of contractility is complicated by the nonlinearity of the ESPVR. Of course, if during an intervention mean arterial pressure does not change (pressure clamped by the baroreflex, [6]), the nonlinearity of the ESPVR does not play a role and the end-systolic volume at this same pressure is moved to smaller volumes with increased contractility. If arterial pressure changes it is recommended that the changes in mean arterial pressure are accounted for. A control run should be compared in which the mean arterial pressure changes are reproduced with a pure vasoconstrictor or a pure vasodilator.

For the ventricle as a whole the relation between Stroke Work and (diastolic) volume (Fig. 20.5) is straight [1, 7] and is called Preload Recruitable Stroke Work with slope M_W, a load insensitive index of cardiac contractility. It has subsequently been shown that M_W can be estimated from a single beat [7]. Stroke Work (Chap. 16) can be approximated by Stroke Volume times mean aortic (or carotid) pressure during ejection (systole). Using carotid pressure allows for estimation of M_W from a single beat and noninvasively.

20.1.5   Assessment of Change in Regional Left Ventricular Function

Contractile function variables can be affected both by changes in global contractility and by regional dysfunction, e.g. myocardial infarction. In the latter case, regional contractile function is of clinical importance, but cannot be studied in

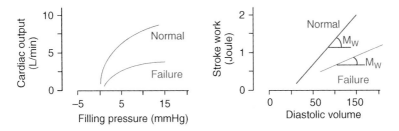

Fig. 20.5 Ventricular function curves under normal conditions, and in heart failure (left). The characterization pertains to ventriculo-arterial interaction and not to the heart alone. Preload recruitable Stroke Work (right) is load-insensitive, and its slope, M_W, a measure of contractility

absolute terms as is the case with global function indices such as the ESPVR and dP_{lv}/dt_{max}. The pragmatic approach therefore is to study local wall movement to see whether it is impaired or, in some cases such as hypertrophic cardiomyopathy, enhanced. Dysfunctional myocardium may respond to a positive inotropic intervention, e.g. post-extra-systolic potentiation or dobutamine infusion. This indicates if the tissue is viable and may improve with reperfusion. This approach is followed in Stress-Echo and Stress-MRI investigations.

20.2   Physiological and Clinical Relevance

The Ventricular Function Curve is very regularly used to demonstrate the effects of therapy on Cardiac Output.

An example is given in Fig. 20.5 (left panel), where the Ventricular Function Curve is shown in control and heart failure. Again, one should be aware of the fact that the graphs do not reflect the differences in the heart alone but also may contain what is changed in the arterial load. However, the slope of the relation between Stroke Work and diastolic volume (Fig. 20.5, right panel) was shown to be load independent and can be used as measure of ventricular contractility [7].

References

1. Glower DD, Spratt JA, Snow ND, Kabas JS, Davis JW, Olson CO, et al. Linearity of the frank-Starling relationship in the intact heart: the concept of preload recruitable stroke work. Circulation. 1985;71:994–1009.
2. Drake-Holland AJ, Mills CJ, Noble MIM, Pugh S. Responses to changes in filling and contractility of indices of human left ventricular mechanical performance. J Physiol Lond. 1990;422:29–39.
3. Zile MR, Baicu CF, Gaasch WH. Diastolic heart failure--abnormalities in active relaxation and passive stiffness of the left ventricle. N Engl J Med. 2004;350:1953–9.
4. Van den Bos GC, Elzinga G, Westerhof N, Noble MIM. Problems in the use of indices of myocardial contractility. Cardiovcvasc Res. 1973;7:834–48.
5. Prinzen FW, Peschar M. Relation between the pacing induced sequence of activation and left ventricular pump function in animals. J Pacing Clin Electrophysiol. 2002;25:484–98.
6. Brooks CI, White PA, Staples M, Oldershaw PJ, Redington AN, Collins PD, et al. Myocardial contractility is not constant during spontaneous atrial fibrillation in patients. Circulation. 1998;98:1762–8.
7. Karunanithi MK, Feneley MP. Single-beat determination of preload recruitable stroke work relationship: derivation and evaluation in conscious dogs. J Am Coll Cardiol. 2000;35:502–13.

Part III
Arterial Hemodynamics

Chapter 21
Wave Travel and Pulse Wave Velocity

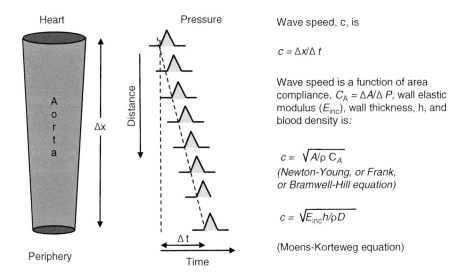

Heart

Pressure

Wave speed, c, is

$$c = \Delta x / \Delta t$$

Distance

Wave speed is a function of area compliance, $C_A = \Delta A / \Delta P$, wall elastic modulus ($E_{inc}$), wall thickness, h, and blood density is:

$$c = \sqrt{A / \rho\, C_A}$$

(Newton-Young, or Frank, or Bramwell-Hill equation)

$$c = \sqrt{E_{inc} h / \rho D}$$

(Moens-Korteweg equation)

Δx

A o r t a

Periphery

Δt

Time

Waves generated by the heart travel down the aorta and major conduit arteries. These waves may be pressure waves, flow or velocity waves or diameter waves. The ratio of the distance Δx, and the time it takes for the wave to travel over this distance, Δt, gives the wave speed or pulse wave velocity, PWV = $\Delta x / \Delta t$. The same wave speed applies to pressure, flow and diameter waves. The wave speed depends on vessel size and the elastic properties of the arterial wall. In the aorta of a healthy subject the wave speed is typically 4–5 m/s. In stiff aortas, having a low compliance (C_A) and a high wall elastic modulus (E_{inc}) the wave speed may be two times higher, implying a four-fold decrease in aortic area compliance. The wave speed in peripheral arteries is higher than in central arteries since the wall thickness is higher and the diameter is smaller. By measuring the foot-to-foot PWV its value is close to the true phase velocity c, and the above equations hold.

21.1   Description

The heart generates pressure and flow waves. Because of the elastic properties of the aorta and the major conduit arteries, the pressure and flow waves are not transmitted instantaneously to the periphery, but they propagate through the arterial tree with a certain speed, which we call wave speed (c) or pulse wave velocity (PWV). In analogy to waves created by a stone dropped in a lake, the waves seen on the surface travel with a speed that is measured by the time it takes for the disturbance (wave) to cover a certain distance. The distance traveled by the wave over the time delay gives the wave speed, $c = \Delta x / \Delta t$ as schematically shown in the Figure in the Box. Also, in analogy with the stone dropped in the lake, the wave transmission takes place even in the absence of blood flow. When a stone is dropped in a river, the waves superimpose on the water flow, and the (flow) waves traveling downstream go faster than the waves that move upstream. In other words, the velocity of the blood adds to the wave speed. However, since the blood flow velocity is much (more than 20 times) smaller than the PWV this effect is usually neglected.

21.1.1   Wave Speed Depends on Vessel Elastic Modulus and on Compliance

This equations for wave speed, called phase velocity, are derived for non-viscous fluid and a purely elastic wall; they hold in good approximation for uniform conduit arteries filled with blood (see Chap. 12). The wave speed can be related to the elastic modulus of the wall material via the Moens-Korteweg equation:

$$c = \sqrt{\frac{h \cdot E_{inc}}{2 \cdot r_i \cdot \rho}} = \sqrt{\frac{h \cdot E_{inc}}{D_i \cdot \rho}}$$

where E_{inc} is the incremental elastic (Youngs) modulus, ρ the blood density, h the wall thickness and r_i and D_i the lumen radius and diameter. The Moens-Korteweg equation allows estimation of a material property of the arterial wall, E_{inc}.

Wave speed derived by Frank in 1920, [1] and Bramwell and Hill in 1929 [2] expresses the wave speed as function of arterial compliance.

$$c = \sqrt{\frac{A}{\rho C_A}} = \sqrt{\frac{V \Delta P}{\rho \Delta V}} = \sqrt{\frac{BM}{\rho}} = \sqrt{\frac{1}{\rho K}}$$

with A the lumen area, the area compliance $C_A = \Delta A / \Delta P$ and $A/C_A = V \Delta P / \Delta V$ with length assumed constant, the ρ is blood density and BM and K are Bulk Modulus and distensibility, respectively (Chap. 11). Newton and Young derived this equation first, and Frank introduced it in hemodynamics. This equation allows estimation of structural properties, C_A, BM or K.

21.1.2 *Phase Velocity and Apparent Phase Velocity*

The phase velocity is the wave speed determined by the properties of the vessel wall and blood density as presented above, i.e., wave reflections are assumed not to exist. When two arterial pressures are measured to derive wave speed, these waves include the effect of reflections and with reflections the formulas for PWV become more complex. When Fourier analysis is performed (Appendix 1) on two pressure waves measured a distance Δx apart, the wave speed for each harmonic can be obtained by using the time difference, called phase lag for sine waves, $\Delta \varphi$, between the two harmonics. The phase lag is $\Delta \varphi = 2\pi \, \Delta t / T = 2\pi f \Delta t$, with T the duration of one sinewave period, the inverse of the frequency, f, of the sine wave. The apparent wave velocity, c_{app}, is then calculated for each harmonic as.

$$c_{app,i} = \frac{2\pi \cdot \Delta x}{T_i \cdot \Delta \phi_i} = \frac{2\pi \cdot f_i \cdot \Delta x}{\Delta \phi_i}$$

with i signifying the ith harmonic. If the frequency is given in Hz, Δx in cm, and $\Delta \varphi$ in radians, c_{app} will be in cm/s. Thus, the apparent wave velocity includes the effect of reflections and is therefore not a good measure of vessel compliance. Figure 21.1 shows the apparent wave velocity as a function of frequency. For high frequencies, the apparent wave velocity approaches the true phase velocity because for high frequencies reflections become negligible (Chap. 12).

When the wave speed is determined from the foot of the wave (Fig. 21.2) the value is close to the apparent wave velocity at high frequencies, and thus close to the phase velocity, and the equations above can be applied to derive area compliance or incremental modulus of the wall material. However, the Moens-Korteweg and the Frank/Bramwell-Hill wave speed both pertain to uniform tubes only. When wave speed is measured over the entire aorta the assumption of a uniform tube is obviously not correct.

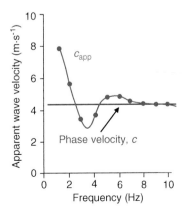

Fig. 21.1 The apparent wave velocity, c_{app} is the speed measured when reflected waves play a role. For high frequencies reflections are small and c_{app} is close to the phase velocity c, the velocity without reflections present

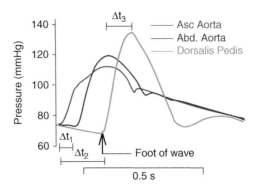

Fig. 21.2 Pressure waves at different locations of the human arterial tree. The distance divided by the time delay of the foot of the waves gives the pulse wave velocity (foot-foot pulse wave velocity). It is assumed that the foot of the wave is determined by high frequencies and therefore the 'foot-to-foot' PWV is close to the phase velocity. The time difference between pressure maxima is not a good measure of the phase velocity c. (Adapted from Ref. [3], by permission)

21.1.3   Methods to Obtain Wave Speed

A number of methods have been developed to derive Pulse Wave Velocity.

Time delay or foot-to-foot method This is the most direct method. Wave speed is estimated from the time it takes for the foot of the pressure, diameter, or blood velocity wave, to travel between two sites a known distance apart. The so calculated foot-to-foot wave velocity is close to the phase velocity and can be used to derive vessel compliance or incremental Youngs modulus E_{inc}. Figure 21.2 shows realistic time delays for pressure waves recorded in the human aorta and the lower limbs [3]. For instance, the delay of the foot of the wave between ascending and thoracic aorta is $\Delta t_1 = 0.056$ s, and the distance is $\Delta x_1 = 0.25$ m. Thus, the proximal aortic wave speed, equals 0.25/0.056 m/s and PWV $= c = 4.5$ m/s. The average wave speed from the aorta to the lower limb is $\Delta x_2/\Delta t_2 = 1.25$ m/0.175 s and PWV $= 7.1$ m/s. Peripheral arteries are smaller, have relatively larger wall thickness, and are stiffer (higher E_{inc}). Therefore, by virtue of the Moens-Korteweg equation, they have a higher wave speed. Note that the estimated aorta-to-dorsalis pedis wave speed (8.5 m/s) is an average wave speed for the entire arterial pathway traveled by the wave (aorta, iliac, femoral, popliteal), and this arterial section is not even close to a uniform tube. If one had used the time delay based on peak systolic pressure ($\Delta t_3 = 0.102$ s, in Fig. 21.2), the estimated wave speed would have been 1.25 m/0.102 s = 12.3 m/s. This speed is much higher than the foot-to-foot estimate of 7.1 m/s. The overestimation is attributed partly to the fact that the artery is stiffer at higher distending pressures but is also partly attributed to wave reflections that contribute to peak systole. It is therefore generally accepted that the time delay should be calculated from the foot or the early up-slope of the wave rather than the systolic part.

Three-pressure method By measurement of three pressures some centimeters apart, reflections can be accounted for and the phase velocity can be derived [4].

Temporal and spatial derivative method For a uniform artery without reflections wave speed can be calculated using the time derivative and spatial derivative of pressure [5]: c = (dP/dt)/(dP/dx).

Wave speed derived from pressure and diameter measurements It holds in approximation that area compliance $C_A = (A_s - A_d)/(P_s - P_d)$. Local systolic (s) and diastolic (d) pressure can be measured using Oscillometry, and local diameters with US and so that mean, systolic and diastolic areas can be calculated. Wave speed then can be derived using the Frank formula for wave speed, and using this approach PWV can be estimated as a function of pressure [6].

Wave speed from flow and diameter measurements Flow or flow velocity and diameter or area can be measured noninvasively by means of MRI and allows estimation of central PWV noninvasively [7].

Method based on differences Differences of velocity, dv, and pressure, dP, as defined in Wave Intensity (Chap. 23), allow the calculation of PWV at a single location. The basic equation is [8]:

$$c^2 = 1/\rho^2 \Sigma dP^2 / \Sigma dv^2$$

The advantage of the method is that determination can be done at a single location. The method has been applied to the coronary circulation, but it has been criticized [9].

Wave speed derived from flow and area measurements This method [10], see Fig. 21.3, uses noninvasive flow and area measurements by MRI or ultrasonic technologies, thus making it possible to derive wave speed noninvasively. Imagine that the heart ejects into the aorta a certain volume ΔV over a period Δt. The ejected volume will be 'accommodated' in the aorta by means of an increase in the aortic cross-sectional area ΔA over a certain length Δx. The wave speed is the speed with which the perturbation in area, ΔA, has traveled in the aorta, which is $\Delta x/\Delta t$. The

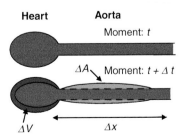

Fig. 21.3 Area and flow changes as related to the wave speed (see text)

volume ejected in the aorta is $\Delta V = \Delta A \cdot \Delta x$ or $\Delta x = \Delta V / \Delta A$. Dividing by Δt, we obtain:

$$c = \frac{\Delta x}{\Delta t} = \frac{\Delta V}{\Delta t \cdot \Delta A}$$

and since $\Delta V / \Delta t$ is equal to the volume flow ΔQ it follows that

$$c = \Delta Q / \Delta A$$

From this relation, we see that when ejection takes place in a stiff artery where the change in area, ΔA, will be small, the wave speed will be high.

The method assumes negligible reflections in early ejection and relates to the calculation of characteristic impedance in early ejection (Chaps. 12 and 23)

$$dQ / dA = dQ / dP \cdot dP / dA = 1 / Z_c \cdot C_A = \text{SQRT}\left[1 / \left(L'C_A\right)\right] = \text{PWV}.$$

The advantage of the method is that both ΔQ and ΔA can be obtained noninvasively by MRI and thus suited for pulmonary and intrathoracic arteries (Chap. 28) [11].

21.1.4   Amplification of Pressure Waves

As can be seen in Fig. 21.2 the systolic pressure increases while travelling towards the periphery. Diastolic pressure changes little or decreases, and mean pressure is practically the same in all conduit arteries (Chap. 6). Therefore, the increase in Pulse Pressure mainly results from the increased systolic pressure. This phenomenon is called Pulse Pressure amplification. In aging amplification decreases [12] as a result of the increased wave speed as has been discussed in Chap. 12.

Amplification and the change in pressure wave shape implies that the calculation of mean pressure from systolic and diastolic pressures depends on the location where pressure is measured. For instance, in the brachial artery mean pressure is close to $(P_s + 2P_d)/3 = P_d + \text{PP}/3$. If in the proximal aorta with a lower systolic pressure the mean pressure also would be calculated with the same formula, mean aortic pressure would be lower than in the brachial artery, which is clearly impossible. In the proximal aorta, a good estimate of mean pressure can be calculated as $P_m = (P_s + P_d)/2 = P_d + \text{PP}/2$. The 1/3 and 1/2 are so-called pressure form factors (Chap. 12).

21.2   Physiological and Clinical Relevance

The above equations show that from wave speed the vessel wall elasticity (E_{inc}) and area compliance C_A can be derived if the artery's geometry (diameter and wall thickness) are known, thus, giving a good estimation of large vessel elasticity.

21.2.1   Carotid-Femoral PWV

The wave speed between carotid artery and iliac or femoral artery, c_{c-f} or CF-PWV, can be measured noninvasively and is accepted as representative for aortic wave velocity. The wave speed allows estimation of aortic elasticity, and this noninvasive method is often used in hypertension research. Some limitations need to be mentioned. The estimation of length should account for the distance between the arch and the location of measurement in the carotid artery where the signal is measured. The ascending aorta is not included while changes in elasticity there may be considerable. With aging the aorta becomes tortuous which results in an underestimation of length and thus an underestimation in wave speed. Recently the intra-arterial and noninvasive determination of PWV have been compared [13].

Other locations for determination of wave speed, such as Carotid to Radial artery wave speed, CR-PWV have been used. Time delay between Brachial artery pressure and Tibial artery pressure is used as heart-to-ankle delay and used to calculate the Cardio-Ankle Vascular Index, CAVI [14]. The CAVI is based on two assumptions, namely Frank's equation for wave speed and the β introduced by Hayashi (Chap. 11) to make the CAVI pressure-independent [15]. The pressure-independent character has, of course advantages for comparison between different patients. However, stiffness of aorta, leg and upper arm arteries are all contributing. Also, the equation for wave speed is strictly speaking only applicable to uniform blood vessels without reflections. Later Spronck et al. introduced a new reference point to make the pressure dependence even smaller [16].

21.2.2   Wave Speed Depends on Pressure

The foot-to-foot PWV is determined at diastolic pressure [6], but the pressure wave spans the range from diastole to systole and in systole wave speed is higher (Fig. 21.4). Wave speed is a function of pressure, due to the nonlinear elastic properties of the arterial wall. Based on compliance and area using the Frank/Bramwell-Hill equation, wave speed can be derived as a function of pressure. The wave speed, in combination with pressure measurement allows to obtain β-stiffness (see Chap. 11) as [15, 16]:

$$\beta = 2\rho \cdot \ln\left(P_s / P_d\right) \cdot \text{PWV}^2 / \left(P_s - P_d\right)$$

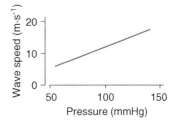

Fig. 21.4 Wave speed increases with pressure in the human brachial artery

Fig. 21.5 Aortic pulse wave velocity as a function of age in individuals with low prevalence of atherosclerosis in urban China. Note the increase by almost a factor of 2 corresponding with a four fold decrease in aortic compliance (for fold increase in aortic stiffness). (From Ref. [17], by permission)

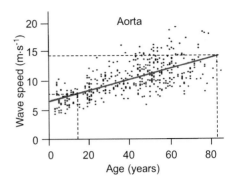

21.2.3 Wave Speed Depends on Age

With age, wave speed increases as shown in Fig. 21.5 where data were measured in normal human subjects, in the absence of atherosclerosis [17]. The increase in wave speed by about a factor two between the ages 15 and 80 years implies a decrease in compliance by a factor four. The increase in aortic stiffness with age is primarily attributed to a progressive thinning, fraying and fracture of elastic laminae, likely due to repetitive cyclic stretch of the pulsating pressure. Changes in aortic wave speed with age depend on location [7].

Although all wall constituents are subjected to the same Pulse Pressure and thus to the same cyclic stretch, it is mainly the elastin that cannot be re-synthesized sufficiently rapidly [18]. The net result is gradual replacement of elastin with collagen. The stiffer aorta implies reduced Windkessel function and higher Pulse Pressure (Chap. 25). The higher Pulse Pressure, in turn, may cause extra wear of the vessel wall resulting in more breakdown of elastin. It has been shown that Pulse Pressure is a strong indicator of cardiovascular mortality and morbidity [19].

References

1. Frank O. Die Elastizität der Blutgefässe Z Biol. 1920;71:255–72.
2. Bramwell JC, Hill AV. The velocity of the pulse wave in man. Proc Roy Soc Lond [Biol]. 1922;93:298–306.
3. Remington JW, Wood EH. Formation of peripheral pulse contour in man. J Appl Physiol. 1956;9:433–42.
4. Taylor MG. An experimental determination of the propagation of fluid oscillations in a tube with a visco-elastic wall; together with an analysis of the characteristics required in an electrical analogue. Phys Med Biol. 1959;4:63–82.
5. Fry DL, Casper AG, Mallos AJ. A catheter tip method for measurement of the instantaneous aortic blood velocity. Circ Res. 1956;4:627–32.
6. Hermeling E, Vermeersch SJ, Rietzschel ER, de Buyzere ML, Gillebert TC, van de Laar RJ, et al. The change in arterial stiffness over the cardiac cycle rather than diastolic stiffness is

independently associated with left ventricular mass index in healthy middle-aged individuals. J Hypertens. 2012;30:396–402.

7. Hickson SS, Butlin M, Graves M, Taviani V, Avolio AP, Mceniery CM, et al. The relationship of age with regional aortic stiffness and diameter. JACC Cardiovasc Imaging. 2010;3:1247–55.

8. Davies JE, Whinnett ZI, Francis DP, Willson K, Foale RA, Malik IS, et al. Use of simultaneous pressure and velocity measurements to estimate arterial wave speed at a single site in humans. Am J Phys. 2006;290:H878–85.

9. Rolandi MC, De Silva K, Lumley M, Lockie TP, Clapp B, Spaan JA, et al. Wave speed in human coronary arteries is not influenced by microvascular vasodilation: implications for wave intensity analysis. Basic Res Cardiol. 2014;109:405.

10. Vulliemoz S, Stergiopulos N, Meuli R. Estimation of local aortic elastic properties with MRI. Magn Reson Med. 2002;47:649–54.

11. Ibrahimel SH, Shaffer JM, White RD. Assessment of pulmonary artery stiffness using velocity encoding magnetic resonance imaging: evaluation of techniques. Magn Reson Imag. 2011;29:966–74.

12. Pichler G, Martinez F, Vicente A, Solaz E, Calaforra O, Redon J. Pulse pressure amplification and its determinants. Blood Press. 2016;25:21–7.

13. Weber T, Wassertheurer S, Hametner B, Parragh S, Eber B. Noninvasive methods to assess pulse wave velocity: comparison with the invasive gold standard and relationship with organ damage. J Hypertens. 2015;33:1023–31.

14. Saiki A, Sato Y, Watanabe R, Watanabe Y, Imamura H, Yamaguchi T, et al. The role of a novel arterial stiffness parameter, cardio-ankle vascular index (CAVI), as a surrogate marker for cardiovascular diseases. J Atheroscler Thromb. 2016;23:155–68.

15. Spronck B, Heusinkveld MH, Vanmolkot FH, Roodt JO, Hermeling E, Delhaas T, et al. Pressure-dependence of arterial stiffness: potential clinical implications. J Hypertens. 2015;33:330–8.

16. Spronck B, Avolio AP, Tan I, Butlin M, Reesink KD, Delhaas T. Arterial stiffness index beta and cardio-ankle vascular index inherently depend on blood pressure but can be readily corrected. J Hypertens. 2017;35:98–104.

17. Avolio AP, Chen S-G, Wang R-P, Zhang C-L, Li M-F, O'Rourke MF. Effects of aging on changing arterial compliance and left ventricular load in a in a northern Chinese urban community. Circulation. 1983;68:50–8.

18. Martyn CN, Greenwald SE. Impaired synthesis of elastin in walls of aorta and large conduit arteries during early development as an initiating event in pathogenesis of systemic hypertension. Lancet. 1997;3502:953–5.

19. Mitchell GF, Moye LA, Braunwald E, Rouleau JL, Bernstein V, Geltman EM, et al. Sphygmomanometrically determined pulse pressure is a powerful independent predictor of recurrent events after myocardial infarction in patients with impaired left ventricular function. Circulation. 1997;96:4254–60.

Chapter 22
Wave Separation and Waveform Analysis

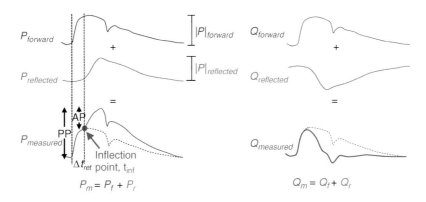

$$P_m = P_f + P_r$$

$$Q_m = Q_f + Q_r$$

Next to systolic, diastolic and mean pressure, separation of pressure into forward and reflected waves and the analysis of the pressure wave shape give hemodynamic information. Pressure and flow waves are waves containing a (compound) wave traveling towards the periphery (forward running wave) and a (compound) reflected wave. Wave separation is the calculation of forward and reflected pressure and flow waves and the calculation can be performed in the time domain (Chap. 12). Forward pressure and flow waves are similar in shape, and the reflected pressure and flow waves are also similar in shape, but the reflected flow wave is inverted with respect to the reflected pressure wave. This difference in polarity of the reflected waves leads to differences in the shape of the measured pressure and flow waves. The separation of the pressure and flow into their forward and reflected components is a useful technique for analyzing and studying wave reflections. The Reflection Magnitude is the ratio of the amplitudes of reflected and forward wave $RM = |P|_{reflected}$ $/|P|_{forward,}$ the Reflection Index is $RI = |P|_{reflected} /(|P|_{forward} + |P|_{reflected})$. In waveform analysis the pressure wave shape is analyzed. The Augmentation Index, is defined as Augmented Pressure over Pulse Pressure: $AIx = AP/PP$. The RI can be compared with the AIx. The return time of the reflected wave is Δt_{ret}, can be compared with the timing of the inflection point, t_{inf}.

22.1   Description

At any location in the arterial tree, the measured pressure and flow waves are the sum of a compound forward wave and a compound reflected wave. Because both forward and reflected wave arise from reflections at the many arterial reflection sites, the compound waves consist of sub-waves, added up to compound waves.

Wave separation analysis is the calculation of compound forward waves P_f, Q_f, and compound reflected waves P_r, Q_r, from the measured pressure and flow. The extra information needed is an estimate of characteristic impedance (Chap. 12).

Waveform analysis pertains to analysis of the pressure waveform itself, such as determination of augmentation index, AIx, and inflection point, t_{inf} (Figure in the Box).

22.1.1   Wave Separation Analysis: Forward and Reflected Components

The visualization of the forward and reflected waves is shown in Fig. 22.1 As discussed in Chap. 12 it holds that

$$P_f = Z_c \cdot Q_f = \left(P_m + Z_c \cdot Q_m\right)/2 \ \ and \ \ P_r = -Z_c \cdot Q_r = \left(P_m - Z_c \cdot Q_m\right)/2$$

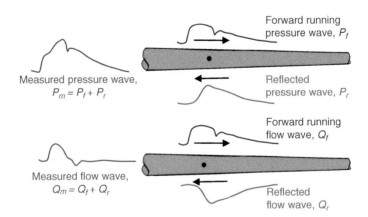

Fig. 22.1 Principle of the separation of pressure and flow waves into their forward and reflected components

with P and Q pressure and flow, and m, f and r measured, forward and reflected waves [1, 2].

From this separation, the oscillatory output power of the heart can be separated in forward and reflected components [3]:

$$\text{Power} = P_m(t) \cdot Q_m(t) = \left(P_f + P_r \right) \cdot \left(Q_f + Q_r \right) = \left(P_f + P_r \right) \cdot \left(P_f - P_r \right) / Z_c$$
$$= \left(P_f(t)^2 - P_r(t)^2 \right) / Z_c$$

Thus when the reflected pressure wave is 30% of the forward wave the oscillatory reflected power is about 10%.

The above formulas are simple to use when the characteristic impedance, Z_c, is a real number, as in large conduit arteries, where blood viscosity can be neglected and the wall is close to purely elastic (Chap. 12).

We may calculate Z_c as:

$$Z_c = \rho \cdot c / A$$

with ρ blood density, c the local phase velocity and A the luminal cross-sectional area (see below).

In practice, the characteristic impedance of large vessels can be determined in two ways, as detailed in Chap. 12. The ratio of the pressure and flow change in early systole or from the high frequency impedance modulus.

In smaller vessels, the same analysis holds and same equations apply, with the exception that the characteristic impedance, Z_c, is a frequency dependent complex number and the equations pertain to individual harmonics of pressure and flow (see Chap. 12). The individual harmonics need to be added to obtain the waves in the time domain.

After the derivation of P_f and P_r the Reflection Magnitude can be calculated from the amplitudes of forward and reflected pressure or forward and reflected flow. $RM = P_r/P_f$. The Reflection Index, $RI = P_r/(P_f + P_r)$. The RM and RI are not equal to the Reflection Coefficient as defined in Chap. 12. The reflection coefficient depends on vascular properties only, while the RI and RM depend on the pressure wave shape and thus contain a cardiac contribution. The arrival time of the reflected wave, Δt_{ret}, can be determined from the foot of the waves (see Figure in the Box) as is done for Pulse Wave Velocity (Chap. 21).

It has been shown that by assuming a triangular wave shape for aortic flow (flow 'triangulation method') and measured pressure, the wave separation can be carried out [4, 5]. Subsequent calculation of RM and RI does not need calibrated pressure and flow since they are pressure ratios [4].

Wave separation can be carried out at all locations. The separation of forward and reflected waves along the aorta was carried out by Davies et al. [6] and Tyberg [7] and it was found that at all locations the time delay between the reflected and forward waves is hardly dependent of location, see Fig. 22.2. In other words the reflected pressure wave appears to run towards the periphery rather than towards the

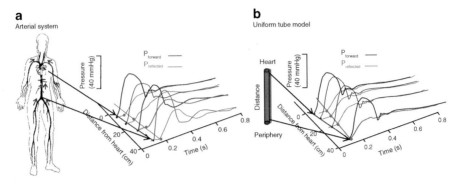

Fig. 22.2 Panel (**a**) Forward and reflected pressure waves in the in-vivo aorta. The reflected and forward waves show similar time delay at the different locations, and the reflected pressure wave appears to run to the periphery, not to the heart. Panel (**b**) Forward and reflected pressures at different locations in a 'loss-less' uniform tube model representing the aorta (Chap. 26). The reflected pressure runs towards the heart. Thus in terms of wave behavior a single tube is not similar to the real arterial system. For explanation see text. (Panel (**a**) adapted in part from Ref. [7], by permission)

heart. The similar time delay between reflected and forward pressure results from the global reflection coefficients at different locations. These reflection coefficients have similar phase angles and thus similar time delays between reflected and forward waves.

If a uniform tube with reflection at its end is used as model of the aorta, the forward wave runs towards the periphery and the reflected wave does run towards the heart. Thus, the *in vivo* data cannot be explained by assuming a uniform tube with a single distal reflection as model of the aorta (see below). Uniform tube models are discussed in Chap. 26.

22.1.2   Waveform Analysis

Waveform analysis is based on the pressure wave shape and mainly pertains to description by the Augmentation Index (AIx) and the timing of the infection point, t_{inf} (Figure in the Box). The AIx does not require calibration of pressure and is therefore ideal for noninvasive studies.

The AIx has been related to the amount of reflection expressed as Reflection Index and Reflection Magnitude (See Figure in Box) but the relations are not tight [8, 9], in part due to the fact that the AIx depends not only on the magnitude of the reflected wave but also on its time of return. Also, the AIx cannot be related with the forward and reflected waves as may be seen in Fig. 22.3 where a negative AIx does not imply a reflected pressure wave that is negative. Similarly, it holds that a negative AIx does not mean negative reflection.

The inflection point is defined as $d^2P/dt^2 = 0$ [10] and its timing, t_{inf}, has been used as arrival time of the reflected wave, t_{ret}. A shoulder point has been defined as

Fig. 22.3 Separation of measured aortic pressure waves (red) into their forward (blue) and reflected waves (green). The Type C beat pertains to a young adult and the Type A beat to an old subject. From C to A type the Augmentation Index, AIx = AP/PP, changes from negative to positive, and the Reflection Magnitude is larger in Type A than Type C. The return time of the reflected wave differs little between A and C beats

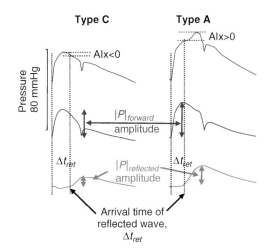

the second zero crossing of $d^4P/dt^4 = 0$ and also has been suggested as arrival time of the reflected wave [11]. Segers has discussed the timing of the inflection point and the shoulder points [10]. The inflection and shoulder points differ from the return time of the reflected wave and differ from each other [8, 9].

Disagreement between the tube model and actual data was observed in several studies, an example being the return time of the reflected wave in aging. With age aortic PWV may increase by a factor 3, but the return time of the pressure wave, determined as t_{inf}, decreases little [12]. Thus, the arrival time of the reflected wave at the heart not simply depends on the wave speed and the distance of a single distal reflection site. Many reflection sites are present in the arterial system leading to a compound reflected wave. The many reflection sites explain the discussion on the 'illusive reflection site' (Chap. 26) and the 'horizon effect' (Chap. 12). The calculation of wave speed from the shoulder point, the inflection point or the return time of the reflected wave, assumes the aorta to be a uniform tube and thus leads to errors [13].

Both Wave Separation and Wave Form Analysis thus show that a tube with a single reflection site at its distal end is not a good model of the aorta (or arterial system). Already in the 1930s this so-called 'uniform tube' model was suggested, and attempts were made to underpin that model by suggesting that at the single reflection site the waves can be reflected 'out of phase' so that an apparent distance is introduced [6, 14, 15]. The uniform tube is discussed in Chap. 26.

22.2   Physiological and Clinical Relevance

The analysis of arterial pressure and flow waves into their forward and reflected running components can be used to quantify the role of wave reflections in physiological and pathological situations. Figure 22.3 shows the aortic pressure waves measured in young healthy adult, type C beat, and an older subject, type A beat [16].

For the type C beat we observe that the amplitude of the reflected wave is smaller than the reflected wave of the A beat, but the return times differ little. The addition of the reflected wave onto the forward wave does not lead to a significant increase in late systolic pressure in the C beat, but does so in the A beat (Fig. 22.3), resulting in a positive Augmentation Index in the A beat. The increased reflection magnitude in the A beat also corresponds with a larger oscillation of the modulus of the input impedance [16]. However, the hemodynamic parameters mean pressure, systemic vascular resistance, Pulse Wave Velocity, and Cardiac Output are not different between the group C beats (n = 4) and group A beats (n = 7).

22.2.1 Reflections and Arterial Stiffness

During vasodilation reflections decrease and pressure and flow in the aorta become more alike. With vasoconstriction the reflections increase and pressure and flow become less alike in shape [17]. With the Valsalva maneuver (Fig. 22.4) the transmural pressure in thoracic and abdominal aorta decreases, but the systemic vascular resistance increases by about 25% [2]. The lower transmural pressure results in a more compliant aorta and a lower wave speed. The compound reflected wave is small and measured pressure and flow become similar in shape. This finding shows

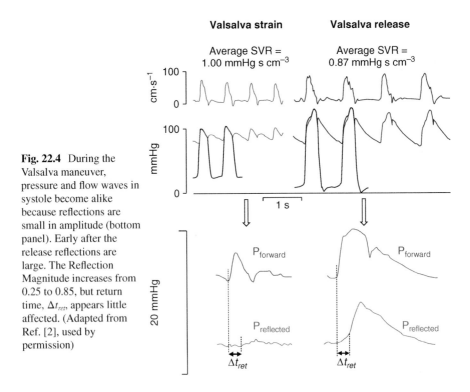

Fig. 22.4 During the Valsalva maneuver, pressure and flow waves in systole become alike because reflections are small in amplitude (bottom panel). Early after the release reflections are large. The Reflection Magnitude increases from 0.25 to 0.85, but return time, Δt_{ret}, appears little affected. (Adapted from Ref. [2], used by permission)

that the magnitude of the reflected wave does not directly relate with vascular (peripheral) resistance but rather to arterial stiffness and wave speed. Thus, the vasoconstriction and vasodilation of the peripheral vascular bed affect the mean pressure and mean pressure determines arterial stiffness. The arterial stiffness rather than the resistance determines reflections. In a model of the systemic arterial system it was indeed found that a change in microvascular resistance hardly affects reflections.

Pulse Pressure amplification decreases with age mainly as a result of the increased arterial stiffness, rather than a changed reflection at the microcirculation (Chap. 12). The increased Pulse Pressure amplification with decreased PWV (Fig. 12.7) and also during the Valsalva maneuver, show the role of arterial stiffness (Fig. 22.5) [18]. Thus, Pulse Pressure amplification decreases with arterial stiffness and thus also with age.

In systemic hypertension, wave speed is increased and thus the many local reflections arrive more simultaneously so that total reflection is increased. This results in an increased reflected pressure wave arriving at the heart in systole, adding to the forward wave, increasing Augmentation Index, Pulse Pressure and systolic pressure [19]. The reflected flow wave is also large but subtracts from the forward flow wave resulting in a smaller net flow.

An experiment where the distinct reflection is increased is shown in Fig. 22.6. When both iliac arteries are manually occluded, the distinct reflection coefficient increases and the reflected wave is increased resulting in a large Augmentation Index [16].

With increased reflection, and thus a higher Augmentation Index, the so-called supply-demand ratio of the cardiac muscle is negatively affected (see Chap. 17).

In peripheral arteries reflections cause a reflected flow wave that may result in a reversal of the measured flow wave, see Fig. 22.7. The negative part of the flow wave disappears in vasodilation, when the reflection and thus the reflected flow wave is smaller, and mean flow increases.

Fig. 22.5 Amplification over the human aorta in control and the Valsalva maneuver

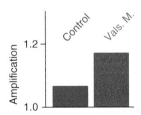

Fig. 22.6 Augmentation Index and Reflection Magnitude in the ascending aortic pressure are increased by mechanical compression of both iliac arteries. (Adapted from Ref. [16], used by permission)

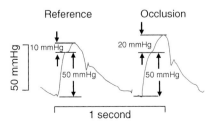

Fig. 22.7 Negative blood flow in part of the cardiac cycle while pressure is still positive results from inertia and reflections. With vasodilation the reflections decrease and flow reversal disappears (femoral artery). (Adapted from Ref. [20], by permission)

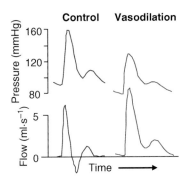

References

1. Westerhof N, Sipkema P, van den Bos GC, Elzinga G. Forward and backward waves in the arterial system. Cardiovasc Res. 1972;6:648–56.
2. Murgo JP, Westerhof N, Giolma JP, Altobelli SA. Manipulation of ascending aortic pressure and flow wave reflections with the Valsalva maneuver: relationship to input impedance. Circulation. 1981;63:122–32.
3. Mynard JP, Smolich JJ. Novel wave power analysis linking pressure-flow waves, wave potential, and the forward and backward components of hydraulic power. Am J Physiol Heart Circ Physiol. 2016;310:H1026–38.
4. Westerhof BE, Guelen I, Westerhof N, Karemaker JM, Avolio A. Quantification of wave reflection in the human aorta from pressure alone: a proof of principle. Hypertension. 2006;48:595–601.
5. Mitchell GF. Triangulating the peaks of arterial pressure. Hypertension. 2006;48:543–5.
6. Davies JE, Alastruey J, Francis DP, Hadjiloizou N, Whinnett ZI, Manisty CH, et al. Attenuation of wave reflection by wave entrapment creates a "horizon effect" in the human aorta. Hypertension. 2012;60:778–85.
7. Tyberg JV, Bouwmeester JC, Parker KH, Shrive NG, Wang JJ. The case for the reservoir-wave approach. Int J Cardiol. 2014;172:299–306.
8. Westerhof BE, Westerhof N. Magnitude and return time of the reflected wave: the effects of large artery stiffness and aortic geometry. J Hypertens. 2012;30:932–9.
9. Westerhof N, Westerhof BE. A review of methods to determine the functional arterial parameters stiffness and resistance. J Hypertens. 2013;31:1769–75.
10. Segers P, Rietzschel ER, De Buyzere ML, De Bacquer D, Van Bortel LM, De Backer G, et al. Assessment of pressure wave reflection: getting the timing right! Physiol Meas. 2007;28:1045–56.
11. Kelly RA, Hayward C, Avolio A, O'Rourke M. Noninvasive determination of age-related changes in the human arterial pulse. Circulation. 1989;80:1652–9.
12. Baksi AJ, Treibel TA, Davies JE, Hadjiloizou N, Foale RA, Parker KH, et al. A meta-analysis of the mechanism of blood pressure change with aging. J Am Coll Cardiol. 2009;54:2087–92.
13. Qasem A, Avolio A. Determination of aortic pulse wave velocity from waveform decomposition of the central aortic pressure pulse. Hypertension. 2008;51:188–95.
14. Sipkema P, Westerhof N. Effective length of the arterial system. Ann Biomed Eng. 1975;3:296–307.
15. Westerhof BE, van den Wijngaard JP, Murgo JP, Westerhof N. Location of a reflection site is elusive: consequences for the calculation of aortic pulse wave velocity. Hypertension. 2008;52:478–83.
16. Murgo JP, Westerhof N, Giolma JP, Altobelli SA. Aortic input impedance in normal man: relationship to pressure wave forms. Circulation. 1980;62:105–16.

17. van den Bos GC, Westerhof N, Randall OS. Pulse wave reflection: can it explain the differences between systemic and pulmonary pressure and flow waves? A study in dogs. Circ Res. 1982;51:479–85.

18. Latham RD, Westerhof N, Sipkema P, Rubal BJ, Reuderink P, Murgo JP. Regional wave travel and reflections along the human aorta: a study with six simultaneous micromanometric pressures. Circulation. 1985;72:1257–69.

19. Fok H, Guilcher A, Brett S, Jiang B, Li Y, Epstein S, et al. Dominance of the forward compression wave in determining pulsatile components of blood pressure: similarities between inotropic stimulation and essential hypertension. Hypertension. 2014;64:1116–23.

20. O'Rourke MG, Taylor MG. Vascular impedance of the femoral bed. Circ Res. 1966;18:126–39.

Chapter 23
Wave Intensity Analysis

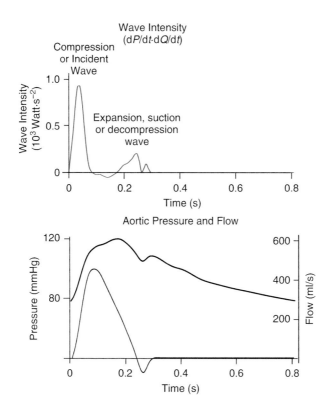

Wave Intensity in the human aorta (top panel) derived from pressure, P, and flow, Q (bottom panel). The main peaks are in early and late ejection. In early ejection both dP/dt and dQ/dt are positive resulting in positive peak, and in late ejection both pressure and flow are decreasing and Wave Intensity is also positive. Wave Intensity

© Springer International Publishing AG, part of Springer Nature 2019   185
N. Westerhof et al., *Snapshots of Hemodynamics*,
https://doi.org/10.1007/978-3-319-91932-4_23

is here calculated from differentiated pressure, dP/dt, and flow, dQ/dt, as $(dP/dt) \cdot (dQ/dt)$, given in Watt s^{-2}, sometimes called 'time normalized Wave Intensity'. Originally Wave Intensity was defined as the product of differences in pressure, $dP = P(t + \Delta t) - P(t)$ and velocity, $dv = v(t + \Delta t) - v(t)$, as $dP \cdot dv$. This implies that both dP and dv and thus also their product, $dP \cdot dv$ in Watt·m^{-2}, depend on the sampling time, Δt, which makes quantitative comparison between studies, when Δt is not reported, difficult. When flow, Q, instead of velocity is used Wave Intensity equals $(dP) \cdot (dQ)$ with units Watt. Flow and velocity are both used and also differentiated and differences in waves have been used. Names of peaks have not been standardized. Wave Intensity Analysis is allowed in nonlinear and time-varying systems. Wave Intensity depends on the interaction of heart and load.

23.1   Description

Wave Intensity Analysis has been developed next to Waveform Analysis and Wave Separation Analysis. While in Waveform and Wave Separation the measured pressure and flow waves are analyzed, Wave Intension Analysis uses 'differences', dP and dQ, and also derivatives, dP/dt and dQ/dt, of pressure and flow. The derivation of Wave Intensity is shown in Fig. 23.1. In this example, the calculations are based on pressure and flow in the aorta. In Panel a the aortic pressure and flow and their forward and reflected components are presented. In panel b, the derivatives of measured pressure and flow are depicted and it may be seen that derivation emphasizes the changes in the original signals, in diastole the derivatives have a small amplitude. The product of the derivatives of pressure and flow, Wave Intensity, is shown in Panel c. It should be noted that the major waves occur in early and late ejection, where changes in the pressure and flow are largest. Wave Intensity is extremely small in diastole, and mid-ejection.

23.1.1   Calculations

Originally Wave Intensity was applied in gas dynamics and sound waves and based on velocity and pressure changes, dv and dP, expressed as *differences*, thus $dP = P(t + \Delta t) - P(t)$ and $dv = v(t + \Delta t) - v(t)$ [1, 2]. Wave Intensity is then $dP \cdot dv$. In hemodynamics flow, Q, instead of velocity has also been used, and Wave Intensity is then calculated as $dP \cdot dQ$. Furthermore, rather than based on differences also *differentials* dP/dt and dQ/dt have been used and Wave Intensity then equals $dP/dt \cdot dQ/dt$ (Fig. 23.1). Instead of pressure the arterial diameter can be used as well, which makes noninvasive determination of Wave Intensity possible [3].

When differences are used the magnitude of WI depends on sample rate. Because sample rate is often not reported quantitative comparison between studies is difficult. Using differentiated signals, the 'time normalized Wave Intensity', $dP/dt \cdot dv/dt$,

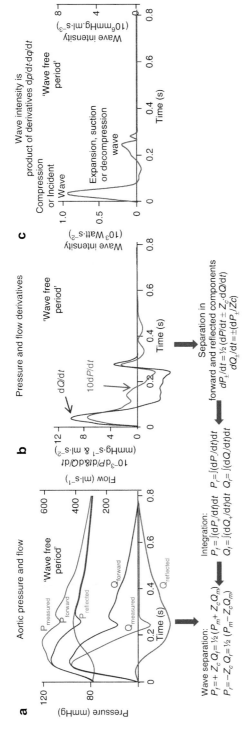

Fig. 23.1 Wave intensity, WI, in the ascending aorta expressed in dP/dt and dQ/dt. In panel (**a**) pressure and flow are presented, with their forward and reflected waves. In panel (**b**) the derivatives of measured pressure and flow are shown and in panel (**c**) their product the 'time normalized Wave Intensity', with units mmHg.ml s^{-2} or Ws^{-2}, is given. In WI several waves may be distinguished (see text). The dP/dt and dQ/dt can be separated in to their forward (+) and reflected (−) components $dP_{\pm}/dt$ and $dQ_{\pm}/dt$, with the same rules as used in wave separation (Chap. 12). Subsequent integration results in the forward and reflected pressure and flow waves as also obtained from Wave Separation (panel **a**). The calculations are similar when differences dP and dQ are used and when velocity rather than flow is used. In the latter part of diastole the WI is small as a result of the differentiation. This has been suggested to be a 'wave free period' indicated by the shaded areas. However, as shown in panel (**a**) forward and reflected waves are present in diastole; reflection against a closed valve, forward and reflected flow wave cancel. Calculation of 'Instantaneous Resistance' in the 'wave free period' violates Ohm's law (Chap. 6)

Table 23.1 Wave intensity units

Parameters	Wave intensity Medical units	Wave intensity SI-units
Wave intensity based on differences		
dP (1 mmHg)·dQ (1 ml·s^{-1})	1 mmHg·ml·s^{-1}	$0.133 \cdot 10^{-3}$ Watt
dP (1 mmHg)·dv (1 cm·s^{-1})	1 mmHg·cm·s^{-1}	$1.33 \cdot$Watt·m^{-2}
Wave intensity based on derivatives		
dP/dt (1 mmHg·s^{-1})·dQ/dt (1 ml·s^{-2})	1 mmHg·ml·s^{-3}	$0.133 \cdot 10^{-3}$·W·s^{-2}
dP/dt (1 mmHg·s^{-1})·dv/dt (1 cm·s^{-2})	1 mmHg·cm·s^{-3}	$1.33 \cdot$W·(m^{-2}·s^{-2})

Table 23.2 Wave intensity waves [1]

	dP/dt	dQ/dt	Wave Intensity
Forward	>0 compression	>0 acceleration	>0 positive
	<0 decompression	<0 deceleration	
Reflected	>0 compression	<0 deceleration	<0 negative
	<0 decompression	>0 acceleration	

For detailed explanation see Ref. [1]

allows for quantitative comparison [4]. Both differences and differentiation amplify noise and in practice filtering is necessary [5]. When volume flow and pressure are used the different methods, $dP \cdot dQ$ and $dP/dt \cdot dQ/dt$, lead to different dimensions of the calculated Wave Intensity (Table 23.1).

Wave Intensity Analysis may be performed in nonlinear and time-varying systems like the coronary arterial system. It may be seen that the Wave Intensity contains many peaks. In general, more distinguishable peaks are found in the coronary arteries than in the aorta. Parker distinguishes four possible sub-waves [2] (see Table 23.2) while Davies et al. shows six peaks in the coronary circulation [6]. In the present literature no standardization of names of peaks, and number of waves exists.

23.1.2   Forward and Reflected Waves

Like in Wave Separation Analysis (Chap. 12) the dP/dt and dQ/dt can be separated into their forward and reflected components dP_+/dt, dP_-/dt, dQ_+/dt, and dQ_-/dt, respectively. Subsequent integration results in the forward and reflected pressure and flow waves obtained from Wave Separation Analysis directly, see Fig. 23.1 [7, 8].

To separate waves into their forward and reflected components the characteristic impedance (Z_c, when flow is used) or the local wave speed (ρc with ρ blood density and c phase velocity, when velocity is used) of the vessel under study is required. Both Z_c and ρc are local parameters and assumed not to be affected by reflections. Two methods to derive them have been proposed (Chap. 12). The Z_c can be calculated from the high-frequency information of the input impedance and ρc from the slope of the pressure-velocity relation in early ejection [9, 10]. The first method is mainly used in wave separation analysis and the second one is mostly used in the separation of forward and reflected dP/dt and dQ/dt [10]. This has led to the idea that the wave separation method is a frequency domain method and the wave intensity method a time domain method. However, both calculations (in conduit vessels) are performed in the time domain [7].

In coronary arteries, characteristic impedance and local wave speed may vary over the cardiac cycle, and an estimate of ρc at a single location was suggested by using the sum of squares method (over the cardiac cycle): $\rho^2 c^2 = \Sigma \Delta P^2 / \Sigma \Delta v^2$ [11]. However, this single point wave speed method has limitations [12].

23.1.3 Interpretations of Wave Intensity

From wave separation analysis it may be seen (Box Figure) that forward and reflected pressure waves are equal in size in diastole, i.e., both contribute equally to measured pressure, while flow waves cancel making flow zero in diastole. This has led to the so-called 'wave free' period concept (Chap. 12). Figure 23.1 also suggests that the latter part of diastole is 'wave free' [13]. However, more accurately formulated, the amplitude of the waves calculated by Wave Intensity are small in diastole with respect to their maximum values as a result of the differentiation. The measured pressure and velocity waves are present over the whole cardiac cycle (Fig. 23.1 panel a), and diastole (or part of diastole) is not wave free.

The assumption of a 'wave free' period was subsequently used as argument that an 'Instantaneous Resistance' could be calculated [13]. In Chap. 6 it has been discussed why resistance can only be calculated from averaged pressure and flow over the entire cardiac cycle.

Two recently proposed methods to analyze arterial function, the Reservoir Wave Concept and the Instantaneous wave Free (pressure-pressure) Ratio (iFR) are, in part, based on the assumption of a 'wave free' period [8].

23.1.4 The Reservoir-Wave Concept

The Reservoir-Wave Concept has been applied to aortic pressure and flow and was first introduced by Wang et al. [14]. The diastolic pressure in the aorta decays almost exponentially and Frank's two-element Windkessel mimics pressure and flow well in diastole. However, Frank's Windkessel does not describe pressure in systole correctly. The three-element Windkessel (Chap. 25) with as third element the aortic characteristic impedance does describe both diastole and systole well [15, 16]. Lighthill introduced an excess pressure, P_{exc}, being the difference between measured aortic pressure and the pressure predicted by Frank's Windkessel [17]. If the three-element Windkessel were a perfect description of the systemic arterial system, the

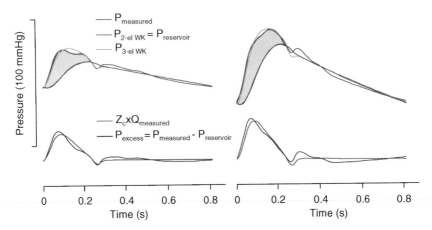

Fig. 23.2 Two examples of the reservoir-wave concept. When measured aortic pressure, $P_{measured}$, is fitted with a two-element Windkessel the reservoir pressure is obtained (dark green). The difference between measured pressure and reservoir or two-element Windkessel pressure is only substantial during ejection (filled area) and their difference is the excess pressure, P_{excess} (blue). The excess pressure is close to aortic characteristic impedance Z_c times flow, $Z_c \cdot Q_{measured}$ (red) as shown in the bottom panels. If the arterial system would be a perfect three-element Windkessel $P_{excess} = Z_c \cdot Q_{measured}$. The seemingly negligible wave intensity in diastole, suggesting a 'wave free period', has been used to propose that the reservoir pressure is not a wave and that wave phenomena are contained in the P_{excess}

excess pressure would be exactly equal to the product of aortic flow and aortic characteristic impedance. However, the arterial system is not exactly a three-element Windkessel and $P_{exc}(t) \approx Z_c \cdot Q(t)$ (Fig. 23.2). The Reservoir-Wave concept adapted the Lighthill approach by assuming that measured aortic pressure is the sum of a two-element Windkessel or reservoir pressure ($P_{reservoir}$) plus the excess pressure, P_{exc}. The $P_{reservoir}$ is a volume related quantity and assumed not due to waves and its shape to be independent of location. The wave-related pressure is assumed to be the excess (or wave pressure), P_{exc} [18, 19]. It was subsequently shown theoretically and experimentally that the Reservoir Wave equals twice the reflected pressure wave: $P_{reservoir} = 2P_{reflected}$ [8, 20]. In other words, the reservoir wave travels over the aorta and is by definition a wave. Mynard et al. have criticized the reservoir wave concept [21].

When P_{exc} is split in its forward and reflected components it is found that the so-calculated reflected wave is small [22], in agreement with the observation that $P_{exc} = Z_c \cdot Q_{measured}$ and the rules of wave separation (Chap. 12). Later it was accepted that the reservoir wave travels with maintaining its shape along the aorta.

23.1.5   The Instantaneous Wave Free Ratio (iFR)

The instantaneous wave Free Ratio, iFR, is proposed as a method to estimate stenosis severity in the coronary arterial system without the need for vasodilation (see Chaps. 5 and 19), and defined as the ratio of distal and proximal pressures of a stenosis during the latter 75% of diastole, the so-called 'wave free period' [13, 23]. The advantage of using diastole is that the effect of cardiac contraction on the coronary vasculature is small. An extra assumption is that, in this 'wave free period', the ratio of pressure and flow ('instantaneous resistance', or mean 'resistance' over this period) is a measure of minimized resistance, and a vasodilator is not required as in (Fractional) Flow Reserve studies (see Chap. 5). This calculation of 'resistance' is erroneous. The iFR is relatively easy to measure, but has been criticized [8, 24]. Recently it has been shown experimentally that the 'instantaneous resistance' is not minimal [25].

23.2   Physiological and Clinical Relevance

23.2.1   *Wave Intensity*

Wave Intensity Analysis represents the high frequency information of pressure and flow waves. Since pressure and flow(velocity) waves depend on heart and arterial load Wave Intensity depends on both as well. However, Wave Intensity may be applied to nonlinear and time varying systems. Clinical usefulness was first published by Sugawara who showed a relation between left ventricular contractility (dP_{lv}/dt), and left ventricular relaxation and Wave Intensity [4]. Fok et al. showed that changes in cardiac pump function contribute to changes in Wave Intensity [26]. Wave Intensity has led to accurate ways to determine local wave speed and characteristic impedance [10].

   Wave intensity has been applied to the whole systemic and pulmonary arterial trees, to the carotid artery in studies on brain perfusion and the coronary system (see also iFR). Ventricular filling and the effect of counter-pulsation have been studied with Wave Intensity Analysis. Exercise effects on Wave Intensity have been reported as well [27]. Changes in Wave Intensity before and after aortic valve replacement also have been reported [28]. Aortic and peripheral arteries can be studied by Wave Intensity noninvasively using MRI-obtained flow velocity and vessel diameter as surrogate of pressure [3].

   A limitation of Wave Intensity is the often-missing information on calibration when differences rather than differentials are used.

23.2.2   *Reservoir-Wave Concept*

The separation of pressure into a wave-less reservoir pressure and a wave related excess pressure, P_{exc}, is artificial and has been seriously criticized [8, 21]. Nevertheless, it has been shown that the reservoir wave changes with age and predicts cardiovascular events [22, 29]. The reflected pressure wave predicts events as well [30], which is not surprising because reservoir pressure equals twice the reflected pressure wave. The excess pressure, when integrated over the cardiac cycle predicts long-term all-cause mortality in stable heart failure [31] in agreement with role of characteristic impedance [32]. The strong relation between excess pressure and characteristic impedance explains this.

23.2.3   The iFR

The instantaneous wave free ratio was introduced as a method to quantify a (coronary) stenosis by only measuring the (diastolic) pressure ratio over a stenosis, without the need for maximal vasodilatation. Although easy to use, it has also been criticized on physical grounds [8] and it has been questioned if it approximates fractional flow reserve [24]. Nijjer et al. showed that coronary 'microvascular resistance' calculated over the 'wave free' period decreases with vasodilation (hyperemia) [25].

References

1. Parker KH, Jones CJ. Forward and backward running waves in the arteries: analysis using the method of characteristics. J Biomech Eng. 1990;112:322–6.
2. Parker KH. An introduction to wave intensity analysis. Med Biol Eng Comput. 2009;47: 175–88. Review
3. Borlotti A, Khir AW, Rietzschel ER, De Buyzere ML, Vermeersch S, Segers P. Noninvasive determination of local pulse wave velocity and wave intensity: changes with age and gender in the carotid and femoral arteries of healthy human. J Appl Physiol (1985). 2012;113:727–35.
4. Sugawara M, Niki K, Ohte N, Okada T, Harada A. Clinical usefulness of wave intensity analysis. Med Biol Eng Comput. 2009;47:197–202.
5. Rivolo S, Nagel E, Smith NP, Lee J. Automatic selection of optimal Savitzky-Golay filter parameters for coronary wave intensity analysis. Conf Proc IEEE Eng Med Biol Soc. 2014; 2014:5056–9.
6. Davies JE, Whinnett ZI, Francis DP, Manisty CH, Aguado-Sierra J, Willson K, et al. Evidence of a dominant backward-propagating suction wave responsible for diastolic coronary filling in humans, attenuated in left ventricular hypertrophy. Circulation. 2006;113:1768–78.
7. Hughes AD, Parker KH. Forward and backward waves in the arterial system: impedance or wave intensity analysis? Med Biol Eng Comput. 2009;47:207–10.
8. Westerhof N, Segers P, Westerhof BE. Wave separation, wave intensity, the reservoir-wave concept, and the instantaneous wave–free ratio: presumptions and principles. Hypertension. 2015;66:93–8. (and *Hypertension* 2015;66:e21)
9. Dujardin JP, Stone DN. Characteristic impedance of the proximal aorta determined in the time and frequency domain: a comparison. Med Biol Eng Comput. 1981;19:565–8.
10. Khir AW, O'Brien A, Gibbs JS, Parker KH. Determination of wave speed and wave separation in the arteries. J Biomech. 2001;34:1145–55.
11. Davies JE, Whinnett ZI, Francis DP, Willson K, Foale RA, Malik IS, et al. Use of simultaneous pressure and velocity measurements to estimate arterial wave speed at a single site in humans. Am J Physiol Heart Circ Physiol. 2006;290:H878–85.
12. Kolyva C, Spaan JA, Piek JJ, Siebes M. Windkesselness of coronary arteries hampers assessment of human coronary wave speed by single-point technique. Am J Phys. 2008;295:H482–90.
13. Sen S, Escaned J, Malik IS, Mikhail GW, Foale RA, Mila R, et al. Development and validation of a new adenosine-independent index of stenosis severity from coronary wave-intensity analysis: results of the ADVISE (ADenosine vasodilator independent stenosis evaluation) study. J Am Coll Cardiol. 2012;59:1392–402.

14. Wang JJ, O'Brien AB, Shrive NG, Parker KH, Tyberg JV. Time-domain representation of ventricular-arterial coupling as a windkessel and wave system. Am J Physiol Heart Circ Physiol. 2003;284:H1358–68.
15. Westerhof N, Elzinga G, Sipkema P. An artificial arterial system for pumping hearts. J Appl Physiol. 1971;31:776–81.
16. Westerhof N, Lankhaar JW, Westerhof BE. The arterial Windkessel. Med Biol Eng Comput. 2009;47:131–41.
17. Lighthill MJ. Waves in fluids. Cambridge: Cambridge University Press; 1978.
18. Tyberg JV, Davies JE, Wang Z, Whitelaw WA, Flewitt JA, Shrive NG, et al. Wave intensity analysis and the development of the reservoir-wave approach. Med Biol Eng Comput. 2009;47:221–32.
19. Tyberg JV, Shrive NG, Bouwmeester JC, Parker KH, Wang JJ. The reservoir-wave paradigm: potential implications for hypertension. Curr Hypertens Rev. 2008;4:203–13.
20. Hametner B, Wassertheurer S, Hughes AD, Parker KH, Weber T, Eber B. Reservoir and excess pressures predict cardiovascular events in high-risk patients. Int J Cardiol. 2014;171:31–6.
21. Mynard JP. Assessment of conceptual inconsistencies in the hybrid reservoir-wave model. Conf Proc IEEE Eng Med Biol Soc. 2013;2013:213–6.
22. Davies JE, Baksi J, Francis DP, Hadjiloizou N, Whinnett ZI, Manisty CH, et al. The arterial reservoir pressure increases with aging and is the major determinant of the aortic augmentation index. Am J Physiol Heart Circ Physiol. 2010;298:H580–6.
23. Sen S, Asrress KN, Nijjer S, Petraco R, Malik IS, Foale RA, et al. Diagnostic classification of the instantaneous wave-free ratio is equivalent to fractional flow reserve and is not improved with adenosine administration. Results of CLARIFY (Classification Accuracy of Pressure-Only Ratios Against Indices Using Flow Study). J Am Coll Cardiol. 2013;61:1409–20.
24. Johnson NP, Kirkeeide RL, Asrress KN, Fearon WF, Lockie T, Marques KM, et al. Does the instantaneous wave-free ratio approximate the fractional flow reserve? J Am Coll Cardiol. 2013;61:1428–35.
25. Nijjer SS, de Waard GA, Sen S, van de Hoef TP, Petraco R, Echavarría-Pinto M, et al. Coronary pressure and flow relationships in humans: phasic analysis of normal and pathological vessels and the implications for stenosis assessment: a report from the Iberian-Dutch-English (IDEAL) collaborators. Eur Heart J. 2016;37:2069–80.
26. Fok H, Guilcher A, Brett S, Jiang B, Li Y, Epstein S, et al. Dominance of the forward compression wave in determining pulsatile components of blood pressure: similarities between inotropic stimulation and essential hypertension. Hypertension. 2014;64:1116–23.
27. Schultz MG, Davies JE, Roberts-Thomson P, Black JA, Hughes AD, Sharman JE. Exercise central (aortic) blood pressure is predominantly driven by forward traveling waves, not wave reflection. Hypertension. 2013;62:175–82.
28. Davies JE, Sen S, Broyd C, Hadjiloizou N, Baksi J, Francis DP, et al. Arterial pulse wave dynamics after percutaneous aortic valve replacement: fall in coronary diastolic suction with increasing heart rate as a basis for angina symptoms in aortic stenosis. Circulation. 2011;124:1565–72.
29. Narayan O, Davies JE, Hughes AD, Dart AM, Parker KH, Reid C, et al. Central aortic reservoir-wave analysis improves prediction of cardiovascular events in elderly hypertensives. Hypertension. 2015;65:629–35. Erratum in: Hypertension 2015;66:e28
30. Weber T, Wassertheurer S, Rammer M, Haiden A, Hametner B, Eber B. Wave reflections, assessed with a novel method for pulse wave separation, are associated with end-organ damage and clinical outcomes. Hypertension. 2012;60:534–41.
31. Davies JE, Lacy P, Tillin T, Collier D, Cruickshank JK, Francis DP, et al. Excess pressure integral predicts cardiovascular events independent of other risk factors in the conduit artery functional evaluation substudy of Anglo-Scandinavian cardiac outcomes trial. Hypertension. 2014;64:60–8.
32. Mitchell GF, Gudnason V, Launer LJ, Aspelund T, Harris TB. Hemodynamics of increased pulse pressure in older women in the community-based age, gene/environment susceptibility-Reykjavik study. Hypertension. 2008;51:1123–8.

Chapter 24
Arterial Input Impedance

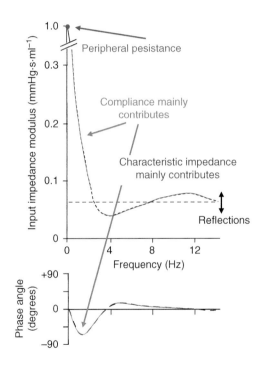

Input impedance completely and comprehensively describes an arterial system. Here the input impedance of the human systemic arterial tree is shown in schematic form. The ratio of the mean arterio-venous pressure drop and mean flow is systemic vascular resistance or peripheral resistance, R_p. To obtain information about the oscillatory aspects of the arterial system wave shapes of pressure and flow are used. To derive this information sinusoidal pressures and flows as obtained by Fourier analysis (see Appendix 1) are related. The amplitude ratio and the phase difference

© Springer International Publishing AG, part of Springer Nature 2019
N. Westerhof et al., *Snapshots of Hemodynamics*,
https://doi.org/10.1007/978-3-319-91932-4_24

of the sine waves of pressure and flow are calculated, giving the modulus and phase angle of the impedance (application of Ohm's law). The impedance modulus and phase are plotted as a function of the frequency, with at zero frequency systemic vascular resistance. For intermediate frequencies the impedance modulus decreases precipitously and the phase angle is negative. This shows the contribution of (total) arterial compliance, C. For high frequencies the modulus approaches a constant value and the phase angle is close to zero. This is the contribution of the aortic characteristic impedance, Z_c, which is a real quantity for large vessels. Thus the three elements R_p, C, and Z_c together give a good description of the input impedance. Without reflections in the arterial system, the input impedance would be equal to aortic characteristic impedance and the pressure and flow would have the same wave shape. For low frequencies the reflections at the many discontinuities, 'diffuse reflections', add and cause the impedance to be high. At high frequencies local, reflected waves return with different phases and contribute less causing the impedance to be close to the characteristic impedance. The oscillations about the characteristic impedance are related to distinct reflections, and depend on local geometry. The frequency of the minimum of the impedance modulus and the zero crossing of the phase angle have been used to calculate the effective reflection site (the quarter wave length rule). This calculation is often inaccurate. Input impedance can be derived for any (sub) section of the arterial system, but the present chapter mainly concentrates on the systemic arterial system as a whole.

24.1   Description

24.1.1   Definition of Impedance

Impedance is the relation between the pressure difference over and flow through a linear system, for sinusoidal signals. Impedance completely describes the whole system at its entrance, and therefore often called input impedance. Input impedance derivation is performed from the pulsatile pressure difference and pulsatile flow by applying of Fourier analysis and calculation of their harmonics (Appendix 1). Inversely, when the impedance is known, a given flow allows for the calculation of pressure in terms of magnitude and wave shape and vice versa. Systemic arterial and pulmonary arterial input impedance are a comprehensive description of the systemic and pulmonary arterial tree. Input impedances of organ systems may be derived as well.

24.1.2   Derivation of Input Impedance

In the calculations of input impedance, Z_{in}, we use both the mean values and the pulsatile part of the pressure and flow waves. We apply Fourier analysis of the aortic pressure and flow because impedance calculations can only be performed for sinusoidal signals (in the frequency domain). Fourier analysis is only permitted for a full beat, or a series of full beats. The details and limitations of Fourier analysis are discussed in Appendix 1. To derive impedance Ohm's law is applied as is done for the calculation of resistance from mean pressure and mean flow (Chap. 6). As discussed in Chap. 6, Ohm's law may only be applied to full beats and this also holds for the calculation of impedance. For each pair of sine waves of pressure and flow (called harmonics) we calculate the ratio of the amplitudes (impedance modulus) and the difference in phase angle (impedance phase angle). It is only allowed to perform these calculations if the system is in the steady state, time-invariant, and linear. Steady state means that the arterial system may not vary in time over the study period, e.g., vasomotor tone should be constant. Linearity in this context implies that if a sine wave of pressure is applied a sine wave of flow results. The calculation of impedance of a time-varying system does not lead to interpretable results. An example is the coronary circulation, where resistance and arterial compliance are time-varying over the heartbeat. For a nonlinear system the calculation of impedance also does not lead to interpretable results. An example is the calculation of 'impedance' from ventricular pressure and aortic flow, where the aortic valves make the system nonlinear, and the result is not meaningful. The arterial system is not perfectly linear but the variations of pressure and flow over the heartbeat are sufficiently small so that linearity is approximated and the derived input impedance is a meaningful description. The limitations of linearity and time-invariance also hold for the calculation of peripheral resistance, see Chap. 6. It has been shown that some of the scatter of the input impedance data (Fig. 24.1) results from nonlinearity [1, 2].

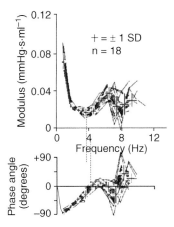

Fig. 24.1 Input impedance calculated from 18 heart beats. The scatter in the input impedance is caused, in part, by noise on the pressure and flow signals especially affecting the small amplitudes of high harmonics. Non-linearity of the arterial system also contributes to the scatter. The blue line is drawn through the averaged values. The vertical dashed lines indicate that the modulus minimum and phase zero crossing are not at the same frequency, implying that a single tube with real, in phase reflection is not a good model of the entire arterial tree and the quarter wave length rule may not be applied. Impedance of a patient with type A beat. (Adapted from Ref. [1], by permission)

Fourier analysis and subsequent calculation of the input impedance only gives information at frequencies that are multiples of the Heart Rate, i.e., the harmonics (Appendix 1). Because the information contained in the signals for high frequencies is small, the higher harmonics (Appendix 1) are subject to noise, so that the impedance at high frequencies often scatters considerably (Fig. 24.1). Analyzing multiple heartbeats and averaging the results decreases noise [1]. By pacing the heart at different rates or by analyzing long stretches of data in a steady state, the frequency resolution can be increased.

In the systemic circulation venous pressure may be neglected (Chap. 6), so that Fourier analysis of aortic pressure and flow gives a sufficiently accurate approximation of the input impedance. However, in the analysis of the pulmonary circulation venous pressure cannot be neglected (Chap. 28).

In Appendix 2 the basic hemodynamic elements are discussed. For a resistor, it holds that the sine waves of pressure and flow are in phase, i.e., the phase angle is zero. For compliance the flow is advanced with respect to pressure. This is seen as $-90°$ in the impedance phase angle. For inertance flow is delayed, and shows as $+90°$ for the impedance phase. The modulus of the impedance decreases with frequency, as $1/\omega C$ for compliance, and increases with frequency, as ωL, for the inertance, respectively. In Chap. 12 characteristic impedance is discussed. It is shown that in a large arteries, like the aorta, the mass effects and compliance effects interact in such a way that sinusoidal pressure and flow waves are in phase, and their ratio is constant, this interaction implies that characteristic impedance is a frequency-independent number. This means that the amplitude ratio of pressure and flow is the same for all frequencies and the phase angle is zero. It should be remembered that characteristic impedance is not a simple Ohmic resistor: it is non-existent at zero Hertz and no energy is lost in it. Thus, when modeling characteristic impedance with a resistor this limitation must be kept in mind.

24.1.3   Explanation of Input Impedance

The peripheral resistance, total arterial compliance and characteristic impedance together describe the main features of the input impedance (see Figure in the Box).

24.1.4   Input Impedance and Wave Transmission

From the principles of travelling and reflected waves we can explain input impedance. For a reflection-less system the input impedance equals aortic characteristic impedance. Inversely, the difference between input impedance and characteristic impedance results from reflections. The reflected waves resulting from reflections at bifurcating arteries and other discontinuities return to the proximal aorta. The reflected waves add and result in an impedance that differs from aortic characteristic impedance. For low frequencies, the return times of the reflected waves a small fraction of the period of the wave, all waves add 'in phase' and total reflection is large: input impedance differs from aortic characteristic impedance. For high frequencies, the return times of waves are considerable fraction of the period of the waves and they arrive with different phases, and cancel each other out so that the arterial system appears reflection-less: input impedance differs little from aortic characteristic impedance, i.e. constant modulus and phase angle close to zero. Also damping is stronger for the high frequencies and reduces the magnitude of the reflections. It has been suggested that in the human arterial system distinct (relatively strong) reflections may occur at the aortic bifurcation or at the level of the renal arteries. These distinct reflection sites are possibly leading to the secondary rise in systolic pressure and the pressure augmentation (type A beat, Chap. 22). The ratio of reflected and forward running wave amplitudes (reflection magnitude) is related to the magnitude of the oscillations in the impedance modulus [1].

24.1.5   Impedance and Windkessel

The description of the impedance given in the Box suggests three important parameters describing input impedance. These three parameters form the basis of the Windkessel models (Chap. 25). The original two-element Windkessel, proposed by Frank, consists of peripheral resistance, R_p, and total arterial compliance, C. From the information on input impedance, which became available in the 1960s, the idea of aortic characteristic impedance, Z_c, as third Windkessel element appeared [3]. However, we should keep in mind that when the characteristic impedance is modeled with a resistor the mean pressure over mean flow will be $R_p + R_c$, while it should be R_p only. Although this error is not large for the systemic circulation where R_c is about 7% of R_p, it leads to errors when, for instance the three-element Windkessel is used to estimate total arterial compliance. To correct for these shortcomings, a fourth element, the total arterial inertance (see Chap. 25) was introduced [4].

24.1.6   Effective Length of the Arterial System

The frequencies where the minimum in the input impedance modulus and the zero crossing of the phase angle occur have been used to estimate the 'effective length' of the arterial system (See Chap. 26). The effective length of the arterial system is used as a conceptual description to determine at what distance from the ascending aorta the major reflection arises. In this concept, it is assumed that the arterial system behaves like a single tube, the aorta, with a single resistance, the peripheral resistance or impedance at its distal end. Based on single tube models the 'quarter wave length' principle was introduced. With a distal resistance the frequency of the modulus minimum and the zero crossing of the phase angle are found for a tube

Fig. 24.2 Types of beats relate to input impedance. In subjects with Type A beats a distinct reflection returns in systole and pressure augmentation is high. The impedance oscillates about the characteristic impedance. In Type C beats, reflections are smaller augmentation is negative and the impedance oscillates less than in the Type A beat. (Adapted from Ref. [1], by permission)

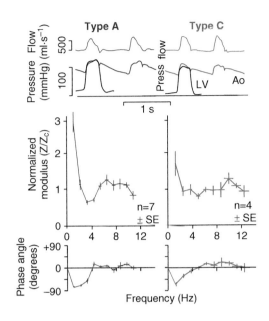

length $l = c_{phase}/(4f_{min}) = \lambda/4$. Quantitatively we describe this phenomenon as follows. The wave speed, c_{phase}, equals wavelength, λ, times frequency, f, thus, $c_{phase} = \lambda \cdot f$. When wave speed $c_{phase} = 600$ cm/s, and the impedance minimum is found at 4 Hz (Fig. 24.1), the wave length $\lambda = c/f = 150$ cm and the 'effective length' of the tube (aorta) is a quarter wave length, $l = \lambda/4 = 38$ cm. Figures 24.1 and 24.2 show that the zero-crossing of the phase angle differs from the impedance minimum. The assumption of a single tube, mimicking the aorta loaded with the peripheral resistance as model of the systemic arterial tree is too simple and often unrealistic [5, 6]. Tube models and their limitations are discussed in Chap. 26.

24.1.7 External Power

The power produced by the heart equals $(1/T) \int P(t) \cdot Q(t) \cdot dt$, with integration over the heart period T, and is called total external power (see Chap. 16). When mean aortic pressure and Cardiac Output are multiplied the mean power is obtained. The difference between total and mean power is called oscillatory or pulsatile power, which is about 15% of total power. Using Ohm's law, mean power can also be calculated from $CO^2 \cdot R_p$. In the frequency domain, we can perform the following calculations. Oscillatory power must be calculated for each harmonic (i) separately as $P_i \cdot Q_i = Q_i^2 \cdot |Z_{in,i}| \cdot \cos\varphi_i$ and then added as: Power $= \Sigma Q_i^2 \cdot |Z_{in,i}| \cos\varphi_i$, with $|Z_{in,i}|$ the impedance modulus and φ_i the impedance phase angle, and i harmonic number. It has been suggested that the minimum of the modulus of the input impedance should relate to Heart Rate since power was then thought to be minimal. However, we see that not the modulus $|Z_{in,i}|$ but the real part of the input impedance (modulus times cosine of the phase angle) determines power. Often the real part of the impedance has no clear minimum and if it does, it is not found at the same frequency as the minimum of the impedance modulus.

How power is related to the forward and reflected pressure and flow waves was shown in Chap. 22. In the frequency domain mean forward and reflected power equal $Q_f^2 R_p$ and $Q_r^2 R_p$, respectively, with their ratio $Q_f^2/Q_r^2 = \Gamma_q^2 = \Gamma_p^2$. With a reflection coefficient at zero Hz the $\Gamma = (R_p - Z_c)/(R_p + Z_c) \approx 0.87$ (Chap. 12), the ratio of forward and reflected mean power is 0.77. Thus about $0.77/(1 + 0.77) = 44\%$ of the mean power reflects. For the oscillatory components, the ratio equals $\Gamma^2(\omega)$ for each harmonic, and these need to be summed. The total oscillatory power is about 15% of total power.

24.1.8 Impulse Response

Conceptually, it is rather awkward that while pressure and flow are functions of time, the input impedance is expressed as a function of frequency. There exists a characterization of the arterial system in the time domain. This characterization is the so-called impulse response function, which is the pressure that results from an impulse of flow. The impulse should be a short-lasting flow, i.e., short with respect to all travel times and characteristic times of the arterial system, and typically about 1–5 ms in duration. Because the impulse has a height with dimension ml^{-1} and the duration is in seconds, the area under the impulse is ml. The pressure response resulting from this impulse is normalized with respect to the volume of the impulse and the units of the impulse response are therefore mmHg/ml. The calculation of the impulse response function from measured pressure and flow is complicated but straightforward [7]. When the measured flow is broken up in a number of short impulses following each other, the proper addition of the impulse responses leads to the pressure as a function of time.

The input impedance and impulse response function form a 'Fourier pair'. Fourier analysis of the impulse response function leads to the input impedance and inverse transformation of input impedance leads to the impulse response function [7].

If the impulse response is short in duration with respect to the time constant of variation of the time varying system, it may be used to obtain a characterization of that system as a function of time. For example, if the duration of the impulse response is less than 100 milliseconds, and the system under study varies with a typical time of a few hundred milliseconds, the system can be characterized by the impulse response. In this way input impedance of the coronary arterial system was derived in systole and diastole [8].

24.2 Physiological and Clinical Relevance

Although the input impedance gives a comprehensive description of the arterial system its practical use is limited. As discussed above, derivation of input impedance requires Fourier analysis of pressure and flow waves and the data show scatter

(Fig. 24.1), and interpretation requires models. Thus, routine clinical applications are seldom carried out. However, impedances calculated in the human and animals have led to a much better understanding of arterial function. For instance, the input impedance of the arterial system, when normalized to peripheral resistance, is similar in mammals [9]. This explains, in part, why aortic pressures and flows are of similar in shape in mammals (Chap. 32).

Also, derivation of arterial compliance from impedance is of limited accuracy since the modulus is already decreased to near characteristic impedance values for the first or second harmonics (Figure in the Box). Nevertheless, the knowledge of the function the arterial system has greatly helped its function and can serve as quantitative tests of arterial models (Chaps. 25 and 26).

The arterial system can be described in terms of Windkessel models and distributed models. The main arterial parameters describing input impedance are peripheral resistance, total arterial compliance and aortic characteristic impedance (Figure in the Box). Arterial function is often easier to understand when the three Windkessel parameters are given as description of the arterial system. With the modern computing techniques, the calculation of the parameters of the Windkessel model can be performed rapidly and gives directly interpretable results (Chap. 25). For instance, the effect of a change in total arterial compliance on aortic pressure, which is often not obvious from the impedance plot, can be obtained directly by means of the Windkessel, and the impedance calculation can be avoided.

24.2.1   *Characteristic Differences in Pressure Wave Shapes*

The examples shown in Figs. 24.2 and 24.3, make clear that, although the pressure and flow waves result from the interaction of the heart and arterial load, major features of the pressure wave shape arise from the arterial system and can therefore be related to aspects of the input impedance.

In older subjects, where arterial compliance is decreased the Pulse Wave Velocity and reflections are increased. The larger compound reflected wave adds to the forward pressure wave resulting in an increase in Pulse Pressure, Augmentation Index and systolic pressure, a Type A wave (Chap. 22). As a result of the increased reflection the input impedance oscillates around the characteristic impedance. In subjects with small reflections, the pressure shows an early maximum, with negligible or negative augmentation, and the impedance oscillates only little.

Fig. 24.3 Valsalva strain increases intra-thoracic and intra-abdominal pressures. The thus lower transmural pressure increases arterial compliance and lowers pulse wave velocity. Reflections decrease. An almost reflection-less situation appears where pressure and flow resemble each other (left, top) and input impedance is close to aortic characteristic impedance. In the release phase the reverse is true, reflections are large, pressure and flow wave shapes differ strongly and input impedance oscillates. (Adapted from Ref. [10], by permission)

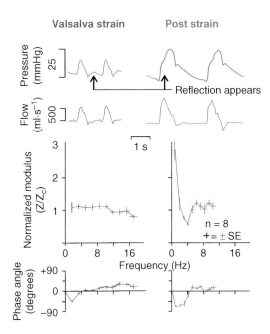

24.2.2   Changes in Reflection

In the Fig. 24.3 (left side) we see that during the Valsalva maneuver aortic pressure resembles aortic flow in terms of wave shape [10]. During the Valsalva maneuver, intra-thoracic and intra-abdominal pressures increase. The transmural pressure of the aorta decreases and the aortic compliance increases leading to a decreased pulse wave velocity [11]. Waves from different reflection sites arrive more at random in the proximal aorta and reflections smaller. As a result pressure and flow become similar in shape and the input impedance is close to the characteristic impedance of the aorta. After the release of the Valsalva maneuver, cardiac filling and transmural pressure are increased, wave speed is increased as well and reflections increase, and a large augmentation in the pressure is seen (Fig. 24.3 right side). It should be mentioned that during the Valsalva Maneuver arterial stiffness is decreased but peripheral resistance is somewhat increased and not decreased, from 1045 ± 48 to 1342 ± 141 dyne·s·cm^{-5} [10]. From this experiment we have to conclude that reflections at the periphery contribute little to overall reflections, but it is the (many) local reflections at all discontinuities in the major conduit arteries that are of primary importance.

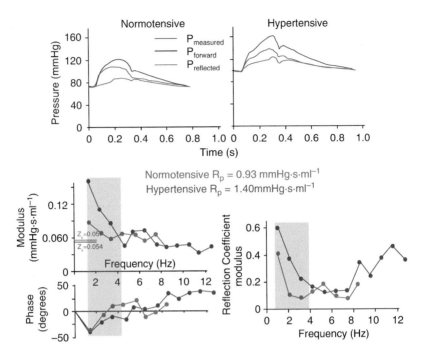

Fig. 24.4 Hemodynamics of hypertension. In the top panel the aortic pressure with its forward and reflected waves of a normotensive and a hypertensive subject are shown. Data in the other panels are averaged, normotensives (n = 14) and hypertensives (n = 12). The mean pressure is increased due to the resistance increase. The reflection magnitude is increased from 0.43 to 0.63. Group-averaged input impedance modulus and phase at low frequencies differ considerably as a result of the decreased in arterial compliance. The reflection coefficient is also increased for the low frequencies. The relative increase in resistance and decrease in compliance are about 50%. Colored areas indicates harmonics 1–3 the major determinants of wave shapes. (Based on data by Ref [12])

24.2.3 Hypertension

Figure 24.4 shows an example of the changes in pressure, input impedance and reflection coefficient. Peripheral resistance is increased by about 50%, and arterial compliance is decreased about 50% [12]. Mean pressure is higher because peripheral resistance is increased. The Pulse Pressure is mainly increased as a result of the decrease in compliance. It may be seen that for the first three harmonics the input impedance modulus is larger in hypertension than normotension, implying a decrease in compliance and higher reflection coefficient.

With increasing age systolic pressure increases and diastolic pressure may even decrease somewhat. Figure 24.5 schematically shows the changes in input impedance with age. Resistance increases in aging but the magnitude of the increase is relatively small. In aging the wave speed increases strongly up to a factor two, and aortic compliance may decrease by a factor 3–4. Characteristic impedance is

Fig. 24.5 In hypertension peripheral resistance and thus mean pressure is increased are increased with a limited amount (4). Compliance is decreased resulting in a larger pulse pressure, PP, and in a less rapid decrease in impedance modulus with frequency (1), and a higher characteristic impedance (2). Reflections are increased, the impedance oscillates more about the characteristic impedance (3), and the wave is augmented (3). (Adapted from Ref. [13], by permission)

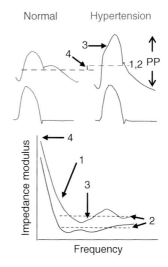

increased due to the aortic stiffening. The decrease in aortic compliance is the main reason why pulse pressure increases.

In essential hypertension both resistance and compliance change by similar amounts, but in old age hypertension the main parameter of the arterial system that changes is compliance.

References

1. Murgo JP, Westerhof N, Giolma JP, Altobelli SA. Aortic input impedance in normal man: relationship to pressure wave forms. Circulation. 1980;62:105–1116.
2. Stergiopulos N, Meister J-J, Westerhof N. Scatter in the input impedance spectrum may result from the elastic nonlinearity of the arterial wall. Am J Phys. 1995;269:H1490–5.
3. Westerhof N, Elzinga G, Sipkema P. An artificial system for pumping hearts. J Appl Physiol. 1971;31:776–81.
4. Stergiopulos N, Westerhof BE, Westerhof N. Total arterial inertance as the fourth element of the windkessel model. Am J Phys. 1999;276:H81–8.
5. Sipkema P, Westerhof N. Effective length of the arterial system. Ann Biomed Eng. 1975;3:296–307.
6. Westerhof BE, van den Wijngaard JP, Murgo JP, Westerhof N. Location of a reflection site is elusive: consequences for the calculation of aortic pulse wave velocity. Hypertension. 2008;52:478–83.
7. Sipkema P, Westerhof N, Randall OS. The arterial system characterized in the time domain. Cardiovasc Res. 1980;14:270–9.
8. Van Huis GA, Sipkema P, Westerhof N. Coronary input impedance during the cardiac cycle as obtained by impulse response method. Am J Phys. 1987;253:H317–24.
9. Westerhof N, Elzinga G. Normalized input impedance and arterial decay time over heart period are independent of animal size. Am J Phys. 1991;261:R126–33.
10. Murgo JP, Westerhof N, Giolma JP, Altobelli SA. Manipulation of ascending aortic pressure and flow reflections with the Valsalva maneuver: relationship to input impedance. Circulation. 1981;63:122–32.

11. Latham RD, Westerhof N, Sipkema P, Rubal BJ, Reuderink P, Murgo JP. Regional wave travel and reflections along the human aorta: a study with six simultaneous micromanometric pressures. Circulation. 1985;72:1257–69.
12. Ting CT, Chen JW, Chang MS, Yin FC. Arterial hemodynamics in human hypertension. Effects of the calcium channel antagonist nifedipine. Hypertension. 1995;25:1326–32.
13. O'Rourke MF. Pulsatile arterial haemodynamics in hypertension. Aust N Z J Med. 1976;6(Suppl 2):40–8.

Chapter 25
The Arterial Windkessel

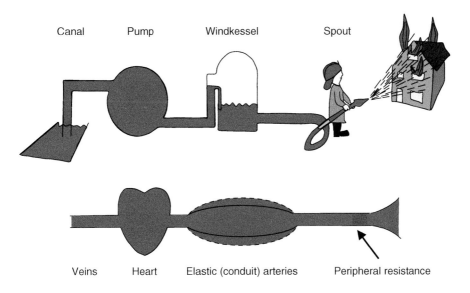

The analogy between the fire engine with the heart and arterial system modeled with a Windkessel. The peripheral resistance is the summed resistance of all small arteries, arterioles and capillaries. Total arterial compliance is the sum of the compliances of all arteries, mainly the aorta and conduit arteries. The Windkessel model can help us to understand how the arterial system functions, it can be used as a realistic load in isolated heart studies, it can be used in modeling, and it can form the basis for estimating arterial system parameters. The Windkessel is a 'lumped model' and does not take into account pressure and flow waves. Adapted from Ref. [1], by permission.

© Springer International Publishing AG, part of Springer Nature 2019
N. Westerhof et al., *Snapshots of Hemodynamics*,
https://doi.org/10.1007/978-3-319-91932-4_25

25.1   Description

Otto Frank, 1899, popularized the original two-element Windkessel, consisting of a compliance, equal to total arterial compliance, C, and a resistance representing total resistance of the microcirculation, R_p. He reasoned that the decay of ascending aortic diastolic pressure, when flow is zero, can be described by an exponential curve, $P(t) = P_o \cdot e^{-t/RpC} = P_o \cdot e^{-t/\tau}$. The time constant,$\tau$, i.e., the time for pressure to decrease to 37% of its starting pressure, is given by the product of peripheral resistance, R_p, and total arterial compliance, C, (Fig. 25.1). The blood ejected into the compliant conduit vessels (mainly aorta) leaves the system through the peripheral resistance. A greater resistance causes a slower discharge of the stored blood from the compliant vessels and the time constant is larger. Also, in a larger compliance more blood is stored, and a longer time constant results.

Frank's objective was to derive Cardiac Output from aortic pressure. By measuring the pulse wave velocity of the aorta (carotid to femoral) together with averaged aortic cross-sectional area, and using the Moens-Korteweg equation (Chap. 12) area compliance, C_A, can be derived. When aortic length, L, is also known volume compliance, $C = C_A \cdot L$, is calculated. Using C and the estimate τ from the diastolic pressure decay, the peripheral resistance can be obtained from $R_p = \tau/C$. Finally from mean pressure and resistance, using Ohm's law, mean flow, CO, can be calculated. The assumption that all compliance is located in the aorta, thus neglecting the compliance of the smaller conduit vessels, is not correct, in health about 2/3 of total arterial compliance is found in the aorta. After pulsatile flow measurement became available, and arterial input impedance could be determined (Chap. 24), the shortcomings of the two-element Windkessel became clear.

Figure 25.2 shows three Windkessels and their input impedances [1]. The input impedance of the two-element Windkessel exhibits a continuously decreasing modulus and a phase angle that approaches minus 90° for high frequencies, while

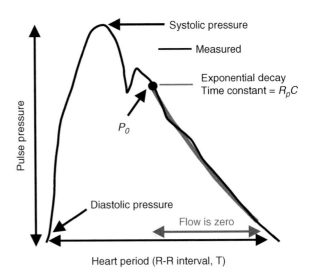

Fig. 25.1 Windkessel models predict an exponential decay of aortic pressure when flow is zero, i.e., in diastole. This decay is characterized by the decay time that equals R_pC, with R_p peripheral resistance and C total arterial compliance, and described by $P(t) = P_0 e^{-t/RpC}$

Systolic pressure

Measured

Exponential decay
Time constant = R_pC

Pulse pressure

P_0

Diastolic pressure

Flow is zero

Heart period (R-R interval, T)

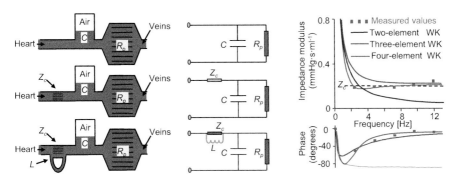

Fig. 25.2 Left: The three Windkessels. The hydraulic version (left) and electrical representation (right). The two-element Windkessel (Frank) contains total peripheral resistance (R_p), and total arterial compliance (C). The three-element Windkessel results from adding aortic characteristic impedance, (Z_c). The characteristic impedance accounts for blood mass ($L' = \rho/A$) ejected in a compliant aorta (C_A), and equals wave speed over aortic area, A. The four-element Windkessel contains total arterial inertance, L, playing a role at the very low frequencies. This fourth element also solves the problem that characteristic impedance, although having the dimension resistance, is not a real resistor and therefore, in the three-element Windkessel model mean pressure over mean flow equals $Z_c + R_p$ instead of R_p. Right: Input impedances of the three Windkessels compared with the measured input impedance. The two-element Windkessel clearly falls short, especially in the high frequency range. The three-element Windkessel is less accurate at very low frequencies. This is the result of the representation of the characteristic impedance by a resistance. (Adapted from Ref. [1], used by permission)

the actual input impedance at high frequencies shows a constant impedance modulus and a phase angle of about zero degrees (Chap. 24).

The three-element Windkessel is based on Frank's two-element Windkessel with the addition of the (aortic) characteristic impedance [2]. From a wave transmission and reflection standpoint, it can be reasoned that for high frequencies reflections in the proximal aorta cancel out and for an aorta without reflected waves the input impedance equals its characteristic impedance (Chap. 24). Or, in other words, for high frequencies the input impedance equals the characteristic impedance of the proximal aorta. The input impedance of the three-element Windkessel is

$$Z_{in} / Z_c = \left[1 + R_p / Z_c + i \cdot \omega R_p C \right] / \left[1 + i \cdot \omega R_p C \right]$$

Aortic characteristic impedance is a real number, i.e., its modulus is constant with a value $Z_c = \sqrt{\rho \cdot \Delta P / (\Delta A \cdot A)}$ and its phase angle is zero (Chap. 12). This behavior is similar to that of a resistance. Therefore, a resistor is often used to mimic the characteristic impedance of the proximal aorta. The introduction of the characteristic impedance or characteristic resistance as the third element of the Windkessel can be seen as bridging the lumped models and the transmission line models. However, the characteristic impedance is only present for oscillatory pressure and flow and does not dissipate energy while a resistor does. The approximation of characteristic impedance by a resistor leads to errors in the low frequency range. When, for instance, total arterial compliance is determined from aortic pressure and flow by

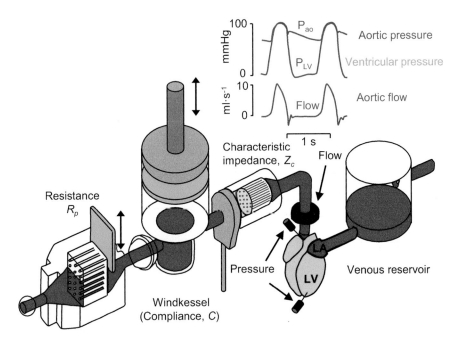

Fig. 25.3 The three-element Windkessel is a lumped model of the entire systemic arterial tree and mimics the load on the heart. Its three parameters have a physiologic meaning (see Chap. 24). The peripheral resistance, R_p, equals the resistance of all small arteries, arterioles and capillaries. The total arterial compliance, C, equals the sum of the compliances of all arteries, with most of the compliance in the aorta and conduit arteries. The characteristic impedance of the proximal aorta, Z_c, forms the link of the Windkessel and transmission line models. When the three-element Windkessel model is used to load an isolated heart, the pressures and flow generated by the model are similar to those found in vivo (top inset)

parameter estimation of the three elements of the Windkessel, the compliance is consistently overestimated. To overcome the low-frequency errors of the three-element Windkessel, a fourth element was introduced to circumvent the inconsistency resulting from modeling the characteristic impedance by a resistance [3], and its input impedance is shown in Fig. 25.2. It has been established that the inertance term equals total inertance of the arterial system. Using this four-element Windkessel model, total arterial compliance is estimated accurately from pressure and flow.

It is possible to construct a hydraulic version of the three-element Windkessel as shown in Fig. 25.3 [2]. When this hydraulic model is loading a real heart, the combination results in ventricular and aortic pressures and aortic flow that are in wave shape and magnitude similar to those measured *in-vivo* as shown in Fig. 25.4 [4].

When flow is zero, as in diastole, the decrease of aortic pressure, is characterized by the decay time (Fig. 25.1), which equals R_pC for all three Windkessel models. To calculate the decay-time one starts with some delay after valve closure, about 10% of the heart period.

The Windkessel models only mimic the behavior of the entire arterial system, or sub-systems, at their entrance. This lumped description of the system means that pressures within these models, such as pressures distal of the characteristic impedance,

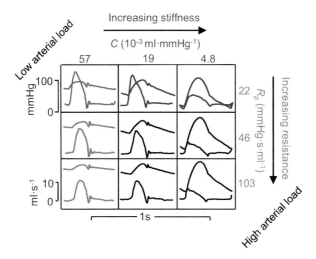

Fig. 25.4 Aortic pressure and flow resulting from an isolated cat heart pumping into a three-element Windkessel. The effect of changes in peripheral resistance (increasing downwards, green) and arterial compliance (decreasing to the right, blue) are shown. The control condition is the left top panel (red). The advantage of the use of such a model is that all venous and cardiac parameters can be kept constant while a single parameter of the load, here resistance or compliance can be varied. (Adapted from Ref. [4], by permission)

have little meaning, and do not represent the pressure in the more distal arterial system. Windkessels do not in any way model wave travel and wave reflection.

25.1.1   How the Arterial Tree Reduces to a Windkessel

For higher Pulse Wave Velocity thus larger wave lengths the arterial system is relatively short with respect to wave length. This implies that pressures at different locations vary more simultaneously, and the system reduces to a (two-element) Windkessel with all waves assumed to be simultaneous. Segers et al. have shown that the three-element Windkessel is a better arterial model in when arterial stiffness is high as in older subjects with high Pulse Wave Velocity, than in young subjects [5]. This effect is known as 'Windkesselness' of the arterial system.

25.1.2   Limitations of the Windkessel

The Windkessel is a simplified description of the arterial system.

- The decrease of (aortic) pressure in diastole is not following a single exponential decay. In general the decay time is longer in the later part of diastole. This is in part due to the increase in compliance with lowering pressure, but linear 1-D

Fig. 25.5 Two examples how the three-element Windkessel can describe the gross wave shape of aortic pressure. Details, such as augmentation and inflection point are not represented well

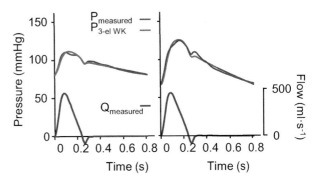

models show this effect as well, indicating that the reflected waves do not necessarily add to a single exponential pressure decay.

- In systole the three-element Windkessel pressure does not necessarily result in the measured pressure wave as shown in Fig. 25.5. Inversely when the pressure predicted by the two-element is subtracted from the measured pressure the difference is not necessarily equal to $Z_c \cdot Q$ (Chap. 23).
- Input impedance of the three-element Windkessel is a smoothed version of the actual impedance implying that detailed features of the pressure are not represented (see Figures in Chap. 24).

25.1.3   Other Lumped Models

Other lumped models are partly Windkessel models with more elements and partly tube models. More Windkessel-like elements in series may evolve to transmission line models, but often the parameters lose their physiologic meaning. Input impedance and wave travel of tube models are discussed in Chap. 26.

25.2   Physiological and Clinical Relevance

Windkessel models, especially the three-element Windkessel, can explain the behavior of the input impedance and give a meaning to the three main parameters that describe the arterial system. Windkessel models also find their use as load for the isolated ejecting hearts (Figs. 25.3 and 25.4). In such a hydraulic Windkessel parameters may be changed and cardiac pump function studied. Figure 25.4 shows an example, where an isolated heart pumps in a hydraulic Windkessel model. The effects of changes in peripheral resistance and total arterial compliance on pressure and flow can be studied while cardiac contractility, Heart Rate and cardiac filling are maintained constant [4].

Figure 25.5 shows the magnitude and wave shape of aortic pressure resulting from flow and the three-element Windkessel. Since three-element Windkessel impedance is a smoothed version of the real impedance the details of the pressure wave are not exactly represented. However, systolic and diastolic pressures predicted by the three-element Windkessel model under varying conditions, including the Valsalva maneuver, compare well with measured pressures as: $P_{systolic,predicted} = 1.034 \cdot P_{systolic,measured} - 3.12$ ($R^2 = 0.97$) and $P_{diastolic,predicted} = 0.997\ P_{diastolic,measured} - 1.63$ ($R^2 = 0.99$) [6]. Thus, the Windkessel model represents systolic and diastolic pressures well but is of limited accuracy regarding the pressure wave shape (Fig. 25.5).

Figure 25.6 shows the effect of aging on pressure as predicted by the Windkessel. In aging the peripheral resistance increases more than Cardiac Output decreases, resulting in the small increase in mean pressure. Total arterial compliance decreases considerably (factor ~2) and causes the increase in Pulse Pressure.

An important use of the Windkessel models is the estimation of arterial parameters. Several methods have been proposed for arterial compliance derivation [7]. These methods are (see Fig. 25.7):

The Stroke Volume over Pulse Pressure Method This method is rather old [8] but has been reintroduced recently [9, 10]. The method assumes that Stroke Volume is ejected in the conduit vessels (aorta) and that there is no run-off through the periphery. Therefore, this ratio overestimates compliance [11] and should be used in comparisons only. Also, the method is not reliable under extreme changes. During the Valsalva maneuver SV decreases from 89 to 32 ml and Pulse Pressure from 34 to 20 mmHg [12], predicting a compliance *de*crease from 2.6 to 1.6 ml/mmHg, while compliance measured in other ways including the decay time method described above shows a two-fold *in*crease.

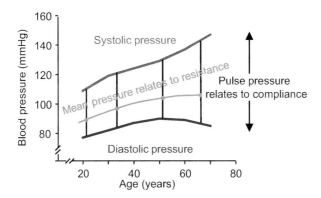

Fig. 25.6 Proximal aortic pressure as a function of age. While systolic pressure continuously increases with age (red), diastolic pressure even decreases at higher ages (blue). Mean pressure (green) increases initially but hardly changes at higher ages. The increase in mean pressure mainly relates to an increase in peripheral resistance, while the increase in pulse pressure (vertical black lines) mainly results from the decrease in total arterial compliance

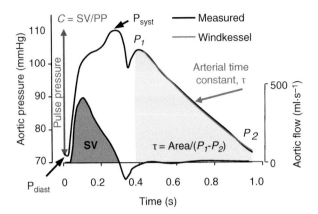

Fig. 25.7 Methods to estimate total arterial compliance: (1) Stroke volume (blue) divided by Pulse Pressure, P_s-P_d. (2) The decay time of diastolic aortic pressure, $\tau = R_pC$ (green) and $R_p = P_{mean}$ /Q_{mean}. (3) Area method: The area (A) under the diastolic aortic pressure (yellow) divided by the pressure difference in diastole $\tau = A/(P_1$-$P_2)$, plus method 2

The decay time method described above.

The area method, where the area under the diastolic aortic pressure divided by the pressure difference between start and endpoint is set equal to decay time.

$$RC = \int_{t_1}^{t_2} \frac{P(t)}{P_1 - P_2} dt$$

Knowing the R_pC time and calculating R_p, i.e., the ratio of mean pressure and mean flow, the compliance can be derived [13].

The two-area method is based on the following equation:

$$\int_{t_1}^{t_2} Q(t) dt = C \cdot (P_2 - P_1) + \frac{1}{R_p} \int_{t_1}^{t_2} P(t) dt$$

The equation is applied to two periods of the cardiac cycle; the period of onset of systole to peak systole and the period from peak systole to the end of diastole. Thus, two equations with two unknowns, R_p and C, are obtained [14].

The Pulse Pressure method is based on fitting the systolic and diastolic pressures predicted by the two-element Windkessel with measured aortic flow as input, to the measured values of systolic and diastolic pressure. Although the two-element Windkessel does not produce correct wave shapes, the low frequency input impedance is very close to the actual impedance and systolic and diastolic pressure are mainly determined by low frequencies [15]. The method is practical when flow can be measured noninvasively (e.g., MRI, US) and aortic systolic and diastolic pressures can be derived from noninvasive pressures (via Brachial of Carotid artery, see Chap. 27).

The parameter estimation method fits the three-element or four-element Windkessel using pressure and flow as a function of time. When aortic flow is fed into the Windkessel the pressure is predicted. This pressure can be compared to the measured pressure. By minimization of the Root Mean Square Errors, RMSE, of the difference between measured and predicted pressures the best Windkessel parameters are obtained. In this way, all the Windkessel parameters can be derived including a good estimate of characteristic impedance. Using the three-element Windkessel compliance is overestimated [11], but this is not the case using the four-element Windkessel [3]. Also, inversely, pressure may be used as input and minimization of flow errors is then performed [7].

The transient method can be applied when pressure and flow are not in the steady state. Peripheral resistance can then not be calculated from mean pressure and mean flow, because aortic flow is not equal to peripheral flow. Using the three-element Windkessel with flow as input, pressure may be calculated while storage of blood in the large conduit arteries is accounted for. By curve fitting of the Windkessel parameters to obtain minimal difference between measured and predicted pressure the Windkessel parameters can be estimated accurately [16].

The input impedance method fits the input impedance of the three-element of four-element Windkessel model to the measured input impedance, by minimization of the RMSE, in a way similar to method mentioned above.

The wave velocity method is not based on the Windkessel but on transmission of waves (Chaps. 12 and 21). This method estimates the compliance of the section over which the pressures are measured, e.g. brachial-femoral artery wave speed.

It should be emphasized that all Windkessel-based methods require accurate pressure measurement in the proximal aorta. The first three methods require measurement of Cardiac Output only, while the next 5 methods require ascending aortic flow wave shape. The wave velocity method requires two accurate measurements of pressure, of flow, or of diameter, in terms of time (Chap. 12).

Finally, the three- or four-element Windkessel models can be used in lumped models of the arterial system and heart to predict the contribution of heart and load on pressure and flow under different conditions [17, 18].

References

1. Westerhof N, Lankhaar JW, Westerhof BE. The arterial Windkessel. Med Biol Eng Comput. 2009;47:131–41.
2. Westerhof N, Elzinga G, Sipkema P. An artificial system for pumping hearts. J Appl Physiol. 1971;31:776–81.
3. Stergiopulos N, Westerhof BE, Westerhof N. Total arterial inertance as the fourth element of the windkessel model. Am J Phys. 1999;276:H81–8.
4. Elzinga G, Westerhof N. Pressure and flow generated by the left ventricle against different impedances. Circ Res. 1973;32:178–86.
5. Segers P, Rietzschel ER, De Buyzere ML, Vermeersch SJ, De Bacquer D, Van Bortel LM, et al. Noninvasive (input) impedance, pulse wave velocity, and wave reflection in healthy middle-aged men and women. Hypertension. 2007;49:1248–55.

6. Westerhof N, Westerhof BE. A review of methods to determine the functional arterial parameters stiffness and resistance. J Hypertens. 2013;31:1769–75.
7. Stergiopulos N, Meister J-J, Westerhof N. Evaluation of methods for estimating total arterial compliance. Am J Phys. 1995;268:H1540–8.
8. Hamilton WF, Remington JW. The measurement of the stroke volume from the pressure pulse. Am J Phys. 1947;148:14–24.
9. Randall OS, Esler MD, Calfee RV, Bulloch GF, Maisel AS, Culp B. Arterial compliance in hypertension. N Z J Med. 1976;6:49–59.
10. Chemla D, Hébert JL, Coirault C, Zamani K, Suard I, Colin P, et al. Total arterial compliance estimated by stroke volume-to-aortic pulse pressure ratio in humans. Am J Phys. 1998;274:H500–5.
11. Segers P, Brimioulle S, Stergiopulos N, Westerhof N, Naeije R, Maggiorini M, et al. Pulmonary arterial compliance in dogs and pigs: the three-element windkessel model revisited. Am J Phys. 1999;277:H725–31.
12. Murgo JP, Westerhof N, Giolma JP, Altobelli SA. Manipulation of ascending aortic pressure and flow wave reflections with the Valsalva maneuver: relationship to input impedance. Circulation. 1981;63:122–32.
13. Liu Z, Brin KP, Yin FCP. Estimation of total arterial compliance: and improved method and evaluation of current methods. Am J Phys. 1986;251:H588–600.
14. Self DA, Ewert RD, Swope RP, Latham RD. Beat-to-beat estimation of peripheral resistance and arterial compliance during +Gz centrifugation. Aviat Space Environ Med. 1994;65:396–403.
15. Stergiopulos N, Meister J-J, Westerhof N. Simple and accurate way for estimating total and segmental arterial compliance: the pulse pressure method. Ann Biomed Eng. 1994;22:392–7.
16. Toorop GP, Westerhof N, Elzinga G. Beat-to beat estimation of peripheral resistance and arterial compliance during pressure transients. Am J Phys. 1987;252:H1275–83.
17. Segers P, Stergiopulos N, Westerhof N. Quantification of the contribution of cardiac and arterial remodeling in hypertension. Hypertension. 2000;36:760–5.
18. Maksuti E, Westerhof N, Westerhof BE, Broomé M, Stergiopulos N. Contribution of the arterial system and the heart to blood pressure during normal aging – a simulation study. PLoS One. 2016;11:e0157493.

Chapter 26
Distributed Models and Tube Models

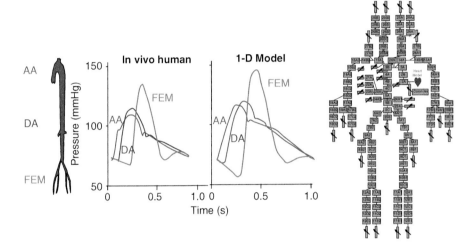

The distributed, or 1-D model, of the human systemic arterial tree shown here accounts for the morphology, oscillatory flow theory, and viscoelastic properties of the arterial wall. The left panel shows pressures measured in the human *in vivo*, ascending aorta, descending aorta, and femoral artery The right figure shows pressures predicted by the model at the three same locations. It may be seen that peripheral pressures arrive later, are smoother, and have a larger pulse pressure (pressure amplification). Distributed models allow the study of input impedance, wave travel, reflections, and wave shapes of pressure and flow at different locations in the arterial tree. In short, the distributed models allow insight into phenomena the Windkessel models do not describe. Several geometrically very accurate distributed models have been published, even (3-D models) that show flow patterns in the vessels. Simpler models such as single (sometimes tapering) tubes, or two tubes in parallel are discussed in the text. Adapted from Ref. [1], by permission.

© Springer International Publishing AG, part of Springer Nature 2019
N. Westerhof et al., *Snapshots of Hemodynamics*,
https://doi.org/10.1007/978-3-319-91932-4_26

26.1 Description

Distributed models (1-D) that account for arterial geometry, such as the one shown in the Figure in the Box can help in the understanding of the load on the heart and wave transmission and reflection. The construction of distributed models implies breaking up the arterial tree into short segments, accounting for geometry (vessel radius and wall thickness etc.) and mechanical properties (compliance etc.), see Appendix 3. The wave transmission characteristics of each arterial segment can be described by Womersley's oscillatory flow theory, longitudinal impedance, and wall properties formulated by the transverse impedance (Chap. 12).

Distributed models of the arterial tree also can be constructed based on the (simplified) form of the blood flow equations describing the conservation of mass and momentum:

$$\partial Q / \partial x + \partial A / \partial t = 0$$

$$\partial Q / \partial t + \partial \left(Q^2 / A \right) / \partial x = -\left(1 / \rho \right) \cdot A \cdot \partial P / \partial x - 2\pi r \cdot \tau / \rho$$

where A is the vessel cross-sectional area and τ is wall shear stress, usually estimated using Poiseuille's law. The two equations above have three variables: pressure P, flow Q, and area A. Therefore, a constitutive law relating cross-sectional area, A, to pressure, P, is needed to form a system of 3 equations with 3 unknowns, which can be easily solved using different numerical techniques (i.e., finite differences, or method of characteristics). The cross-sectional area-pressure relation gives this information as described by area compliance (Chap. 11).

While the Figure in the Box contains 121 segments [1], models of fewer elements as the one by Alastruey [2] and more elements by Reymond et al. [3] have been proposed. With modern high-powered computing techniques patient-specific models, based on MRI patient data, can be constructed thereby predicting the pressure and flow wave shapes of individuals [3]. The periphery, i.e. vessels beyond the conduit arteries have been modeled by resistances [1], by (local) Windkessels and more detailed descriptions of the periphery [4]. The differences have been discussed by Guan and turn out to have little effect on central hemodynamics [5].

The 3-D models have been constructed accounting for flow profiles and fluid-wall interaction [6, 7]. The 3-D models predict pressure and flow waves shapes only slightly better that the 1-D models, but are required if wall shear and flow profiles are to be described. Distributed models have been extensively used to study arterial input impedance (Chap. 24) and aspects of pressure and flow propagation, such as the effects of viscoelasticity [8], the effects of different forms of arterial disease and the relation of peripheral to central pressure waves [9, 10]. Taylor has shown that a randomly distributed model (in terms of vessel lengths) resembles arterial input impedance and wave travel [11, 12], suggesting that detailed information on arterial geometry is not of great importance to describe input impedance. Also the pulmonary arterial system, although very different in geometry from the systemic arterial tree shows qualitatively similar input impedances (Chap. 28).

26.1.1 Distributed Models

Distributed models predict pressure and flow waves that compare well to actual waves measured in the human [13], as shown in Figure in the Box. Beyond an apparently good qualitative agreement, well known aspects of pressure wave propagation in arteries, such as the systolic pressure amplification, the smoothening of the pressure pulse towards the periphery, and the appearance of a secondary reflection in the diastolic part of a pressure wave in a peripheral artery are well predicted. Figure 26.1 shows the modulus and phase of the input impedance derived from a distributed human systemic arterial model in comparison with the input impedance measured in a young healthy adult [14]. The distributed model predicts all the typical features of the arterial input impedance: the rapid drop in modulus for the first few harmonics, the relatively flat modulus in the medium and high frequency range, and the negative phase values for low frequencies returning to small values at higher frequencies.

26.1.2 Single Tube and Two-Tube Models

Distributed models offer a complete representation of the arterial tree in terms of hemodynamics, but they require a large number of parameters, namely geometry and elasticity of all arterial segments. Also, the distributed models make it difficult to glean information of the main factors that contribute to the wave shapes of pressure and flow. Given these limitations, several researchers have proposed models that are relatively simple but yet allow for the phenomena of wave travel and reflections.

Single uniform tube models have been proposed as representative of the aorta, with a single reflection site at its distal end [15, 16]. These models are based on the assumption that reflections occur at the periphery or aortic bifurcation possibly leading to a 'standing wave' [17]. Two peripheral loads for uniform tube models

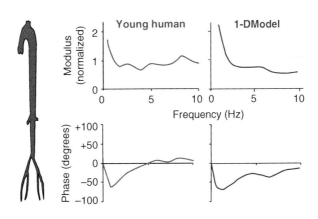

Fig. 26.1 Input impedance measured in a young healthy adult (left), compared with the input impedance of a distributed model (right). The impedance modulus is normalized to aortic characteristic impedance to facilitate comparison

have been proposed, a resistor and a Windkessel representing the microcirculation. The simplest, with a resistive load which is taken equal to systemic vascular resistance, R_p, has a strongly oscillating input impedance. The large oscillations in impedance result from the large reflection coefficient at the distal site since R_p is about 15 times larger than the characteristic impedance of the tube giving a reflection coefficient of 0.88. The uniform tube with Windkessel load with characteristic impedance equal to the characteristic impedance of the tube has a much smaller distal reflection and introduces a time delay, Δt_{refl}, between reflected and forward waves at the reflection site (Fig. 26.2). If the tubes are modeled without viscous blood losses and wall losses oscillations in impedance increase.

All uniform tube models show that the reflected wave runs towards the heart and its arrival time (return time), $t_{ret} = 2\ l/\text{PWV} + \Delta t_{refl}$, with l tube length (Fig. 26.2, left panel). Only in the lossless case with a resistor as load the frequency of first minimum of the impedance modulus, f_{min}, and first zero crossing of the phase angle $f_{phase} = 0$ allow the calculation of effective length via the 'quarter wavelength rule': when the pressure has travelled half a wave length, thus one quarter wavelength forward and one quarter wavelength backward, the pressure waves cancel. This 'quarter wavelength rule', $f_{min} = \text{PWV}/(4\cdot l)$ is based on the standing wave concept [17] and appears often in the older literature. However, it should be realized that these relations hold for $\Delta t_{refl} = 0$ only. With Δt_{refl} not zero and unknown, the reflection site is 'illusive' [18, 19]. The main limitation of the uniform tube models is not their impedance but their wave characteristics. Recently it has been reported that in the aorta the reflected wave runs towards the periphery (see Fig. 22.2) and not towards the heart as the uniform tube models predict [19, 20].

The asymmetric T-tube model was originally proposed by O'Rourke [21, 22], and uses a body tube (aorta) and a tube for the head arteries. The length ratio of the two tubes was chosen 2 to 1. This model was tested by Campbell and Burattini [23, 24]. Input impedance is close to reality, but in each tube the reflected waves run towards the heart. The reflected pressure wave in the head tube arrives earlier at the heart than the reflected pressure of the body tube. This shorter return time is comparable with experimental and model data [20, 25] and is of interest since it is often assumed that the aorta plays the major role in the compound reflected wave return.

A tapered tube as arterial model, shown in Fig. 26.2, has been suggested by Segers et al. [26]. The model shows an input impedance that oscillates little and the time difference between forward and reflected pressure is small and similar at several locations, i.e. the reflected wave does not run towards the heart, in agreement the biological data [19, 20].

The 1-D model consists of a tapering aorta with many side branches (Figure in the Box and 26.2). Since tapering and side-branches can both be seen as local reflection sites this model emphasizes that multiple reflection sites rather than a single reflection site explains wave travel and reflection. The effect of aortic tapering in the 1-D model has been quantified [25].

The uniform tube models, T-tube model, by their deficiency of representing wave travel correctly, have taught us the importance of the contribution of many local reflections (taper, side branches, etc.) to wave arterial wave travel and reflection.

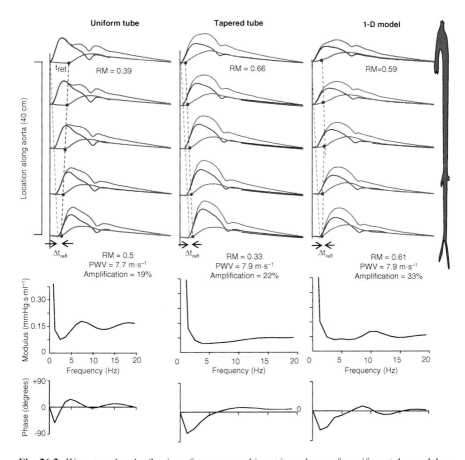

Fig. 26.2 Wave travel and reflection of pressure and input impedance of a uniform tube model, a tapered tube model, and a 1-D arterial model (Figure in the box). Simplified aorta is shown to indicate measurement locations. The single tube and tapered tube model are loaded with a three-element Windkessel with a characteristic impedance equal to the (distal) characteristic impedance of the tube. Systemic Vascular Resistance and total arterial compliance of all models are 1.1 mmHg·s·ml^{-1} and 1.22 ml·mmHg^{-1}, respectively. The choice of a Windkessel as load of the tube models is required to obtain reasonable Reflection Magnitudes (RM) and wave shapes and to limit extreme oscillations in the input impedance. The RM is given at ascending and distal aorta levels. Amplification of pressure is the Pulse Pressure ratio of distal aortic and ascending aortic pressures. In the tube models the reflected wave at the load is delayed with respect to the forward wave, with a time delay ($\Delta t_{refl} = 14$ ms), an effect of the Windkessel load. In the uniform tube model the distally reflected wave travels towards the heart and forward and reflected wave travel with the same wave speed. The return time of the reflected at the heart equals $t_{ret} = 2 \cdot \text{length}/\text{PWV} + \Delta t_{refl}$. This wave travel behavior of the uniform tube is not in line with *in vivo* data (Chaps. 12 and 22). The tapered tube shows a reflected wave running towards the heart and with constant time delay between forward and reflected wave. This is in line with *in vivo* data and results from the many homogeneously distributed reflection sites in the tube. The 1-D model shows a more complex behavior of the reflected wave, since several different reflection sites are present with different reflection coefficients

26.2   Physiological and Clinical Relevance

The comparison of distributed 1-D models and single tube models show that many reflection sites rather than one site are essential in explaining input impedance and wave travel in the arterial system. Single tube models are of limited value since their wave travel characteristics are not realistic. Distributed models have been used mostly for research as analytical tools because they are realistic for simulating a variety of physiological and pathological situations. Although, in principle, distributed models can be used to derive useful parameters of the arterial tree based on *in vivo* measurements, clinical use is difficult because of the large number of parameters required to construct a 'per patient' model. However, the work by Reymond et al. [3, 6] suggest that per patient modeling is becoming feasible.

In arterial modeling the choice of model should depend on the degree of detail required and the focus desired. To understand the effect of total arterial compliance on integrated quantities such as aortic pressure and Cardiac Output, the Windkessel models may suffice as long a one remembers that aspects of waves cannot be considered. To model detailed effects, such a local flows and pressures and their wave transmission, one needs to use distributed models.

References

1. Westerhof N, Bosman F, De Vries CJ, Noordergraaf A. Analog studies of the human systemic arterial tree. J Biomech. 1969;2:121–43.
2. Alastruey J. On the mechanics underlying the reservoir-excess separation in systemic arteries and their implications for pulse wave analysis. Cardiovasc Eng. 2010;10:176–89.
3. Reymond P, Bohraus Y, Perren F, Lazeyras F, Stergiopulos N. Validation of a patient-specific one-dimensional model of the systemic arterial tree. Am J Phys. 2011;301:H1173–82.
4. Olufsen MS. Structured tree outflow condition for blood flow in larger systemic arteries. Am J Phys. 1999;276:H257–68.
5. Guan D, Liang F, Gremaud PA. Comparison of the Windkessel model and structured-tree model applied to prescribe outflow boundary conditions for a one-dimensional arterial tree model. J Biomech. 2016;49:1583–92.
6. Reymond P, Crosetto P, Deparis S, Quarteroni A, Stergiopulos N. Physiological simulation of blood flow in the aorta: comparison of hemodynamic indices as predicted by 3-D FSI, 3-D rigid wall and 1-D models. Med Eng Phys. 2013;35:784–91.
7. Xiao N, Alastruey J, Alberto FC. A systematic comparison between 1-D and 3-D hemodynamics in compliant arterial models. Int J Numer Method Biomed Eng. 2014;30:204–31.
8. Westerhof N, Noordergraaf A. Arterial viscoelasticity: a generalized model. Effect on input impedance and wave travel in the systematic tree. J Biomech. 1970;3:357–79.
9. O'Rourke MF, Avolio AP. Pulsatile flow and pressure in human systemic arteries: studies in man and in a multi-branched model of the human systemic arterial tree. Circ Res. 1980;46:363–72.
10. Stergiopulos N, Young DF, Rogge TR. Computer simulation of arterial flow with applications to arterial and aortic stenosis. J Biomech. 1992;25:1477–88.
11. Taylor MG. The input impedance of an assembly of randomly branching elastic tubes. Biophys J. 1966;6:29–51.

12. Taylor MG. Wave transmission through an assembly of randomly branching elastic tubes. Biophys J. 1966;6:697–716.
13. Remington JW, Wood EH. Formation of peripheral pulse contour in man. J Appl Physiol. 1956;9:433–42.
14. Murgo JP, Westerhof N, Giolma JP, Altobelli SA. Aortic input impedance in normal man: relationship to pressure wave forms. Circulation. 1980;62:105–1116.
15. Sipkema P, Westerhof N. Effective length of the arterial system. Ann Biomed Eng. 1975;3:296–307.
16. Alastruey J, Hunt AA, Weinberg PD. Novel wave intensity analysis of arterial pulse wave propagation accounting for peripheral reflections. Int J Numer Method Biomed Eng. 2014;30:249–79.
17. Hamilton WF, Dow P. An experimental study of the standing waves in the pulse propagated through the aorta. Am J Phys. 1939;125:48–59.
18. Westerhof BE, van den Wijngaard JP, Murgo JP, Westerhof N. Location of a reflection site is elusive: consequences for the calculation of aortic pulse wave velocity. Hypertension. 2008;52:478–83.
19. Davies JE, Alastruey J, Francis DP, Hadjiloizou N, Whinnett ZI, Manisty CH, et al. Attenuation of wave reflection by wave entrapment creates a "horizon effect" in the human aorta. Hypertension. 2012;60:778–85.
20. Tyberg JV, Bouwmeester JC, Parker KH, Shrive NG, Wang JJ. The case for the reservoir-wave approach. Int J Cardiol. 2014;172:299–306.
21. O'Rourke MF. Pressure and flow waves in systemic arteries and the anatomical design of the arterial system. J Appl Physiol. 1967;23:139–49.
22. O'Rourke MF. Vascular impedance in studies of arterial and cardiac function. Physiol Rev. 1982;62:570–623. Review
23. Campbell KB, Burattini R, Bell DL, Kirkpatrick RD, Knowlen GG. Time-domain formulation of asymmetric T-tube model of the arterial system. Am J Phys. 1990;258:H1761–74.
24. Burattini R, Knowlen GG, Campbell KN. Two arterial reflecting sites may appear as one to the heart. Circ Res. 1991;68:85–99.
25. Westerhof BE, Westerhof N. Magnitude and return time of the reflected wave: the effects of large artery stiffness and aortic geometry. J Hypertens. 2012;30:932–9.
26. Segers P, Verdonck P. Role of tapering in aortic wave reflection: hydraulic and mathematical model study. J Biomech. 2000;33:299–306.

Chapter 27
Transfer of Pressure

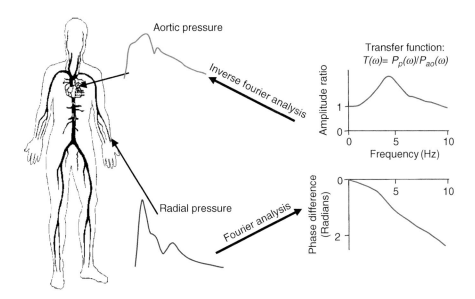

Aortic (systolic) pressure, together with cardiac dimensions defines cardiac afterload (wall stress), and is a better predictor of cardiovascular mortality and morbidity
than peripheral pressures. Aortic pressure is also essential in the estimation input
impedance and reflections. However, aortic pressure cannot be measured noninvasively. Peripheral pressures, such as finger pressure or radial pressure, shown in
the figure, can be measured noninvasively, but peripheral and central pressures differ significantly in both shape and magnitude. Estimates of aortic pressure can be
obtained by 'transferring' the peripheral pressure to aortic pressure. It is most convenient to do the transfer of pressure in the frequency domain, where for each harmonic we define the transfer function as the ratio of the amplitudes and the phase

© Springer International Publishing AG, part of Springer Nature 2019
N. Westerhof et al., *Snapshots of Hemodynamics*,
https://doi.org/10.1007/978-3-319-91932-4_27

lag between peripheral and aortic pressure. This way of representation is shown in the figure. The amplitude is, in general, higher than unity for medium range frequencies, reflecting the increase in pulse pressure between aorta and peripheral artery (Amplification). The phase is negative as a result of the time lag between the two pressure waves, a direct consequence of the time of travel. Discussion exists if a generalized transfer function, applicable to all patients and healthy subjects can be used, or if individualized transfer functions are required. Parameters like body size, arterial elasticity and amount of reflections may vary from patient to patient.

27.1 Description

Peripheral pressures can be measured noninvasively by different techniques. For example, (calibrated) finger pressure can be reliably measured by photoplethysmography [1], and (un-calibrated) radial artery [2] and carotid artery pressure waveforms can be obtained with applanation tonometry [3]. These techniques are commercially available. However, most clinicians and family physicians use brachial pressure obtained with the classical sphygmomanometer allowing for systolic and diastolic values only, with mean pressure calculated as $(P_{syst} + 2P_{diast})/3$, (Chap. 12). These pressures are then used as a substitute for aortic pressure, or, even more so, as a global arterial pressure indicator. However, peripheral and central aortic pressures are not the same. The pressure waveform and the systolic and diastolic pressures can be substantially different between locations (see Chap. 12 and Figure in the Box). In general, systolic pressure increases as we move from central to peripheral sites, a phenomenon called 'systolic peaking' or amplification. Diastolic pressure tends to be slightly lower in peripheral vessels than in central arteries. Thus Pulse Pressure increases towards the periphery and called Pulse Pressure amplification. Obviously mean pressure decreases toward the periphery but the decrease is small, a few mmHg only. It has been suggested that aortic pressure is a better indicator of cardiac morbidity and mortality than peripheral pressure [4, 5] but whether central pressure rather than peripheral pressure is useful in clinical risk stratification is still under discussion [6].

In Chap. 12 it is shown that amplification is mainly determined by vessel stiffness (Pulse Wave Velocity), rather than by peripheral resistance. This stiffness effect explains why in aging, where PWV is increased amplification is decreased [7]. The effect of blood pressure lowering appears to have different effects on aorta and peripheral pressures [8].

27.1.1 Definition of Transfer Function

One way to obtain aortic pressure in magnitude and wave shape from a noninvasively measured peripheral pressure wave is to apply the so-called pressure transfer function. In essence, we define a transfer function, T, which is the ratio of the peripheral pressure wave, P_p, to the aortic pressure wave, P_{ao}. The two pressures can only be related to each other in the frequency domain. Therefore, we have to apply Fourier analysis (see Appendix 1), and for each harmonic the transfer function is defined as the ratio of amplitudes of the peripheral and aortic pressure sine wave and the phase difference between them. The approach is similar to the derivation of input impedance (Chap. 24), where pressure and flow are related. The transfer function, T, can be derived in several ways, but is mathematically expressed as [9–14]:

$$T(\omega) = P_{peripheral}(\omega) / P_{ao}(\omega)$$

The amplitude and the phase of the transfer function between the radial artery and the aorta is shown schematically in the Figure in the Box. The zero-frequency value of the transfer function is the ratio of mean peripheral arterial pressure to mean aortic pressure. Because of the small drop in mean pressure between the aorta and the peripheral artery, this ratio is slightly lower than 1. The amplitude of the transfer function is, in general, higher than unity for medium range frequencies, reflecting the increase in Pulse Pressure (Pulse Pressure Amplification) at the peripheral site. For high frequencies the modulus of the transfer function decreases to negligible values because high frequencies are damped while traveling. The phase is negative, as a result of the phase lag between the two waves, a direct consequence of the time it takes for the wave to travel towards the periphery. The mean slope of the phase of the transfer function is determined by the wave speed.

Several techniques are commercially available to obtain central from peripheral pressures. These methods use a 'generalized transfer function', which is the average of a (large) number of transfer functions measured in a group of human subjects.

27.1.2 Calibration of Noninvasively Determined Pressure Wave Shapes

Applanation tonometry [2], and echo tracking of wall motion [15] are ways to obtain peripheral pressure wave shapes noninvasively, but calibration is not included. Sphygmomanometrically obtained, and thus quantitative values of systolic, $P_{syst,bra}$ and diastolic, $P_{diast,bra}$ pressure, in the peripheral artery, can help in the calibration of noninvasively obtained carotid artery pressure a surrogate of aortic pressure. For instance, the transfer function allows the calculation of the aortic or carotid pressure wave shape and the subsequent calibration is discussed in Chap. 12 [16]. The so-calibrated aortic pressures are:

$$P_{systolic,ao} = 2P_{mean,bra} - P_{diastolic,bra} \text{ and } P_{diast,ao} = P_{diast,bra}$$

When wave shape is not of interest the equations suffice to obtain estimates central diastolic, systolic and mean pressures.

27.1.3 Physical Basis and Simple Mathematical Model for Transfer Function

A simple approach, which helps to understand the physical basis of the transfer function, is to consider forward and reflected waves. When the peripheral pressure wave is separated into its forward and reflected components the aortic pressure wave can be seen as an advanced reflected wave and a delayed forward wave. This simple model gives a reasonable prediction of the transfer function between the aorta and the brachial artery, as shown Fig. 27.1 [11].

27.2 Physiological and Clinical Relevance

Figure 27.2 shows aortic pressure and brachial pressure measured in an individual under control conditions as well as after administration of nitroglycerin [8]. Figure 27.2 also shows that the transfer of pressure depends on the state of the vascular tree. Under control conditions, systolic brachial pressure is approximately 150 mmHg, and systolic aortic pressure about 140 mmHg. Under nitroglycerin,

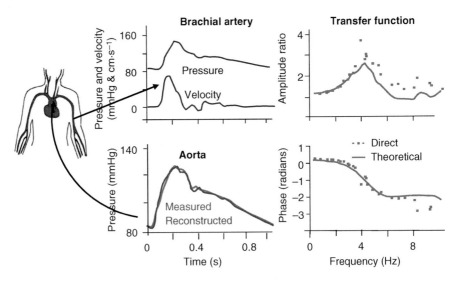

Fig. 27.1 Aorta pressure can be derived from brachial pressure and velocity or flow waves and the travel time of the waves between these two sites. The brachial pressure and flow (or velocity) can be used to calculate forward and reflected pressures. When the reflected pressure wave is advanced and the forward pressure wave is delayed in time, subsequent addition results in aortic pressure. The theoretical transfer function is close to the measured data. (Adapted from Ref. [11], by permission)

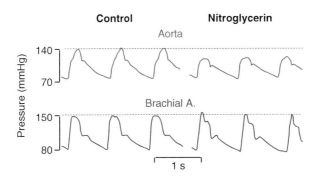

Fig. 27.2 Simultaneous recordings of aortic and brachial pressure waves under control conditions and after administration of nitroglycerin. During vasodilation systolic blood pressure in the brachial artery is not affected while systolic aortic pressure is lowered. Thus, with vasodilation pulse Pressure amplification increases. (Adapted from Ref. [4], by permission)

systolic pressure in the aorta drops significantly and systolic pressure and Pulse Pressure amplification increase. Brachial systolic pressure, remains practically unchanged, now overestimating aortic pressure by more than 30 mmHg. This example demonstrates that peripheral pressure waves are not a reliable substitute for aortic pressure and their relation may vary depending on different physiological parameters, such as mean pressure and wave speed.

The increase in amplification with vasodilation (Fig. 27.2) agrees with the suggestion that amplification is not a direct effect of peripheral reflection, but the result of the decreased mean pressure giving increased arterial compliance. In Chap. 12 pressure amplification is discussed.

From a clinical standpoint it is thus aortic pressure and not peripheral pressure that is of primary importance in a number of aspects. Aortic systolic pressure is the main determinant of cardiac afterload and wall stress and aortic diastolic pressure drives coronary perfusion. The aortic pressure waveform can be used to derive arterial compliance based on a variety of methods (Chap. 25). During ejection, aortic pressure can be taken as a surrogate of left ventricular pressure and, together with noninvasive measurements of left ventricular volume, can be used to estimate cardiac parameters such as End-Systolic Elastance and oxygen consumption (Chaps. 14 and 17).

A major drawback of the pressure transfer function technique is that, at last in theory, a generalized function does not exist. Parameters like body size, mean pressure, and arterial elasticity (PWV), which vary from patient to patient and vasoactive state, are important determinants of pressure transfer. Indeed limitations have been reported, such as gender-specificity [14], pleading for individualization of the transfer function. Thus, the generalized transfer function may not be precise but is easily applicable, but an individually derived transfer function improves the results only little [12, 13].

References

1. Eeftinck Schattenkerk DW, van Lieshout JJ, van den Meiracker AH, Wesseling KR, Blanc S, Wieling W, et al. Nexfin noninvasive continuous blood pressure validated against Riva-Rocci/Korotkoff. Am J Hypert. 2009;22:378–83.
2. Adji A, O'Rourke MF. Determination of central aortic systolic and pulse pressure from the radial artery pressure waveform. Blood Press Monit. 2004;9:115–21.
3. Van Bortel LM, Balkestein EJ, van der Heijden-Spek JJ, Vanmolkot FH, Staessen JA, Kragten JA, et al. Non-invasive assessment of local arterial pulse pressure: comparison of applanation tonometry and echo-tracking. J Hypertens. 2001;19:1037–44.
4. Williams B, Lacy PS, Thom SM, Cruickshank K, Stanton A, Collier D, et al. Differential impact of blood pressure-lowering drugs on central aortic pressure and clinical outcomes: principal results of the conduit artery function evaluation (CAFE) study. Circulation. 2006;113:1213–25.
5. Kollias A, Lagou S, Zeniodi ME, Boubouchairopoulou N, Stergiou GS. Association of Central Versus Brachial Blood Pressure with Target-Organ Damage: systematic review and meta-analysis. Hypertension. 2016;67:183–90.
6. Kostapanos M, McEniery CM, Wilkinson IB. Clinical relevance of central blood pressure - a critical review. Vasa. 2016;45:451–60. Review.
7. Herbert A, Cruickshank JK, Laurent S, Boutouyrie P, Reference Values for Arterial Measurements Collaboration. Establishing reference values for central blood pressure and its amplification in a general healthy population and according to cardiovascular risk factors. Eur Heart J. 2014;35:3122–33.
8. Kelly RP, Gibbs HH, O'Rourke MF, Daley JE, Mang K, Morgan JJ, et al. Nitroglycerin has more favourable effects on left ventricular afterload than apparent from measurement of pressure in a peripheral artery. Europ Heart J. 1990;11:138–44.
9. Karamanoglu M, O'Rourke MF, Avolio AP, Kelly RP. An analysis of the relationship between central aortic and peripheral upper limb pressure waves in man. Eur Heart J. 1993;14:160–7.
10. Chen CH, Nevo E, Fetics B, Pak PH, Yin FCP, Maughan WL, et al. Estimation of central aortic pressure waveform by mathematical transformation of radial tonometry pressure. Validation of a generalized transfer function. Circulation. 1997;95:1827–36.
11. Stergiopulos N, Westerhof BE, Westerhof N. Physical basis of pressure transfer from periphery to aorta: a model based study. Am J Phys. 1998;274:H1386–92.
12. Hope SA, Tay DB, Meredith IT, Cameron JD. Comparison of generalized and gender-specific transfer functions for the derivation of aortic waveforms. Am J Phys. 2002;283:H1150–6.
13. Westerhof BE, Guelen I, Stok WJ, Lasance HA, Ascoop CA, Wesseling KH, et al. Individualization of transfer function in estimation of central aortic pressure from the peripheral pulse is not required in patients at rest. J Appl Physiol. 2008;105:1858–63.
14. Gao M, Rose WC, Fetics B, Kass DA, Chen CH, Mukkamala R. A simple adaptive transfer function for deriving the central blood pressure waveform from a radial blood pressure waveform. Sci Rep. 2016;6:33230.
15. Hoeks APG, Brands PJ, Smeets FA, Reneman RS. Assessment of distensibility of superficial arteries. Ultrasound Med Biol. 1990;16:121–8.
16. Kelly R, Fitchett D. Noninvasive determination of aortic input impedance and external left ventricular power output: a validation and repeatability study of a new technique. J Am Coll Cardiol. 1992;20:952–63.

Chapter 28
Pulmonary Hemodynamics

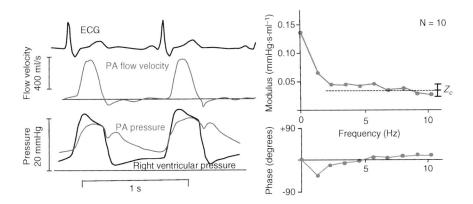

The pulmonary circulation obeys to the same physical laws and principles as the systemic circulation. The main quantitative hemodynamic difference is Pulmonary Vascular Resistance, which is about 7-fold lower than its systemic counterpart, which results in seven times lower mean pulmonary artery pressure. Also, the morphology of the vascular system differs from the systemic vasculature. While the systemic circulation may be approximated by a large reservoir (the aorta) with many conduit and small arteries to provide the different organs with blood, the pulmonary vasculature is more like a system of relatively short tubes that divide with a daughter-mother ratio of about 3 in about 15 generations in arteries and inversely for veins. The venous system has, contrary to the systemic veins, little storage function. Resistance and compliance of the arterial and venous pulmonary vasculature do not differ greatly, while in the systemic circulation arterial resistance is many times larger than venous resistance and arterial compliance many times smaller than venous compliance. The shape of the right ventricle is much more crescent-shape while the left heart is more of an ellipsoidal shape, making estimations of right ventricular wall stress in the right ventricular

N. Westerhof et al., *Snapshots of Hemodynamics*,
https://doi.org/10.1007/978-3-319-91932-4_28

wall inaccurate. Also pulmonary pressure measurement requires catheterization while non-invasive estimates of aortic pressure and (systolic) left ventricular pressure are available. The low pulmonary pressures are subject to noise and catheter movement. The left panel shows an example of Pulmonary Artery Pressure, Right Ventricular Pressure and Pulmonary Artery Flow as measured in the human and the right panel shows input impedance of the pulmonary arterial tree (averaged over 10 heart beats) [adapted from Ref. [1], by permission]. Qualitatively the waves and input impedance are not unlike those of the systemic circulation, only the pressure and impedance modulus magnitude differ.

28.1   Description

The pulmonary circulation obeys to the same laws and physical principles as the systemic circulation. However, not only quantitative differences exist (e.g., pressure) but the morphology of the pulmonary vascular system and the shape of the right heart differ from their systemic counterparts. One major difference is the resistance regulation in the response to oxygen: lowered PO_2 results in pulmonary vasoconstriction but systemic dilatation.

28.1.1   Morphology of the Pulmonary Vasculature

Detailed studies by Horsfield [2] and Huang et al. [3] have reported on quantitative morphology of the human pulmonary vascular system, both arteries and veins. The number of vessels, their diameters and their lengths have been presented based on diameter-defined Strahler orders. Order 1 pertains to arteries and veins of 20 μm, and order 15 to the main pulmonary artery and collecting veins, respectively. Figure 28.1 shows the relation between order number, N_r, and number of arteries, N_a, and veins, N_v. The diameters (D) of arteries and veins relate with order (N_r) as $Log(D_a) = 0.19 \cdot N_r - 1.84$ and $Log(D_v) = 0.20 \cdot N_r - 1.74$, respectively. Artery and vein lengths relate as $Log(l_a) = 0.17 \cdot N_r - 0.95$ and $Log(l_v) = 0.18 \cdot N_r - 0.79$ [3]. Thus, in all orders, except the largest arteries and veins, the number of veins is smaller than the number of arteries but veins have larger diameters and longer lengths than arteries.

The pressure distribution over the entire vascular pulmonary bed has been reported and is shown in Fig. 28.2. It should be noted that there is a considerable pressure drop over the venous part of the vasculature, and that thus venous resistance is a considerable part of the total vascular resistance. This large venous resistance is quite different from the systemic venous resistance which is negligible. Pulmonary arterial compliance is about 40% and venous compliance is about 60%

Fig. 28.1 The Number of
pulmonary arteries and
veins of orders 1–15 of a
(single human) lung. In all
orders (except order 15)
the number of veins is
smaller than the number
of arteries. (Data from
Ref. [3])

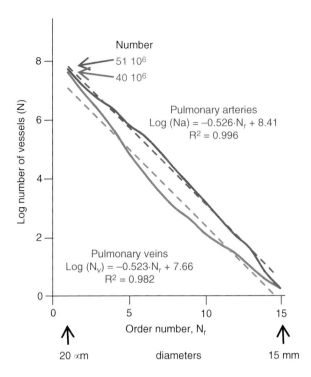

of the total vascular compliance [4]. This ratio is also different from the systemic
vasculature where the venous part acts a reservoir.

28.1.2   *Pressure-Pressure Relations*

Pulmonary Artery Pressure can be characterized by its systolic, diastolic and mean
pressure, *sPAP*, *dPAP* and *mPAP*, their relations are as presented in Fig. 28.3 [8].
Systolic pressure is 1.61 times mean pressure and diastolic pressure is 0.62 times
mean pressure. The proportional relation between *mPAP* and *sPAP* was first reported
by Chemla [9] and relations between *sPAP* and *dPAP* with *mPAP* were shown by
Syyed et al. [10]. The proportional relations imply that the following relation to hold:

$$\text{Pulse Pressure,} PP = sPAP - dPAP \approx mPAP$$
$$\text{and}$$
$$\text{mean Pressure,} mPAP = (sPAP + dPAP)/2$$

Figure 28.4 shows that the proportionalities are independent of Pulmonary
Arterial Wedge Pressure.

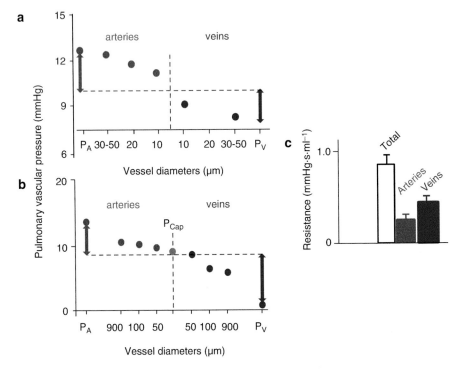

Fig. 28.2 Panels (**a**, **b**). Pressures along the pulmonary vasculature from Pulmonary Artery (PA) to vein (PV) of isolated dog lung. Data of panel (**a**) are measured with micropipette (micropuncture) and those of panel (**b**) averaged data obtained from three methods: retrograde catheters, occlusion technique and micro-puncture. The pressure drop from Pulmonary Artery to capillaries (red arrows) and from capillaries to venous pressure (blue arrows) are indicated. Panel (**c**) shows the resistance of the arterial and venous sections of the vasculature. It should be noted that venous resistance is somewhat higher than arterial resistance. (Figure is a compilation of selected data from Refs. [5–7])

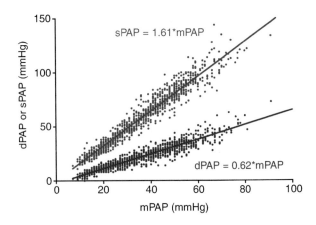

Fig. 28.3 Relation between systolic and diastolic pulmonary artery pressures with mean pulmonary artery pressure. Pulmonary arterial wedge pressure ranged from 1 to 31 mmHg. Normal and hypertensive patients are included, N = 1054. (From Ref. [8], by permission)

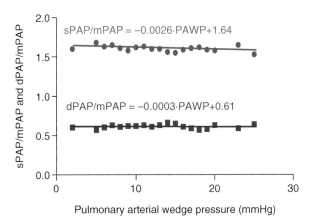

Fig. 28.4 The ratio of Systolic and Mean and Diastolic and Mean Pulmonary Artery Pressure are independent of Pulmonary Arterial Wedge, with ratios 1.64 and 0.61, respectively. It follows that mean pressure is $mPAP \approx (sPAP + dPAP)/2$ and Pulse Pressure, $PP = sPAP - dPAP \approx mPAP$. (From Ref. [8], by permission)

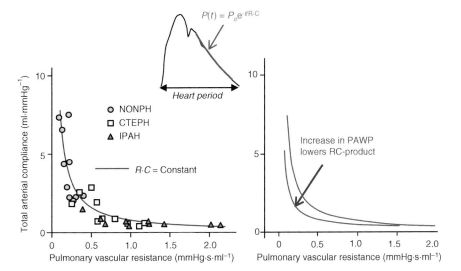

Fig. 28.5 Left panel: The relation between total arterial compliance, C, and Pulmonary Vascular Resistance, R, of three groups of patients. The product RC, describing the exponential decay of pressure in diastole is similar in health and pulmonary hypertension. (From Ref. [11], by permission). Right panel: the RC time depends on Pulmonary Arterial Wedge Pressure

28.1.3 The Relation Between Pulmonary Vascular Resistance and Total Arterial Compliance

Figure 28.5 shows the relation between Pulmonary Vascular Resistance, R and total Arterial Compliance, C [11, 12]. The relation can be described by a hyperbola implying RC, the arterial RC time, is constant. Thus the decay time of pressure in diastole is constant in health and disease. This finding was first reported by Reuben [13]. Tedford et al. [14] showed later that the product depends on Pulmonary Arterial

Wedge Pressure as also shown schematically in Fig. 28.5. Resistance is calculated as $R = (mPAP - PAWP)/Q_{mean}$, and compliance as $C = SV/PP$, with SV Stroke Volume and PP Pulse Pressure (Chap. 25). As discussed in that chapter the derivation of total arterial compliance C may depend on the method used and that the different methods result in different magnitudes of C, leading to different RC-times. However, the hyperbolic relation remains intact using different estimates of C as shown by Lankhaar et al. [11].

Using the information on the pressure-pressure relations, it follows that $C = SV/PP \approx SV/mPAP$. With $Q_{mean} = SV \cdot HR$, where HR is Heart Rate, we obtain

$$R \cdot C = \left[(mPAP - PAWP)/(SV \cdot HR) \right] \cdot \left[SV / mPAP \right] = \left[1 - PAWP / mPAP \right] / HR,$$

showing that increases in $PAWP$ result in lower RC relation (Fig. 28.5).

28.1.4   Input Impedance

Input impedance of the human pulmonary circulation (Figure in the Box), derived from pulmonary artery flow and pressure, has been reported by Murgo et al. [1]. Pagnamenta et al. and Maggiorini et al. showed that dobutamine and embolization have their main effect on the pulmonary vascular resistance and hardly affect the oscillatory components of the input impedance [15, 16]. When we compare pulmonary arterial input impedance with systemic input impedance (Chap. 24) we see that, except for the magnitude, their shapes differ little. The qualitative similarities in impedances can be explained by the work of Taylor who showed that randomly distributed models of tubes also shows similar impedances [17]. In other words, the details on geometry are of little importance.

28.1.5   Wave Travel and Reflection

Determination of pulmonary arterial wave speed from the pressure wave is complicated by the fact that pressure measurements are invasive and distances are short. Use of noninvasive flows (foot-foot) at two locations (MRI) is one feasible approach, provided the time resolution of the flow is sufficiently high. The other method is the one proposed by Vulliémoz et al.: $PWV = \Delta Q/\Delta A$ (see Chap. 21) with both ΔQ and ΔA noninvasively obtainable by MRI [18]. Comparison of the two methods, applied in the pulmonary artery, showed good agreement [19].

Wave transmission time from pulmonary artery to capillaries is about 150 ms at a $mPAP$ of 15 mmHg and reduces to about 50 ms at a $mPAP$ of 50 mmHg [20]. Using invasive pressure measurements in humans, at two locations, the main pulmonary artery and lower lobe branch of the left pulmonary artery, with length estimated from insertion of the catheter, allows estimation of PWV and it was found that PWV is about 3.5 m/s at $mPAP = 13$ mmHg and 10 m/s at $mPAP = 50$ mmHg [21].

Fig. 28.6 Pressure and flow in aorta and common pulmonary artery (red lines) are broken down in their forward (blue) and reflected (green) components. In control reflections in the pulmonary artery are much smaller than in the aorta. With vasodilation and vasoconstriction reflected waves are reduced and increased, respectively. (Adapted from Ref. [22], by permission)

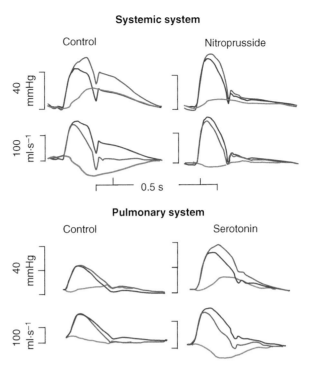

Figure 28.6 shows the Wave Separation Analysis in the pulmonary artery compared with forward and reflected components of the pressure and flow waves in the Aorta. Wave reflections in the pulmonary circulation are smaller than in the systemic arterial tree [22]. When the systemic bed is dilated with nitroprusside reflections decrease, and when the pulmonary arterial system is constricted with serotonin, reflections increase. It should be noticed that the small reflections in the pulmonary artery result in measured pressure and flow waveforms that are of similar shapes. Wave reflections are determined by arterial properties and affect the wave shape of the pressure as shown by Nakayama et al. [23].

Wave Intensity Analysis in the pulmonary arterial system can be carried out using vessel diameter variations, as surrogate of pressure, and noninvasive flow measurement.

Recently Lammers et al. gave a detailed review on impedance and wave travel in the pulmonary arterial system [24].

28.1.6 Pulmonary Vascular Models

The (three-element) Windkessel has been used as model of the pulmonary vasculature [25]. Distributed model approaches can be separated in anatomical [26, 27] models and fractal models based on self-similar vascular properties [28, 29]. The fractal character of the pulmonary arterial tree may be seen from the ratio of ~3.25

daughters per mother vessel for all orders, leading to $3.25^{15} = 48 \cdot 10^6$ arteries of 20 μm, close to the $51 \cdot 10^6$ reported by Huang et al. [3]. For an overview of pulmonary vascular models see [30].

The combined alveolar capillaries have been described as capillary sheets of two endothelial cell layers separated by connective tissue and cellular posts [31]. How much the sheet flow model (over-) simplifies the lung capillary bed is a point of discussion [32].

28.1.7 The Right Heart

Laws and rules discussed for analysis of left heart function apply to the right heart as well. However, the right ventricular shape is more complex than the shape of the left ventricle, making, for instance, the calculation of wall stress from pressure of limited accuracy. The Pressure-Volume analysis has been applied [33] as well as the Pump Function Graph [34]. The relation between oxygen consumption and mechanics appear are not different from what is found in the left heart [35]. Oscillatory power is 23% of total power in control and in hypertension [36], while in systemic hypertension the oscillatory power fraction increases.

Brimioulle et al. have shown that the single beat approach to obtain E_{es} is applicable to the right ventricle as well [37]. Using single beat analysis it was found that ventriculo-arterial coupling was maintained until the end-stage of pulmonary hypertension [38]. Diastolic right ventricular elastance can also be derived from single beats [38, 39].

In summary, the Pressure Volume analysis as discussed in Chap. 14 appears applicable to the right heart, but it should be kept in mind that with the low pressures, noise and distortion may play a greater role than for the left heart.

28.1.8 Ventricular Interaction

Two types of ventricular interaction can be distinguished [40].

1. The systemic and pulmonary circulation are 'in series' implying that mean flow in both systems at least in the steady state is equal. This series arrangement results in mutual effects of left and right heart and is called series interaction. Figure 28.7 shows an example of series interaction in diastolic left heart failure leading to increased pulmonary artery pressure with decreased Stroke Volume.
2. The left and right ventricles share muscle and pericardium. Thus, changes in one ventricle affect the other one depending on the state of the pericardium and muscle mass left and right. This is called direct interdependence or direct interaction. A schematic example of direct ventricular interaction is given in Fig. 28.8, based on data by Janicki and Weber [41].

Fig. 28.7 Example of series interaction of left and right heart in diastolic (left) heart failure

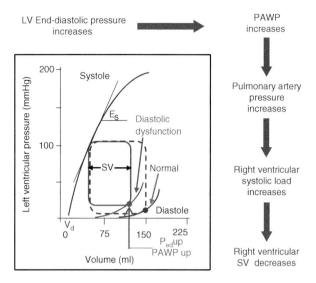

Fig. 28.8 Direct interaction. Increased left ventricular pressure affects both the diastolic and the systolic right ventricular pressure-volume relation (Blue arrows). The effect is larger with intact pericardium. (This schematic presentation is based on data published by Ref. [41])

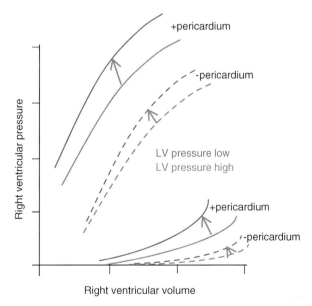

28.2 Physiological and Clinical Relevance

The general relation between *sPAP* and *dPAP* with *mPAP* implies that the measurement of *mPAP* suffices to describe pulmonary hypertension. Use of *sPAP* and *dPAP* as individual carriers of information as is usual in systemic hypertension is not useful in pulmonary hypertension.

28.2.1 Pulmonary Hypertension

With a normal *mPAP* of 15 mmHg, a *mPAP* higher than 25 mmHg is considered Pulmonary Hypertension. Mean pulmonary artery pressure may increase up to about five-fold in pulmonary hypertension. This is a huge increase compared with systemic hypertension where a 50% increase (>160 mmHg, stage 2 hypertension) is considered extreme. This very high pressure causes a large increase in right ventricular load that first results in ventricular adaptation but eventually causes in right heart failure.

Several forms of pulmonary hypertension exist. We here limit the discussion to two major groups of conditions: The first group is labeled as precapillary pulmonary hypertension and is diagnosed when the pulmonary vascular resistance is increased due to increased vascular wall thickness at the expense of the vascular lumen in the small arteries (Pulmonary Arterial Hypertension) or due to chronic emboli in the larger arteries (Chronic ThromboEmbolic Pulmonary Hypertension, CTEPH). The second group is called Postcapillary hypertension and is characterized by pulmonary hypertension due increased Pulmonary Arterial Wedge Pressure, PAWP, as a result of left heart failure. Pre- and postcapillary pulmonary hypertension can occur together and discussion exists how to quantify both effects [8].

In precapillary pulmonary hypertension, next to decreased cross-sectional area of the small arteries [42, 43], venous implications have been suggested since capillary pressures were shown to increase to 29 mmHg with a pulmonary artery pressure of 52 mmHg [44]. Possible rarefaction or pruning, i.e., disappearance of vessels, has been suggested as well [45, 46]. In the rat hypoxia-induced pulmonary hypertension the ratio of alveoli to arteries changed from 22/1 to 38/1 suggesting close to a factor 2 decrease in the number (rarefaction) of small arteries [46]. However, rarefaction is not proven beyond doubt [47]. Nevertheless, loss of vessels could be an explanation why even the best of therapies are not able to bring PVR back to normal values. In a recent experiment Zhou et al. showed in the isolated rat lung perfused with saline that with perfusion from the venous side the perfusate appears in the pulmonary artery. However, in the hypertensive lung the retrograde perfusion leads to fluid leak into the airways rather than backflow to the arteries, indicating the complex changes in the vasculature in pulmonary hypertension [48].

Su et al. showed in the that wave reflection is increased in pulmonary hypertension but the increase hardly depending on severity with PWV increased [49]. In the rat with moderate hypertension (mean pulmonary artery pressure 11–18 mmHg) it was found that wave reflection and PWV were not changed with respect to control [50].

In CTEPH distinct reflection sites exist which may introduce localized reflection possibly seen in the pressure wave shape [23].

In Postcapillary Hypertension defined as mean pulmonary artery pressure >25 mmHg and PAWP >15 mmHg, the pressure is increased as a result of the high filling pressure of the left heart and its high left atrial pressure and PAWP. The effect has been called passive transmission of the high PAWP. When PAWP is above

15 mmHg, defined as diastolic (left) heart failure, and the trans-pulmonary pressure gradient is normal, i.e., less than 12 mmHg, we deal isolated post-capillary hypertension. When the increase in mPAP results from a PAWP >15 mmHg and a trans-pulmonary gradient >12 mmHg (suggesting increased vascular resistance) we speak of Combined post- and pre-capillary PH (CpcPH) [8, 51].

28.2.2 The Right Heart in Pulmonary Hypertension

During the development and progression of pulmonary hypertension the right ventricle and vascular load initially remain coupled; the increase in vascular elastance E_a (Chap. 18) increases pressure and ventricular wall stress. This causes the right ventricle to adapt to preserve flow both by hypertrophy thereby keeping wall stress constant, and changes in cardiac muscle properties together increasing the slope of the End-Systolic Pressure Volume Relation (E_{es}). As a result, the E_{es}/E_a ratio and Stroke Volume are not altered and right ventricular efficiency (ratio of mechanical work and oxygen consumption) is maintained. Diastolic cardiac muscle properties are also changed [39, 52] and, together with the hypertrophy results in increased diastolic stiffness, E_{ed}, (see Chap. 14). In the later phase of the disease the right ventricle will dilate and Stroke Volume starts to decrease. Eventually, the volume increase and the high pressure result in an increase in wall stress, which is only partly counteracted by the hypertrophy. Coupling is not maintained and efficiency decreases [39, 53].

Right ventricular hypertrophy also affects right-left direct interaction, this is resulting in leftward septal bowing due to the lengthened RV contraction duration and hampering left ventricular filling (direct interaction) [54]. The right ventricular decrease in cardiac output may also result in decreased left ventricular filling (series interdependence) and lower systemic pressure. Figure 28.7 shows the result of series interdependence in left heart failure.

References

1. Murgo JP, Westerhof N. Input impedance of the pulmonary arterial system in normal man. Effects of respiration and comparison to systemic impedance. Circ Res. 1984;54:666–7.
2. Horsfield K. Morphometry of the small pulmonary arteries in man. Circ Res. 1978;42:593–7.
3. Huang W, Yen RT, McLaurine M, Bledsoe G. Morphometry of the human pulmonary vasculature. J Appl Physiol. 1996;81:2123–33.
4. Engelberg J, Dubois AB. Mechanics of pulmonary circulation in isolated rabbit lungs. Am J Phys. 1959;196:401–14.
5. Bhattacharya J, Nanjo S, Staub NC. Micropuncture measurement of lung microvascular pressure during 5-HT infusion. J Appl Physiol Respir Environ Exerc Physiol. 1982;52:634–7.
6. Hakim TS, Kelly S. Occlusion pressures vs. micropipette pressures in the pulmonary circulation. J Appl Physiol. 1989;67:1277–85.

7. Michel RP, Hakim TS, Freeman CR. Distribution of pulmonary vascular resistance in experimental fibrosis. J Appl Physiol. 1988;65:1180–90.
8. Handoko ML, De Man FS, Oosterveer FP, Bogaard HJ, Vonk-Noordegraaf A, Westerhof N. A critical appraisal of transpulmonary and diastolic pressure gradients. *Physiol Rep*. 2016;4 pii: e12910.
9. Chemla D, Castelain V, Humbert M, Hébert JL, Simonneau G, Lecarpentier Y, et al. New formula for predicting mean pulmonary artery pressure using systolic pulmonary artery pressure. Chest. 2004;126:1313–7.
10. Syyed R, Reeves JT, Welsh D, Raeside D, Johnson MK, Peacock AJ. The relationship between the components of pulmonary artery pressure remains constant under all conditions in both health and disease. Chest. 2008;133:633–9.
11. Lankhaar J-W, Westerhof N, Faes TJC, Marques KMJ, Marcus JT, Postmus PE, et al. Quantification of right ventricular afterload in patients with and without pulmonary hypertension. Am J Physiol Heart Circ Physiol. 2006;291:1731–7.
12. Lankhaar J-W, Westerhof N, Faes TJC, Gan CT, Marques KM, Boonstra A, et al. Pulmonary vascular resistance and compliance stay inversely related during treatment of pulmonary hypertension European. Eur Heart J. 2008;29:1688–95.
13. Reuben SR. Compliance of the human pulmonary arterial system in disease. Circ Res. 1971;29:40–50.
14. Tedford RJ, Hassoun PM, Mathai SC, Girgis RE, Russell SD, Thiemann DR, et al. Pulmonary capillary wedge pressure augments right ventricular pulsatile loading. Circulation. 2012;125:289–97.
15. Pagnamenta A, Fesler P, Vandinivit A, Brimioulle S, Naeije R. Pulmonary vascular effects of dobutamine in experimental pulmonary hypertension. Crit Care Med. 2003;31:1140–6.
16. Maggiorini M, Brimioulle S, De Canniere D, Delcroix M, Naeije R. Effects of pulmonary embolism on pulmonary vascular impedance in dogs and minipigs. J Appl Physiol. 1998;84:815–21.
17. Taylor MG. The input impedance of an assembly of randomly branching elastic tubes. Biophys J. 1966;6:29–51.
18. Vulliemoz S, Stergiopulos N, Meuli R. Estimation of local aortic elastic properties with MRI. Magn Reson Med. 2002;47:649–54.
19. Ibrahim e-SH, Shaffer JM, White RD. Assessment of pulmonary artery stiffness using velocity encoding magnetic resonance imaging: evaluation of techniques. Magn Reson Imag. 2011;29:966–74.
20. Reuben SR. Wave transmission in the pulmonary arterial system in disease in man. Circ Res. 1970;27:523–9.
21. Kopeć G, Moertl D, Jankowski P, Tyrka A, Sobień B, Podolec P. Pulmonary artery pulse wave velocity in idiopathic pulmonary arterial hypertension. Can J Cardiol. 2013;29:683–90.
22. van den Bos GC, Westerhof N, Randall OS. Pulse wave reflection: can it explain the differences between systemic and pulmonary pressure and flow waves? A study in dogs. Circ Res. 1982;51:479–85.
23. Nakayama Y, Sugimachi M, Nakanishi N, Takaki H, Okano Y, Satoh T, et al. Noninvasive differential diagnosis between chronic pulmonary thromboembolism and primary pulmonary hypertension by means of Doppler ultrasound measurement. J Am Coll Cardiol. 1998;31:1367–71.
24. Lammers S, Scott D, Hunter K, Tan W, Shandas R, Stenmark KR. Mechanics and function of the pulmonary vasculature: implications for pulmonary vascular disease and right ventricular function. Compr Physiol. 2012;2:295–319.
25. Segers P, Brimioulle S, Stergiopulos N, Westerhof N, Naeije R, Maggiorini M, et al. Pulmonary arterial compliance in dogs and pigs: the three-element windkessel model revisited. Am J Phys. 1999;277:H725–31.
26. Tawhai MH, Clark AR, Burrowes KS. Computational models of the pulmonary circulation: insights and the move towards clinically directed studies. Pulm Circ. 2011;1:224–338.

27. Qureshi MU, Vaughan GD, Sainsbury C, Johnson M, Peskin CS, Olufsen MS, et al. Numerical simulation of blood flow and pressure drop in the pulmonary arterial and venous circulation. Biomech Model Mechanobiol. 2014;13:1137–54.

28. Dawson CA, Krenz GS, Karau KL, Haworth ST, Hanger CC, Linehan JH. Structure-function relationships in the pulmonary arterial tree. J Appl Physiol. 1999;86:569–83.

29. Moledina S, de Bruyn A, Schievano S, Owens CM, Young C, Haworth SG, et al. Fractal branching quantifies vascular changes and predicts survival in pulmonary hypertension: a proof of principle study. Heart. 2011;97:1245–9.

30. Tawhai MH, Burrowes KS. Modelling pulmonary blood flow. Respir Physiol Neurobiol. 2008;163:150–77. Review

31. Fung YC, Sobin SS. Theory of sheet flow in lung alveoli. J Appl Physiol. 1969;26:472–88.

32. Sobin SS, Fung YC. Response to challenge to the Sobin-Fung approach to the study of pulmonary microcirculation. Chest. 1992;101:1135–43. Review

33. de Man FS, Handoko ML, van Ballegoij JJ, Schalij I, Bogaards SJ, Postmus PE, et al. Bisoprolol delays progression towards right heart failure in experimental pulmonary hypertension. Circ Heart Fail. 2012;5:97–105.

34. Overbeek MJ, Lankhaar JW, Westerhof N, Voskuyl AE, Boonstra A, Bronzwaer JG, et al. Right ventricular contractility in systemic sclerosis-associated and idiopathic pulmonary arterial hypertension. Eur Respir J. 2008;31:1160–6.

35. Wong YY, Westerhof N, Ruiter G, Lubberink M, Raijmakers P, Knaapen P, et al. Systolic pulmonary artery pressure and heart rate are main determinants of oxygen consumption in the right ventricular myocardium of patients with idiopathic pulmonary arterial hypertension. Eur J Heart Fail. 2011;13:1290–5.

36. Saouti N, Westerhof N, Helderman F, Marcus JT, Boonstra A, Postmus PE, et al. Right ventricular oscillatory power is a constant fraction of total power irrespective of pulmonary artery pressure. Am J Respir Crit Care Med. 2010;182:1315–20.

37. Brimioulle S, Wauthy P, Ewalenko P, Rondelet B, Vermeulen F, Kerbaul F, et al. Single-beat estimation of right ventricular end-systolic pressure-volume relationship. Am J Physiol Heart Circ Physiol. 2003;284:H1625–30.

38. Trip P, Rain S, Handoko ML, van der Bruggen C, Bogaard HJ, Marcus JT, et al. Clinical relevance of right ventricular diastolic stiffness in pulmonary hypertension. Eur Respir J. 2015;45:1603–12.

39. Rain S, Handoko ML, Trip P, Gan CT, Westerhof N, Stienen GJ, et al. Right ventricular diastolic impairment in patients with pulmonary arterial hypertension. Circulation. 2013;128:2016–25.

40. Belenkie I, Smith ER, Tyberg JV. Ventricular interaction: from bench to bedside. Ann Med. 2001;33:236–41. Review

41. Janicki JS, Weber KT. The pericardium and ventricular interaction, distensibility, and function. Am J Phys. 1980;238:H494–503.

42. Stacher E, Graham BB, Hunt JM, Gandjeva A, Groshong SD, McLaughlin VV, et al. Modern age pathology of pulmonary arterial hypertension. Am J Respir Crit Care Med. 2012;186:261–72.

43. Chazova I, Loyd JE, Zhdanov VS, Newman JH, Belenkov Y, Meyrick B. Pulmonary artery adventitial changes and venous involvement in primary pulmonary hypertension. Am J Pathol. 1995;146:389–97.

44. Kafi SA, Mélot C, Vachiéry J-L, Brimioulle S, Naeije R. Partitioning of pulmonary vascular resistance in primary pulmonary hypertension. J Am Coll Cardiol. 1998;31:1372–6.

45. Reid LM. Structure and function in pulmonary hypertension: new perceptions. Chest. 1966;89:279–88.

46. Rabinovitch M, Gamble W, Nadas AS, Miettinen OS, Reid L. Rat pulmonary circulation after chronic hypoxia: hemodynamic and structural features. Am J Phys. 1979;236:H818–27.

47. Hopkins N, McLoughlin P. The structural basis of pulmonary hypertension in chronic lung disease: remodelling, rarefaction or angiogenesis? J Anat. 2002;201:335–48.

48. Zhou C, Crockett ES, Batten L, McMurtry IF, Stevens T. Pulmonary vascular dysfunction secondary to pulmonary arterial hypertension: insights gained through retrograde perfusion. Am J Physiol Lung Cell Mol Physiol. 2018;314:L836–45.

49. Su J, Manisty C, Parker KH, Simonsen U, Nielsen-Kudsk JE, Mellemkjaer S, et al. Wave Intensity Analysis Provides Novel Insights Into Pulmonary Arterial Hypertension and Chronic Thromboembolic Pulmonary Hypertension. *J Am Heart Assoc.* 2017;6i:e006679.

50. Su J, Logan CC, Hughes AD, Parker KH, Dhutia NM, Danielsen CC, et al. Impact of chronic hypoxia on proximal pulmonary artery wave propagation and mechanical properties in rats. Am J Physiol Heart Circ Physiol. 2018;314:H1264–78. https://doi.org/10.1152/ajpheart.00695.2017.

51. Vachiéry JL, Adir Y, Barberà JA, Champion H, Coghlan JG, Cottin V, et al. Pulmonary hypertension due to left heart diseases. J Am Coll Cardiol. 2014;62:D100–8.

52. Rain S, Bos Dda S, Handoko ML, Westerhof N, Stienen G, Ottenheijm C, et al. Protein changes contributing to right ventricular cardiomyocyte diastolic dysfunction in pulmonary arterial hypertension. J Am Heart Assoc. 2014;3:e000716.

53. Vonk Noordegraaf A, Westerhof BE, Westerhof N. The relationship between the right ventricle and its load in pulmonary hypertension. J Am Coll Cardiol. 2017;69:236–43. Review

54. Marcus JT, Gan CT, Zwanenburg JJ, Boonstra A, Allaart CP, Götte MJ, et al. Interventricular mechanical asynchrony in pulmonary arterial hypertension: left-to-right delay in peak shortening is related to right ventricular overload and left ventricular underfilling. J Am Coll Cardiol. 2008;51:750–7.

Chapter 29
Mechanotransduction and Vascular Remodeling

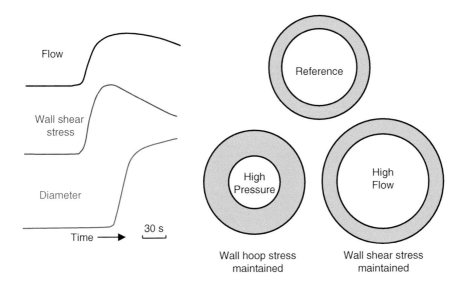

Blood vessels respond to pressure and flow, more exactly to hoop stress and wall shear.

Short term. A pressure increase results in a smooth muscle contraction and thus in a diameter decrease, so that hoop stress normalizes (myogenic response, see Chap. 19). A flow increase implies an increase in wall shear stress, which is sensed by the endothelium (glycokalix). The endothelium liberates relaxing factors (e.g., NO) causing dilatation. The increase in diameter reduces the wall shear stress. This is called Flow Mediated Dilation (left panel).

Long term. Sustained high blood pressure implies a high wall hoop stress that leads to wall thickening (hypertrophy), and normalization of hoop stress. Increased flow gives increased wall shear stress and leads to increase in vessel diameter. In general, vascular remodeling leads to a restoration to control levels of hoop stress and wall shear stress (right panel).

© Springer International Publishing AG, part of Springer Nature 2019
N. Westerhof et al., *Snapshots of Hemodynamics*,
https://doi.org/10.1007/978-3-319-91932-4_29

29.1 Description

One of the fundamental characteristics of living tissues is their ability to respond to changes in their mechanical environment.

Although often referred to the macroscopic quantities of pressure and flow, vascular responses are better associated with wall hoop stress and wall shear stress. We recall that wall hoop stress (σ) is related to transmural pressure through the law of Laplace, $\sigma = P/h$ (see Chap. 9), and that wall shear stress (τ) is related to flow, or axial pressure drop, $\Delta P/l$, through the law of Poiseuille, $\tau = 4\eta \cdot Q/\pi r_i^3 = (\Delta P/l)/(r_i/2)$ (Chap. 2).

29.1.1 Short Term Arterial Adaptation

Pressure Effects In the short term, under physiologic conditions, an increase in transmural pressure increases hoop stress, and, via the myogenic response (Chap. 19) of the smooth muscle, vessel diameter decreases and hoop stress is normalized. Thus the increase in vascular tone counterbalances the increased pressure.

Flow Effects Acute changes in blood flow lead to adjustments in vessel caliber, via endothelium-dependent vasodilation or vasoconstriction. A flow increase, leads to an increase in wall shear stress, which is sensed by the endothelium, and followed by vasodilation. Vasodilators, e.g., NO, are released and the smooth muscle relaxes. Muscle relaxation results in vasodilation and increase in vessel diameter, thereby normalizing the shear stress. In Chap. 2 we mentioned that wall shear stress is neither the same in similar vessels in different mammals, nor the same in different vessels in a single animal. Yet it appears that local endothelial cells have a desired set-point of shear stress.

Axial Effects The mechanical behavior of the arterial wall is dominated by three stresses: flow induced wall shear stress and the circumferential and axial components of the pressure-induced intramural stress. These stresses regulate the three most important geometric properties of an artery: its luminal radius, its wall thickness, and its axial length. But while radius and wall thickness are relatively easy to measure *in vivo*, axial length is more difficult to pin down. Nevertheless, an increasing amount of evidence seems to indicate that the arterial wall compensates an increase in intramural pressure not only via circumferential remodeling but also via a reduction in axial stretch, thus increasing its unloaded length [1].

29.1.2 Mechanotransduction

Mechanotransduction refers to the many mechanisms by which cells convert mechanical stimuli into chemical activity. One such mechanism is flow-induced vasorelaxation, whereby increased wall shear stress causes smooth muscle relaxation, (Figure in the Box, at left).

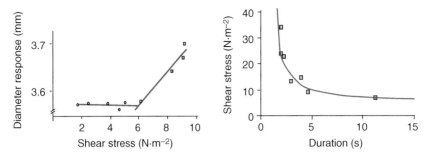

Fig. 29.1 The diameter response relates linearly with shear stress, above a threshold value (left panel). Strength (stress magnitude) and duration of the stress determine the response to shear stress. They relate inversely, like a strength-duration curve (right panel). (Adapted from [4], by permission)

Fig. 29.2 An increase mean flow (top trace) induces an increase in diameter (bottom trace), as shown in the early part of the tracings. The subsequent increase in the pulsatility of flow, at the same mean flow, has no detectable effect on diameter. A further increase in mean flow induces the final increase in the diameter (last part of the tracings). (Adapted from Ref. [4], by permission)

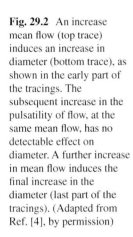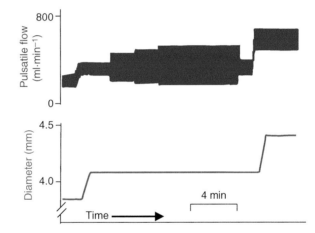

This aspect of mechanotransduction only takes place when the endothelium is intact. The search for the mechanism was based on the finding by Furchgott that Acetylcholine, ACh, only relaxes the smooth muscle if the vascular endothelium is intact [2]. The factor liberated by the endothelium was named Endothelium Derived Relaxing Factor, EDRF [2]. Palmer et al. showed that EDRF is Nitric Oxide NO, a small molecule that also plays a role in synaptic transmission [3]. Thus in shear rate dependent dilation NO plays a major role as a dilating factor. The shear stress needs to be higher than a certain threshold value before diameter changes occur (Fig. 29.1, left). The level of the stress, and its duration, need to be of sufficient magnitude to elicit a response (Fig. 29.1, right). This is a relation akin to the strength-duration curve defining the response of nerve tissue. Also it has been shown that it is mainly the mean shear stress that causes vasodilation and not the magnitude of oscillations about the mean stress (Fig. 29.2). Shear stress dependent arterial dilatation is abolished by the NO synthesis inhibitor L-NAME, by hyaluronidase, and by intraluminal hyperglycemia.

At present, it is accepted knowledge that the glycocalyx (a gel layer 0.5 μm thick between the endothelium and the blood in the lumen) is the main sensor of changes

in shear stress. However, many different transmembrane and intracellular mecha-
nosensors have been reported, including G protein–coupled receptors, ion chan-
nels, plasma membrane phospholipids, receptor tyrosine kinases, caveolae,
integrins and their basal adhesion complex or platelet endothelial cell adhesion
molecule-1 (PECAM-1) and its associated intercellular junction complex [5, 6].
Mechanotransduction of shear force is not restricted to the luminal membrane but
has also been observed at remote sites via propagation of forces through the cyto-
skeleton [7].

29.1.3 Long Term Vascular Adaptation

Growth and remodeling are processes that allow the living tissue to maintain an
optimal environment under physiological development (Chap. 2) as well as under
various pathologic conditions. The arterial wall responds to prolonged changes in
transmural pressure or flow by means of geometrical adaptation (e.g., hypertrophy),
structural adaptation (e.g., change in scleroprotein content, stiffening) and functional adaptation (e.g., changes in endothelial function or vascular smooth muscle
tone).

Pressure Effects In the long term an increase in pressure leads to a thickening of the
arterial wall (hypertrophy). Wall thickening lowers wall hoop stress down to control
(normotensive) levels, thus counterbalancing the increase in pressure. An example
of such adaptation is shown in Fig. 29.3.

Flow Effects Chronic changes in flow lead to remodeling. Long-term, flow-induced
remodeling implies reorganization of cellular and extracellular wall components.
The adaptive response to changes in blood flow has been studied in various animals
and it was found that the vessel inner diameter adapts to preserve the level of wall
shear at the intimal surface. Kamiya and Togawa [9] first demonstrated that the
adaptive response to an increase in flow leads to normalization in wall shear stress.
They constructed an arterio-venous shunt between the carotid artery and jugular

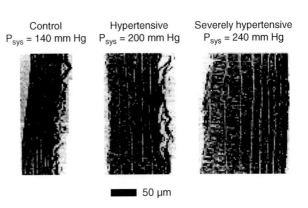

Fig. 29.3 Thoracic aortas
of rats fixed under their
in vivo pressure and
stained with Azan.
Sections are parallel to the
longitudinal axis of the
vessel with the intimal
surface facing leftward.
(Adapted from Ref. [8], by
permission)

Control
$P_{sys} = 140$ mm Hg

Hypertensive
$P_{sys} = 200$ mm Hg

Severely hypertensive
$P_{sys} = 240$ mm Hg

■ 50 µm

vein of a dog, which led to a significant increase in blood flow in the ipsilateral carotid and a decrease in blood flow in the contralateral one. Six to eight months after the operation, carotid diameter was increased in the segment with high flow and decreased in the segment with low flow. The diameter change preserved wall shear stress within 15% of the pre-operation levels, despite the severe increase or decrease in flow. Similar findings were reported by Langille [10] on the rabbit carotid artery, where a reduction in flow led to a reduction in internal diameter and restoration of wall shear stress (see Fig. 29.4). Remodeling in response to increased flow appears to be associated with cell hyperplasia, structural changes in internal elastic lamina and adventitia as well as with the contractile properties of the artery. The endothelium and nitric oxide synthesis are the main mediators in the vessel adaptation to flow. For example, inhibition of nitric oxide synthesis totally abolishes the capacity of the pig carotid artery to remodel and maintain control levels of wall shear in the presence of an arterio-venous shunt [11].

Axial Effects Van Loon et al. [12] showed that during *ex vivo* experiments the axial force increases with pressure if the artery is held at an axial stretch above its *in vivo* value and decreases with pressure if the artery is stretched less than it was *in vivo*. However, when the artery is stretched exactly as it was *in vivo*, the axial force needed to keep it in place does not depend on pressure. This discovery demonstrated for the first time that axial stress is inherent to the microstructure of the artery and is not governed by peripheral tethering [1, 12]. The adaptive axial response to changes in blood flow or pressure has been investigated in several animal studies. When rabbit cerebral arteries [13] or carotid arteries [14] are exposed to a sustained increase in blood flow they respond with a significant lengthening that can result in gross tortuosity. Jackson et al. showed that an artificially imposed extension of the

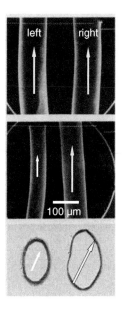

Fig. 29.4 Scanning Electron micrographs of methacrylate casts of left and right common carotid arteries of a normal rabbit (top) and after 2 weeks after left carotid flow was reduced (middle), as indicated by white arrow. Cross-sections after 2 weeks of left common carotid flow reduction are given in the bottom panel. (Adapted from Ref. [10], by permission)

carotid artery in rabbits results in adaptive *in vivo* remodeling, with synthesis of additional extracellular matrix until the original *in vivo* stretch has been restored [15]. Eberth et al. used a model in which the aortic arch was transversally banded in order to induce a local increase in pulse pressure in the right but not the left common carotid artery. Biaxial force-length tests showed that the *in vivo* axial stretch was significantly lower in the right carotid artery than in the left while circumferential stress-stretch behavior was similar in both carotids, thus providing indirect evidence for an effective axial compensation mechanism [16].

29.1.4   Residual Stress in Relation to Growth and Remodeling

In Chap. 10 it was mentioned that both cardiac tissue and vascular tissue are not at a zero stress state when all loads are removed [17]. It was also postulated that residual stresses help maintain a uniform stress distribution across the wall (Chap. 10). When, for different physiological or pathological reasons, the biomechanical environment to which the wall is subjected is changed, mechanical stresses within the arterial wall will also be altered and their distribution will not be uniform. A remodeling process will likely take place in order to restore stresses and strain to control levels.

Remodeling leads to changes in geometry and structure, with addition or resorption of mass. Consequently, the zero stress state will change. Changes in the zero stress state, or changes in the opening angle allow for the monitoring of arterial wall remodeling. Figure 29.5 shows changes in wall thickness and opening angle in various positions along the aorta of rats, which received a very tight banding of the thoracic aorta just below the diaphragm. For the aorta above the banding site, which was exposed to higher pressure, we observe a progressive thickening of the aortic wall during the entire post-surgery period (normalization of hoop stress). The opening angle, however, shows a non-monotonic evolution. Initially, the opening angle increases, indicative of higher growth in the internal wall layers. Later, as the wall thickens and stress levels are restored, the opening angle returns to control levels as

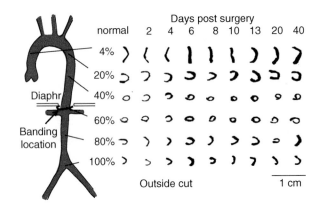

Fig. 29.5 Photographs of aortic rings cut open radially to reveal their zero stress state (ZSS). The first column shows the ZSS in normal rats. The other columns show the change in ZSS after hypertension was induced by banding of the aorta above the coeliac trunc. (Adapted from Ref. [17], by permission)

well. The initial higher growth in the internal wall layers is reflected by the increase in opening angle. This demonstrates that remodeling is dependent on the local stress distribution and also that wall remodeling affects the residual stress distribution within the arterial wall.

29.2 Physiological and Clinical Relevance

29.2.1 Arterial Remodeling in Hypertension

In presence of essential hypertension, vascular resistance increases due to alterations in resistance vessel architecture, decrease in lumen diameter and increase in media thickness/lumen diameter ratio. This corresponds to an inward eutrophic remodeling, as schematically shown in Fig. 29.6. The type of remodeling in resistance vessels depends on the type of hypertension and treatment. Human renal hypertension leads to inward hypertrophic remodeling. During anti-hypertensive treatment the situation is often reversed and outward eutrophic remodeling and hypertrophic remodeling is observed. Figure 29.6 shows the different types of remodeling that can be distinguished, as suggested by Mulvany [18].

29.2.2 Arterial Remodeling in Hypertension: Large Arteries

Remodeling due to hypertension is known to increase wall thickness and restore wall hoop stress. In terms of compliance and elastic properties, arterial remodeling tends to be vessel specific. Aortic and carotid artery compliances are reduced in

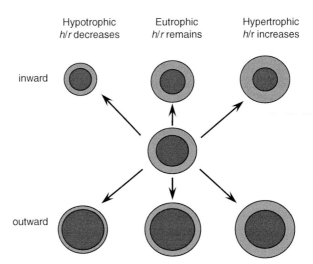

Fig. 29.6 Classification of different types of arterial remodeling, i.e. a structurally determined change. (Adapted from Ref. [18], by permission)

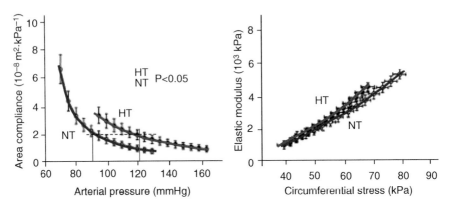

Fig. 29.7 Radial artery area compliance (left) and elastic modulus (right) measured in vivo in a group of normotensive (NT, n = 22) and hypertensive subjects (HT, n = 25). When compared at their corresponding mean operating pressures (NT: 90 mmHg; HT: 121 mmHg) area compliance was similar despite significant concentric hypertrophy (left panel). In normotensive subjects wall thickness is 0.28 mm compared to 0.40 mm in hypertensive patients. Internal diameter is the same and equal to 2.50 mm in both groups. The incremental elastic modulus-stress curve (right panel) was essentially the same in normotensives and hypertensives, suggesting similar tissue material properties in the two groups. (Adapted from Ref. [19], by permission)

hypertension. Radial artery compliance and incremental elastic modulus (Fig. 29.7), however, seem to be preserved in hypertensive patients [19]. It is important here to acknowledge the nonlinear nature of the compliance and elastic modulus curves. Compliance is expressed as a function of pressure (structural property) and elastic modulus as a function of stress or strain (material property). We observe that at their corresponding operating pressure, normotensive and hypertensive radial arteries exhibit the same compliance, which is indicative of some kind of structural remodeling aiming to maintain normotensive compliance levels. Further, the incremental modulus-stress curve is identical in normotensive and hypertensive patients, which means that the intrinsic elastic properties of the wall material remained the same. This example demonstrates nicely the capacity of the radial artery to remodel in hypertension in a manner that normalizes wall stress by thickening, maintains control compliance levels despite exposure to higher pressure and preserves the intrinsic elastic properties of the arterial tissue.

29.2.3   Flow Mediated Dilatation, FMD, as a Means to Evaluate Endothelial Function

Metabolic vasodilatation within an organ supplied causes a fall in peripheral resistance so that blood flow in the artery supplying the organ increases (Figure in the Box, top trace). The increased flow causes an increase in wall shear stress (middle trace). The mechano-sensor within the arterial wall, the endothelium, detects the wall shear and produces arterial dilatation, so that the increased flow required down-stream is accommodated and wall shear stress normalized. The vasodilation is mediated by the endothelium-dependent relaxing factor nitric oxide (NO). The response is abolished if the animal is pretreated with a NO synthase inhibitor or when the endothelium is removed or made nonfunctional. The increase in diameter in the supply artery is called Flow Mediated Dilatation (FMD).

Flow Mediated Dilatation can be studied noninvasively in arteries. For instance, brachial artery diameter can be measured during control and during post-occlusion reactive hyperemia where flow is increased. The increased wall shear stress causes endothelium dependent dilation which can be measured noninvasively (Ultrasound, Wall tracking). An endothelium independent vasodilator, (e.g., sublingual glyceryl trinitrate, GTN), is used to test muscle relaxation of the artery without involvement of the endothelium [20, 21].

29.2.4 Low Shear and Atheroma

According to Caro [22], and substantial subsequent literature, atheromatous plaques develop preferentially at sites with low shear. Different hypotheses as to why this is the case have been debated, but it is generally accepted that shear responsive genes are upregulated at low shear regions, thus making these regions more welcoming for inflammatory cells through an increased expression of adhesion factors [23]. A more detailed analysis of the role of shear stress in atherosclerosis is discussed in Chap. 30.

It can also be appreciated why diabetic patients and people with glucose intolerance have accelerated athero-thrombotic disease, as the hyperglycemia inhibits the production of NO in response to shear stress [24]. Hyperinsulinaemia occurs in patients pre-disposed to type-2 diabetes (metabolic syndrome or insulin resistance) and may occur with excess insulin administration in type 1 diabetes. The hyperinsulinaemia results in more dilated arteries than normal, and therefore shear stress is lower than normal (shear stress is inversely related to the radius to the third power, see Chap. 2). Thus diabetic hyperinsulinaemia creates an arterial tree with overall low shear stresses, predisposing to atheroma, and the accompanying diabetic hyperglycemia also inhibits the response to increased shear as generated by exercise, further predisposing the patient to arterial lesions.

Axial stress and bypass grafts The fact that it is near impossible to estimate axial quantities from *in vivo* makes it difficult to illustrate the effect of axial stress on arterial remodeling with clinically relevant examples. One potentially important application is the fact that an artery that has been bypassed by a graft, e.g. after surgical intervention due to aortic aneurysm or coronary artery disease, will usually experience an altered axial stretch. A computational model of a bypassed graft has demonstrated that abnormal circumferential and axial stresses in the vicinity of the stent-graft anastomosis cause wall thickening that tends to restore the stress state such that it approaches the stress state existing further from the clamped area [25].

References

1. Humphrey JD, Eberth JF, Dye WW, Gleason RL. Fundamental role of axial stress in compensatory adaptations by arteries. J Biomech. 2009;42:1–8.
2. Furchgott RF, Zawadzki JV. The obligatory role of endothelial cells in the relaxation of arterial smooth muscle by acetylcholine. *Nature*. 1980;27.;288(5789):373–6.
3. Palmer RMJ, Ferrige AG, Moncada S. Nitric oxide release accounts for the biological activity of endothelium-derived relaxing factor. Nature. 1987;27:524–6.
4. Kelly RF, Snow HM. Characteristics of the response of the iliac artery to wall shear stress in the anaesthetised pig. J Physiol. 2007;582:731–43.
5. Tarbell JM, Simon SI, Curry FR. Mechanosensing at the vascular interface. Annu Rev Biomed Eng. 2014;16:505–32. Review
6. Chatzizisis YS, Coskun AU, Jonas M, Edelman ER, Feldman CL, Stone PH. Role of endothelial shear stress in the natural history of coronary atherosclerosis and vascular remodeling: molecular, cellular, and vascular behavior. J Am Coll Cardiol. 2007;49:2379–793.
7. Davies PF. Hemodynamic shear stress and the endothelium in cardiovascular pathophysiology. Nat Clin Pract Cardiovasc Med. 2009;6:16–26.
8. Matsumoto T, Hayashi K. Stress and strain in hypertensive and normotensive rat aorta considering residual strain. J Biomech Eng. 1996;118:62–73.
9. Kamiya A, Togawa T. Adaptive regulation of wall shear stress to flow change in canine carotid artery. Am J Phys. 1980;239:14–29.
10. Langille BL, O'Donnell F. Reductions in arterial diameter produced by chronic decreases in blood flow are endothelium-dependent. Science. 1986;231:405–7.
11. Tronc F, Wassef M, Esposito B, Henrion D, Glagov S, Tedgui A. Role of NO in flow-induced remodeling of the rabbit common carotid artery. Arterioscler Thromb Vasc Biol. 1996;16:1256–62.
12. Van Loon P. Length-force and volume-pressure relationships of arteries. Biorheology. 1977;14:181–201.
13. Lehman RM, Owens GK, Kassell NF, Hongo K. Mechanism of enlargement of major cerebral collateral arteries in rabbits. Stroke. 1991;22:499–504.
14. Sho E, Nanjo H, Sho M, Kobayashi M, Komatsu M, Kawamura K, et al. Arterial enlargement, tortuosity, and intimal thickening in response to sequential exposure to high and low wall shear stress. J Vasc Surg. 2004;39:601–12.
15. Jackson ZS, Gotlieb AI, Langille BL. Wall tissue remodeling regulates longitudinal tension in arteries. Circ Res. 2002;90:918–25.
16. Eberth JF, Gresham VC, Reddy AK, Popovic N, Wilson E, Humphrey JD. Importance of pulsatility in hypertensive carotid artery growth and remodeling. J Hypertens. 2009;27:2010–21.
17. Fung YC, Liu SQ. Change of residual strains in arteries due to hypertrophy caused by aortic constriction. Circ Res. 1989;65:1340–9.
18. Mulvany MJ. Vascular remodelling of resistance vessels: can we define this? Cardiovasc Res. 1999;41:9–13.
19. Laurent S, Girerd X, Mourad J-J, Lacolley P, Beck L, Boutouyrie P, et al. Elastic modulus of the radial artery wall material is not increased in patients with essential hypertension. Arterioscler Thromb. 1994;14:1223–31.
20. Lambert J, Aarsen M, Donker AJM, Stehouwer CDA. Endothelium-dependent and -independent vasodilation of large arteries in Normoalbuminuric insulin-dependent diabetes mellitus. Arterioscler Thromb Vasc Biol. 1996;16:705–11.
21. Lavi T, Karasik A, Koren-Morag N, Kanety H, Feinberg MS, Shechter M. The acute effect of various glycemic index dietary carbohydrates on endothelial function in nondiabetic overweight and obese subjects. J Am Coll Cardiol. 2009;53:2283–7.
22. Caro C, Fitzgerald J, Schroeter R. Arterial wall shear and distribution of early atheroma in man. Nature. 1969;223:1159–60.

23. Helderman F, Segers D, de Crom R, Hierck BP, Poelmann RE, Evans PC, et al. Effect of shear stress on vascular inflammation and plaque development. Curr Opin Lipidol. 2007;18:527–33. Review

24. Kelly R, Ruane-O'Hara T, Noble MIM, Drake-Holland AJ, Snow HM. Effect of hyperglycaemia on endothelial dependent dilatation in the iliac artery of the anaesthetized pig. J Physiol. 2006;573:133–45.

25. Rachev A, Manoach E, Berry J, Moore JE Jr. A model of stress-induced geometrical remodeling of vessel segments adjacent to stents and artery/graft anastomoses. J Theor Biol. 2000;206:429–43.

Chapter 30
Blood Flow and Arterial Disease

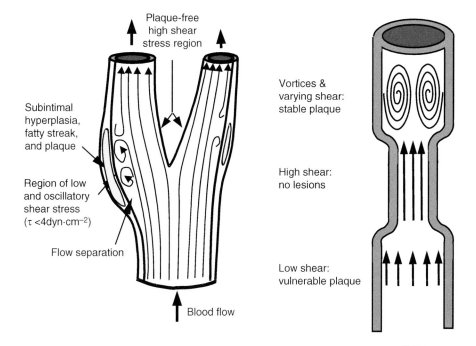

Plaque-free
high shear
stress region

Subintimal
hyperplasia,
fatty streak,
and plaque

Region of low
and oscillatory
shear stress
($\tau < 4\,\text{dyn·cm}^{-2}$)

Flow separation

Blood flow

Vortices &
varying shear:
stable plaque

High shear:
no lesions

Low shear:
vulnerable plaque

Atherosclerosis is a localized disease. It develops near bifurcations and areas where shear stress, the frictional force that the blood flow exerts on the intimal surface, is low (shear stress less than 4 dynes/cm²). A classic example is the carotid sinus, where flow separation takes place in some periods of the cardiac cycle leading to low and oscillatory shear stress. Flow patterns and location of plaques are schematically shown in the left panel. Areas of normal shear stress (>10 dynes/cm²) or areas subjected to high shear, are plaque-free, adapted from Ref. [1], used by

© Springer International Publishing AG, part of Springer Nature 2019
N. Westerhof et al., *Snapshots of Hemodynamics*,
https://doi.org/10.1007/978-3-319-91932-4_30

permission. The right panel shows that low shear results in larger lesions and vulnerable plaque, while in areas with vortices and variable shear more stable plaques develop, composition of these plaques also differs, adapted from Ref. [2], by permission. Wall shear stress not only plays a role in atherosclerosis, but is also a major determinant of graft failure and intima hyperplasia following angioplasty and stenting.

30.1   Description

Hemodynamic forces not only regulate blood vessel geometry and structure, i.e., remodeling, but they can be considered also as main factors influencing the development of different forms of vascular disease, such as atherosclerosis and aneurysms. Of particular importance is the role of shear stress, the minute force resulting from the friction that the flowing blood exerts on the luminal surface, on the localization and development of atherosclerosis.

Atherosclerosis is associated with genetic predisposition and systemic factors such as hypertension, hyperlipidemia, smoking, etc. However, the localized nature of the disease, which occurs principally in areas of disturbed flow such as near bifurcations and curvatures, cannot be explained by systemic factors that apply equally throughout the vasculature. It is recognized today that atherosclerosis develops in areas where shear stress is low, typically less than 4 dyn/cm^2, or 0.4 Pa, and changes direction during the cardiac cycle. An example is the wall of the carotid sinus, where local shear is low and flow separates during the decelerating phase of the heart cycle, leading to flow separation and thus flow reversal and change in shear stress direction (left panel of Figure in the Box). Other areas where low shear stress co-localizes with atherosclerosis are the coronaries, the infrarenal aorta and the femoral artery.

30.1.1   Shear Stress and Endothelial Function

Apart from its non-thrombogenic protective role, the endothelial layer constitutes the mechano-sensing element, which senses the local flow conditions and produces autocrine and paracrine factors for the functional regulation of the arterial wall. Studies of endothelial cells *in vitro* and *in vivo* have revealed the deleterious effect of low and oscillatory, vortex-related, shear stress on endothelial function. Under physiological shear ($\sigma > 10$ dyn/cm^2) endothelial cells align in the direction of flow whereas they do not when exposed to low shear ($\sigma < 4$ dyn/cm^2). Low and oscillatory shear stress lead to inhibition of NO-synthase, greater endothelial cell cycling and increase in apoptosis. Low and oscillatory shear also contribute to local endothelial dysfunction, which may lead to enhanced monocyte adhesion, increased platelet activation, increased vasoconstriction, increased smooth muscle cell proliferation, and increased oxidant activity, thus constituting a likely model for atherogenesis. It has been shown that low shear stress in combination with flow patterns such as vortices determine the type of plaque, both in composition and vulnerability (right panel of Figure in the Box). Low shear results in vulnerable plaque while vortex-based shear results in more stable plaque [2]. High shear stress induces an atheroprotective endothelial phenotype, increases NO production, and decreases the expression of vasoconstrictors, inflammatory response mediators, adhesion molecules and oxidants.

Detailed discussion on the relation between shear stress and endothelial function can be found in the review articles by Davies et al. [3] and Malek et al. [1].

30.2 Physiological and Clinical Relevance

30.2.1 Assessing Risk for Atherosclerosis

Ultrasound measurements in the carotid artery of healthy young adults aged 28–38 years revealed a significant inverse relation between the measured intima-media thickness and local shear stress. This suggests that there is a prognostic value in the assessment of local wall shear levels using noninvasive techniques, such as ultrasound Doppler or MRI.

Since the velocity profile near a bifurcation depends strongly on the geometry, it has been suggested that there exist 'geometrical risk' factors for atherosclerosis. Certain branching geometries, i.e., high curvatures and large angles, may predispose to atherosclerosis because they would lead more easily to flow separation and low shear stress regions [4].

30.2.2 Shear Stress and Intima Hyperplasia in Vein Grafts

Intima hyperplasia in vein grafts is also sensitive to wall shear. Dobrin et al. [5] examined the effect of all mechanical factors (pressure, extension, and shear stress) on intima hyperplasia and medial thickening in autogenous vein grafts in dogs. Autologous vein grafts were used to bypass a segment of the femoral artery. The femoral artery on one side was ligated, so that all femoral blood flow passed through the graft. The femoral artery at the opposite side was left patent, which permitted only part of the flow to pass through the vein graft. A stiff cuff was placed over the middle section of the vein grafts impeding radial expansion. Cross-sectional areas are given in Fig. 30.1. The results show that intima hyperplasia is greater on both sides, in the distended, low shear, regions, than in the regions constrained by the cuffs, thus at high shear. Furthermore, intima hyperplasia was globally lower on the side with high flow, obtained by femoral artery ligation, as compared to the side were femoral artery was left patent, i.e., low flow.

Fig. 30.1 Intimal
hyperplasia in vein grafts.
(Adapted from Ref. [5], by
permission)

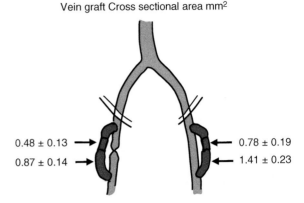

Vein graft Cross sectional area mm²

0.48 ± 0.13 →   ← 0.78 ± 0.19

0.87 ± 0.14 →   ← 1.41 ± 0.23

30.2.3   Shear Stress and Intima Hyperplasia in Bypass Grafts

High shear stress inhibits neointima formation in artificial ePTFE grafts. Animal
experiments have shown that exposure of implanted grafts to higher shear, by means
of distal arterio-venous fistulas, leads to a decrease in the thickness of the already
existing neointima hyperplasia.

Low and oscillatory wall shear stress patterns may also be responsible for the
failure of bypass grafts. In the vicinity of an end-to-side anastomosis, blood flow is
greatly disturbed. This is mainly due to the abrupt change in geometry. For vascular
grafts, intima hyperplasia develops preferentially at the 'toe' and the 'heel' of the
anastomosis. These are exactly the locations where flow separation, low wall shear
stress and large gradients of wall shear stress take place.

30.2.4   Intima Hyperplasia Following Angioplasty and Stenting

Restenosis is an undesirable occlusive response to stent implantation after balloon
angioplasty. In contrast to balloon angioplasty, where acute or sub-acute recoil represents the major mechanism of restenosis, stent restenosis is exclusively attributed
to neointima proliferation, a tissue reaction often termed intima hyperplasia (IH).
Morphological studies have demonstrated that neointima is caused by early smooth
muscle cell ingrowth, which is then gradually replaced by extracellular matrix.

There is a good deal of scientific evidence that intima hyperplasia is sensitive to
flow. Kohler and Jawien [6] studied the effects of flow on intima hyperplasia after
balloon injury of the rat common carotid. Flow was increased, by ~35%, by ligation
of the opposite common carotid artery or decreased, also by ~35%, by ligation of
the ipsilateral internal carotid. Two weeks after the intervention, intima thickness,
indicated by the distance between the artery lumen and arrow, was significantly
smaller in the high flow group (Fig. 30.2a) as compared with the low-flow group
(Fig. 30.2b).

Fig. 30.2 Histological sections of the rat carotid subjected to high flow (**a**) and low flow (**b**) indicating the degree of intimal hyperplasia 2 weeks after balloon injury. (Adapted from Ref. [6], by permission)

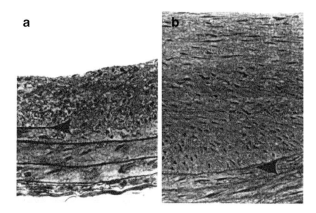

There appears also to be strong clinical evidence for the relation between post interventional flow and patency of balloon angioplasty. If local flow, and thus wall shear stress, after balloon angioplasty is high, the artery is expected to remain patent. This observation, common to many physicians practicing balloon angioplasty, is substantiated by studies reporting increased long-term patency after angioplasty in lower extremity arteries when flows are high. Direct clinical proof of the inverse relationship between wall shear stress and intima thickness was given by Wentzel et al. [7]. Computational fluid dynamics simulations of the flow field within a stented carotid artery have demonstrated that athero-prone regions co-localize with stent mal-apposition and stent strut interconnections [8].

The restenosis problem following stent placement has been drastically reduced with the use of drug-eluting stents. Drug-eluting stents with the capability to deliver anti-inflammatory or anti-proliferative drugs directly to the adjacent arterial tissue, inhibit neointima hyperplasia and restenosis.

30.2.5 Shear Stress and Aortic Aneurysm

Cerebral aortic aneurysms have a saccular, eccentric shape that can be digitally removed to retrieve the aortic geometry prior to disease. Such artificially generated 'baseline' geometries have been used to relate computationally obtained shear stress descriptors with the onset of cerebral aneurysm formation [9]. Long time follow-up of cerebral aneurysms further demonstrated that those areas experiencing lowest time-averaged wall shear stress are also the areas where the aneurysm grows most. Due to the recirculation of blood the dilated zone of the aneurysm experiences locally decreased and oscillatory shear stress that accelerates the local process of inflammation and proteolysis, thus entering into a vicious circle [10]. Abdominal aortic aneurysms on the other hand have a diffuse shape that makes it impossible to retrieve the original, non-diseased geometry. That is why most research on the role of shear stress in aneurysm initiation is performed in mice [11]. Computationally derived wall shear stress patterns have demonstrated a decreased shear stress in patients with spinal cord injury, which may be linked to the higher incidence of aneurysm formation in these patients [12]. Computational models of patient-specific abdominal aortic aneurysms have been used to demonstrate that the deposition of intraluminal thrombus is most likely driven by local hemodynamics [13].

References

1. Malek AM, Alper SL, Izumo S. Hemodynamic shear stress and its role in atherosclerosis. JAMA. 1999;282:2035–42.
2. Cheng C, Tempel D, van Haperen R, van der Baan A, Grosveld F, Daemen MJ, et al. Atherosclerotic lesion size and vulnerability are determined by patterns of fluid shear stress. Circulation. 2006;113:2744–53.
3. Davies PF, Barbee KA, Lal R, Robotewskyj A, Griem ML. Hemodynamics and atherogenesis. Endothelial surface dynamics in flow signal transduction. Ann N Y Acad Sci. 1995;748:86–102. discussion 102-103
4. Goubergrits L, Affeld K, Fernandez-Britto J, Falcon L. Atherosclerosis in the human common carotid artery. A morphometric study of 31 specimens. Pathol Res Pract. 2001;197:803–9.
5. Dobrin PB, Littooy FN, Endean ED. Mechanical factors predisposing to intimal hyperplasia and medial thickening in autogenous vein grafts. Surgery. 1989;105:393–400.
6. Kohler T, Jawien A. Flow affects development of intimal hyperplasia after arterial injury in rats. Arterioscler Thromb. 1992;12:963–71.
7. Wentzel JJ, Krams R, Schuurbiers JC, Oomen JA, Kloet J, Van der Giessen WJ, et al. Relationship between neointimal thickness and shear stress after Wallstent implantation in human coronary arteries. Circulation. 2001;103:1740–5.
8. De Santis G, Conti M, Trachet B, De Schryver T, De Beule M, Degroote J, et al. Impact of stent-vessel (mal) apposition following carotid artery stenting: mind the gaps! Ann Biomed Eng. 2013;16:648–59.
9. Mantha A, Karmonik C, Benndorf G, Strother C, Metcalfe R. Hemodynamics in a cerebral artery before and after the formation of an aneurysm. AJNR Am J Neuroradiol. 2006;27:1113–8.
10. Boussel L, Rayz V, McCulloch C, Martin A, Acevedo-Bolton G, Lawton M, et al. Aneurysm growth occurs at region of low wall shear stress: patient-specific correlation of hemodynamics and growth in a longitudinal study. Stroke. 2008;39:2997–3002.
11. Trachet B, Renard M, De Santis G, Staelens S, De Backer J, Antiga L, et al. An integrated framework to quantitatively link mouse-specific hemodynamics to aneurysm formation in angiotensin II-infused ApoE −/− mice. Ann Biomed Eng. 2011;39:2430–44.
12. Yeung JJ, Kim HJ, Abbruzzese TA, Vignon-Clementel IE, Draney-Blomme MT, Yeung KK, et al. Aortoiliac hemodynamic and morphologic adaptation to chronic spinal cord injury. J Vasc Surg. 2006;44:1254–65.
13. Di Achille P, Tellides G, Humphrey JD. Hemodynamics-driven deposition of intraluminal thrombus in abdominal aortic aneurysms. Int J Numer Method Biomed Eng. 2017;33:e2828.

Part IV
Integration

Chapter 31
Determinants of Pressure and Flow

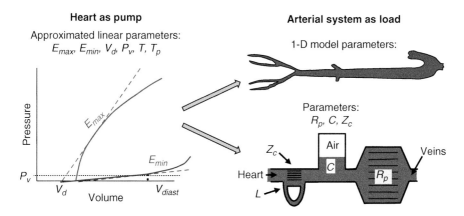

Heart as pump

Approximated linear parameters:
$E_{max}, E_{min}, V_d, P_v, T, T_p$

Arterial system as load

1-D model parameters:

Parameters:
R_p, C, Z_c

Pressure and flow result from the interaction of the heart, the pump, and the arterial system, the load. Understanding the quantitative contribution of the heart and the arterial system to pressure and flow is important in the study of hypertension, cardiac failure and other cardiovascular diseases. The heart can be described on the basis of the pressure-volume relation, left, or from muscle properties. The arterial load, can be described by a Windkessel or 1-D model, right. A simple approach is to use the pressure-volume relation for the heart and the three-element Windkessel for the load. When we linearize the pressure volume relations the total number of parameters to describe cardiac pump function is 6, and for the Windkessel it is 3. Using this limited number of parameters, their quantitative contribution to systolic and diastolic pressure and Stroke Volume can be worked out. Dimensional analysis shows that $R_p \cdot C/T$ and $C \cdot E_{max}$ are parameters that couple the heart and load, and they play an important role in pressure and Stroke Volume. The normalized $E_N(t_N)$ curve describing, the heart and the normalized input impedance, describing the arterial system, are similar in different mammals, explaining the similarities of pressure and flow wave shapes in mammals

© Springer International Publishing AG, part of Springer Nature 2019
265
N. Westerhof et al., *Snapshots of Hemodynamics*,
https://doi.org/10.1007/978-3-319-91932-4_31

31.1 Description

Blood pressure and Cardiac Output result from the interaction of the heart and arterial load. It is also known that changes in cardiac and arterial properties are related as has been shown in aging [1]. However, quantitative information about the contribution of heart and arterial load to pressure and flow under different physiological conditions and during various diseased states is limited. To quantitatively analyze the cardiac and arterial contributions to systolic and diastolic pressure and Stroke Volume models have been developed describing the cardiac pump and the arterial load. Cardiac models are mostly based on the time-varying elastance concept (Chap. 14), and the requires only a limited number of parameters, the diastolic and systolic pressure volume relations, E_{max}, E_{min}, (model terms for linearized E_{es} and E_{ed}, Chap. 14), and the time varying function $E(t)$, which, when normalized in magnitude and timing of the peak, T_p, can be written as $E_N(t_N)$ [2]. This general approach is used by several authors, with differences in the details [3–6]. Other heart models, based on strain modeling, have been used as well [7, 8].

The arterial system can be described by the three-element Windkessel model (Chap. 25) [3] or by 1-D arterial models [4–6]. Below we discuss a model based on the time-varying elastance concept and the three-element Windkessel, where the number of parameters is limited.

31.1.1 Dimensional Analysis

Dimensional analysis, or the concept of similitude, is a powerful method to systematically derive relations of a system and offers two major advantages [9]. First, it reduces the number of variables, and second, it groups the cardiac and arterial parameters in dimensionless terms, which are automatically scaled to Heart Rate and body size. This will be a particularly important issue when we discuss comparative physiology (Chap. 32). The parameters that describe the heart as a pump, including venous filling pressure are E_{max}, E_{min}, V_d, T_p, and venous filling pressure, P_v, and heart period (1/Heart Rate), T. The arterial load is mimicked by the three-element Windkessel, with parameters Z_c, R_p and C (Chap. 25). The total number of parameters is 9, namely 6 for the heart and 3 for the arterial system. Figure in the Box and Fig. 31.1.

The dependent variables systolic and diastolic pressure (P_s and P_d) and Stroke Volume, SV, can be written as a function of these nine cardiac and arterial parameters. Dimensional analysis implies that when the variables and the parameters are non-dimensionalized, the number of non-dimensional parameters can be reduced by three. Three is the number of reference dimensions (time, force and length) describing the variables [9]. Thus six non-dimensional parameters remain. An intelligent choice is the following [3]:

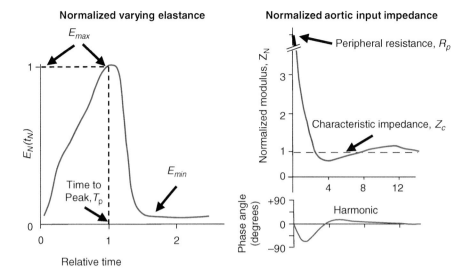

Fig. 31.1 The normalized elastance curve, $E_N(t_N)$, and the normalized input impedance, Z_{in}/Z_c, are independent of animal size, resulting in similar wave shapes of aortic pressure and flow in mammals, and with pressures even having the same in magnitude

$$P_s / P_v = \Phi_1\left(Z_c / R_p, R_p C / T, CE_{min}, E_{max} / E_{min}, E_{min} V_d / P_v, T_p / T\right)$$

$$P_d / P_v = \Phi_2\left(Z_c / R_p, R_p C / T, CE_{min}, E_{max} / E_{min}, E_{min} V_d / P_v, T_p / T\right)$$

$$SV \cdot E_{min} / P_v = \Phi_3\left(Z_c / R_p, R_p C / T, CE_{min}, E_{max} / E_{min}, E_{min} V_d / P_v, T_p / T\right)$$

The next step is to find the dependence of the non-dimensional variables on the non-dimensional parameters. The normalized $E_N(t_N)$ (Fig. 31.1) is fixed [2], and the contribution of T_p/T to P_s/P_v, P_d/P_v, and $SV \cdot E_{min}/P_v$ is small and can be neglected. It turns out experimentally that the parameter $E_{min} \cdot V_d/P_v$ does not contribute to P_s/P_v and P_d/P_v; that Z_c/R_p does not determine P_d/P_v and SV/V_d; while E_{max}/E_{min} does not determine $SV \cdot E_{min}/P_v$. The contribution of Z_c/R_p to P_s/P_v turns out to small and is neglected as well [3]. The relations then can be simplified to:

$$P_s / P_v \approx \Phi_1\left(R_p C / T, CE_{min}, E_{max} / E_{min}\right)$$

$$P_d / P_v \approx \Phi_2\left(R_p C / T, CE_{min}, E_{max} / E_{min}\right)$$

$$SV \cdot E_{min} / P_v \approx \Phi_3\left(R_p C / T, CE_{min}, E_{min} \cdot V_d / P_v\right)$$

In all non-dimensional variables we see that the parameters $R_p C/T$, (arterial time constant and heart period) and $C \cdot E_{min}$ (arterial compliance i.e. 1/arterial stiffness and ventricular diastolic elastance) appear. We call them ventriculo-arterial coupling parameters. This emphasizes the fact that the interaction of pump and load determines pressure and flow.

The Frank-Starling mechanism also emerges from the above equations. Leaving all parameters the same, the pressures are simply proportional to venous pressure, P_v. Stroke Volume is also related to filling pressure, but in a more complex way. In reality the diastolic Pressure-Volume relation is not straight and therefore the effect of filling is in reality more complex than shown here.

The pressures also depend on E_{max}/E_{min} a measure of contractility of the heart. The Stroke Volume is also described by the rather complex term $E_{min} \cdot V_d / P_v$, which is related to diastolic ventricular filling and can be written as $V_d/(V_{diast} - V_d)$, with V_{diast} end-diastolic ventricular volume.

On the basis of the results obtained with the dimensional analysis we can perform a sensitivity analysis of pressure and Stroke Volume to individual parameters. The results are given in the Table 31.1.

We note that the normalized parameters $R_p C/T$, CE_{min}, E_{max}/E_{min} do not depend on body size, (Chap. 32) so that for similar venous pressures, aortic systolic and diastolic pressures will be similar in all mammals. Stroke Volume does depend on body size.

The wave shapes of pressure and flow result from the shape of the $E(t)$-curve describing the pump and the input impedance describing the arterial load, Z_{in}. When both are normalized, $E_N(t_N)$ and $Z_{in,N}$ [10] they are independent of body size, explaining why aortic pressure and flow have similar shapes in mammals (Chap. 32).

31.2   Physiological and Clinical Relevance

The analysis shows in quantitative terms the contribution of cardiac and arterial parameters to blood pressure and Stroke Volume. It may be seen from Table 31.1 that resistance has a much stronger effect on systolic blood pressure than compliance has. However, changes in compliance are often considerably larger than resistance changes. For instance, between the ages of 20 and 80 years PWV may increase a

Table 31.1 Quantitative contribution of heart and arterial system to pressure and Stroke Volume

Parameter	$P_{systole}$	$P_{diastole}$	SV
Z_c	+9	0	0
R_p	+41	+90	−28
C	−10	+22	+5
T	−50	−90	+28
E_{max}	+40	+32	+33
E_{min}	−100	−100	−100
P_v	+100	+100	+100

Percent changes in systolic, diastolic pressure and Stroke Volume, resulting from a 100% increase in a single cardiac or arterial parameter. The minus sign indicates a decrease with an increase in a parameter. Thus, a 20% change in heart period (T) results in a $- (20/100) \cdot 50 = -10\%$ change in systolic pressure and a −18% change in diastolic pressure

factor 2 (Fig. 21.5) implying a compliance decrease by a factor of 3–4, while the resistance increase is about 15%. Thus the decrease in compliance predicts an increase systolic blood pressure by 15%, while the age related resistance increase predicts a systolic pressure increase of slightly over 4%. This prediction is assuming no role of changes in cardiac properties (see below).

On the basis of the dimensionless parameters shown above it may be suggested that E_{max}/E_{min} is a better measure of contractility than E_{max} alone, because this ratio is size independent, while the E_{max} is depending on the ventricular volume.

The theoretical results can be compared with biological data. Experimental data [11] obtained from the isolated heart loaded with a Windkessel model indeed show that compliance changes alone have a small effect on systolic blood pressure and a larger effect on diastolic blood pressure (Chap. 25). When compliance is decreased *in vivo* (Chap. 11) other parameters also change and systolic pressure increases and diastolic pressure decreases [12]. The main difference between the *ex vivo* and *in vivo* results is the adaptation of the heart during the decrease in compliance. The *ex vivo* heart, was unchanged in terms of filling and contractility (Chap. 25), while *in vivo* the heart does adapt and Cardiac Output diminishes less than in the *ex vivo* situation (see Fig. 11.7, Chap. 11). Thus, the changed cardiac function *in vivo* has an effect on blood pressure.

31.2.1 Contribution of Arterial System and Heart in Systolic Hypertension

The contributions of both heart and arterial system to the increase in aortic pressure with age is shown in Fig. 31.2 [13]. In the literature it is well established that hypertension results in ventricular hypertrophy and therefore a higher E_{max} [1]. However, it is often not realized that cardiac hypertrophy causes changes in the properties of the cardiac pump such as increased wall thickness (i.e. increased E_{min} and E_{max}) and that these changes may, in turn, contribute to a further increase in blood pressure. Using the models, as given in the Box, the contributions of the heart and arterial system to systolic aortic pressure in four groups of hypertensive patients were calculated and the results are shown in Fig. 31.3 [14]. It may be seen that in concentric remodeling the increase in systolic blood pressure is mainly the result of the altered arterial system, while in eccentric hypertrophy the contribution to the increased systolic pressure is mainly the result of changed cardiac properties. This example therefore shows that both heart and arterial system need to be considered in hypertension research.

Fig. 31.2 The effect of aging on systolic and diastolic aortic pressure, resulting from arterial changes alone (blue) and from both arterial and cardiac changes (red). (Adapted from Ref. [13], used by permission)

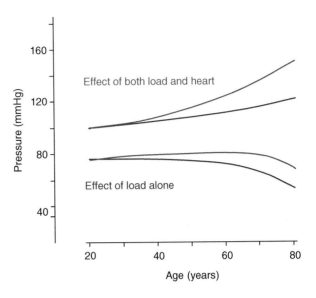

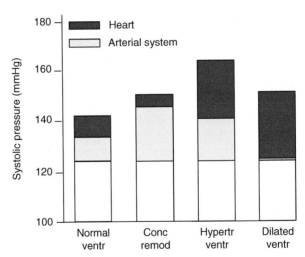

Fig. 31.3 Cardiac and arterial contributions to systolic pressure increase in four groups of hypertensive patients. Several stages in cardiac changes are depicted, (1) Normal ventricle; (2) Concentric remodeling; (3) Hypertrophied left ventricle; and (4) Dilated left ventricle. The white bars give the systolic pressure of the normal cardiovascular system. In concentric remodeling most of the systolic pressure increase results from the change in the arterial system (yellow) while the cardiac change has a small effect (red). When the ventricle is dilated in hypertension most of the pressure increase is caused by the heart. (Adapted from Ref. [14], by permission)

References

1. Redfield MM, Jacobsen SJ, Borlaug BA, Rodeheffer RJ, Kass DA. Age- and gender-related ventricular-vascular stiffening: a community-based study. Circulation. 2005;112:2254–62.
2. Senzaki H, Chen C-H, Kass DA. Single-beat estimation of end-systolic pressure-volume relation in humans: a new method with the potential for noninvasive application. Circulation. 1996;94:2497–506.
3. Stergiopulos N, Meister J-J, Westerhof N. Determinants of stroke volume and systolic and diastolic aortic pressure. Am J Phys. 1996;270:H2050–9.
4. Formaggia L, Lamponi D, Tuveri M, Veneziani A. Numerical modeling of 1D arterial networks coupled with a lumped parameters description of the heart. Comput Methods Biomech Biomed Engin. 2006;9:273–88.
5. Liang F, Takagi S, Himeno R, Liu H. Multi-scale modeling of the human cardiovascular system with applications to aortic valvular and arterial stenoses. Med Biol Eng Comput. 2009;47:743–55.
6. Liang F, Guan D, Alastruey J. Determinant factors for arterial hemodynamics in hypertension: theoretical insights from a computational model-based study. J Biomech Eng. 2018;140:031006. https://doi.org/10.1115/1.4038430.
7. Gao H, Carrick D, Berry C, Griffith BE, Luo X. Dynamic finite-strain modelling of the human left ventricle in health and disease using an immersed boundary-finite element method. IMA J Appl Math. 2014;79:978–1010.
8. Chen WW, Gao H, Luo XY, Hill NA. Study of cardiovascular function using a coupled left ventricle and systemic circulation model. J Biomech. 2016;49:2445–54.
9. Munson BR, Young DF, Okiishi TH. Fundamentals of fluid mechanics. New York: Wiley; 1994.
10. Westerhof N, Elzinga G. Normalized input impedance and arterial decay time over heart period are independent of animal size. Am J Phys. 1991;261:R126–33.
11. Randall OS, van den Bos GC, Westerhof N. Systemic compliance: does it play a role in the genesis of essential hypertension? Cardiovasc Res. 1984;18:455–62.
12. Elzinga G, Westerhof N. Pressure and flow generated by the left ventricle against different impedances. Circ Res. 1973;32:178–86.
13. Maksuti E, Westerhof N, Westerhof BE, Broomé M, Stergiopulos N. Contribution of the arterial system and the heart to blood pressure during normal aging – a simulation study. PLoS One. 2016;11:e0157493.
14. Segers P, Stergiopulos N, Westerhof N. Quantification of the contribution of cardiac and arterial remodeling to hypertension. Hypertension. 2000;36:760–5.

Chapter 32
Comparative Physiology

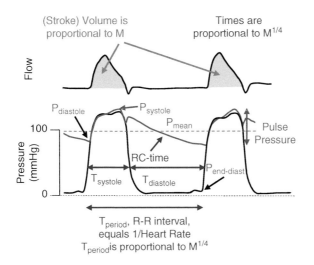

(Stroke) Volume is proportional to M

Times are proportional to $M^{1/4}$

Flow

$P_{diastole}$

$P_{systole}$

P_{mean}

100

Pulse Pressure

Pressure (mmHg)

RC-time

$T_{systole}$ $T_{diastole}$ $P_{end-diast}$

0

T_{period}, R-R interval, equals 1/Heart Rate

T_{period} is proportional to $M^{1/4}$

Cardiac Output and basal metabolism are proportional to $M^{3/4}$

Pressures and wave speed do not depend on body mass M

To compare parameters in different mammals we make use of the so-called allometric equation: $PA = PA_0 M^e$, with PA the parameter of interest, PA_0 a reference value, M body mass, and e the exponent. Aortic and ventricular pressure are similar in shape and magnitude in mammals (exponent $e = 0$). *Heart Rate* (HR, 1/Heart Period, T) depends on body mass as $M^{-1/4}$. The aortic flow wave shape is similar in mammals but its magnitude depends on body size with Cardiac Output proportional to $M^{3/4}$. This strong similarity results from the relations between the basic parameters describing the cardiovascular system (Chap. 31). The R_pC-time of aortic pressure decay in diastole, with R_p peripheral resistance and C total arterial compliance,

© Springer International Publishing AG, part of Springer Nature 2019
N. Westerhof et al., *Snapshots of Hemodynamics*,
https://doi.org/10.1007/978-3-319-91932-4_32

and the heart period, T_{period}, both scale as $M^{1/4}$. The ventriculo-arterial coupling parameter $R_p C/T_{period}$ is independent of body mass and thus the same in mammals. Volume parameters such a heart size and Stroke Volume, SV, are proportional to body mass. Since CO equals HR times SV, it is proportional to $M^{3/4}$. Basal metabolism is proportional to CO, and thus also proportional to $M^{3/4}$. The coupling parameter CE_{min}, and the ratio's E_{max}/E_{min} (Chap. 31) and $T_{diastole}/T_{period}$ are independent of body mass. The limited data available on the $E(t)$ curve, when scaled to its maximum and time of peak suggest similarity as well. The ratio of peripheral resistance and aortic characteristic impedance is independent of animal size, implying that normalized aortic input impedance is similar in mammals. Since all parameters prescribing aortic pressure and flow wave shapes are independent of animal size, the pressure and flow waves are similar in mammals. Pressures even have the same magnitude, while Cardiac Output scales to $M^{3/4}$. Similar mean pressure (at brain level) is probably a necessary condition for brain perfusion, and the similar diastolic pressure and constant fraction of diastole, $T_{diastole}/T_{period}$, are conditions to provide sufficient subendocardial coronary perfusion. The similar pressures in mammals suggest the stringent conditions on pressure control and that even borderline hypertension is abnormal.

32.1   Description

Comparative physiology is based on the allometric equation [1, 2]:

$$PA = PA_0 \cdot M^e$$

with PA the parameter of interest, PA_0 a reference value, M body mass, and e the exponent. When the logarithm of both sides is taken the equation can be rewritten as:

$$\log(PA) = \log(PA_0) + e \log M$$

This equation states that, when a parameter PA is plotted against body mass M, in a double logarithmic plot, a straight line with slope e is obtained. If two parameters have the same slope (same e), the ratio of the parameters does not depend on body mass, i.e., the ratio is independent of the size (mass) of the animal.

Basal Metabolic rate (BMr) was shown to relate to body mass, M, as [2]

$$MBr = MBr_0 \cdot M^{0.756} \approx MBr_0 \cdot M^{3/4}$$

and became known as the ¾ law.

Originally basal metabolic rate was assumed to relate to Body Surface Area (BSA), the so-called body surface law, BSL. The BSL was based on the idea that heat diffusion to the environment depends on body surface area and that exchange of substrates and metabolites, via diffusion, also depends on surfaces. However these surfaces are not proportional. Also BSA is difficult to obtain accurately. The conversion from BSA to body mass is complex and trials to simplify the relation such as by assuming a sphere for the entire body, BSA = Volume$^{2/3} \approx M^{2/3}$ is too inaccurate since the area-mass relation is stature-dependent. More sophisticated estimates are including both body mass and body height [3] and also height plus head circumference for humans [4].

The first researcher, who, by thorough experimentation and reasoning, suggested the ¾ law between Basal Metabolic rate and body mass was Kleiber [2]. The Body Surface Law, although less accurate was only reluctantly abandoned. The arguments regarding the relation BMr and M or BMr and BSA is not closed yet [5] but we will use the ¾ law here. Aortic pressure depends somewhat on body size with $M^{0.05}$, which is much less than one would expect to keep brain pressure similar in mammals, namely a power of 0.3 [5]. We here assume pressure to be independent of body mass.

The ¾ law implies that cellular metabolism decreases with animal size. It has indeed been observed both *in-vitro* and *in-vivo* that metabolism of isolated organs and cells decreases with animal size. The tissue basal metabolic rate per kilogram in the mouse is 30-fold more than that of the cow.

Difference in O_2 content of arterial and venous blood is similar in mammals and blood supply to the tissues is regulated to meet metabolism; therefore BMr is proportional to blood flow. We will see below that Cardiac Output also relates to $M^{3/4}$.

In general Volumes are proportional to total body volume (thus body mass, M) [6, 7].

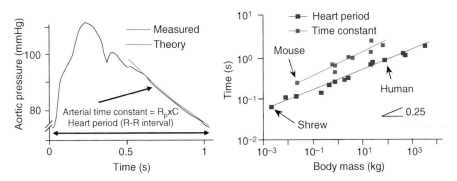

Fig. 32.1 Aortic pressure (left) and a log-log plot of heart period and R_pC-time (right). The aortic pressure shows an exponential decay in diastole, characterized by the arterial parameter R_pC-time, i.e., peripheral resistance, R_p, times total arterial compliance, C. The heart period, T_{period}, is a cardiac parameter. Both times show an increase with body mass with an exponent of ¼. This implies that the ratio of the two, the ventriculo-arterial coupling parameter R_pC/T_{period} is the same in mammals. (Adapted from Ref. [9], used by permission)

32.1.1 Cardiovascular Scaling

Mean systemic arterial blood pressure at brain level is similar in mammals [8].

The ventriculo-arterial coupling parameter $R_p \cdot C/T$ (see Chap. 31) is an example of the study of comparative physiology, where it is shown that the characteristic time of the arterial system, $R_p C$-time, and the characteristic time of the heart, the heart period $T = 1/HR$, have the same exponent, 0.25 (Fig. 32.1). This implies that their ratio is independent of body mass [9]. The similar Pulse Pressure found in mammals can be understood on the basis of this mass-independence as follows. Total arterial compliance, C, is proportional to Stroke Volume divided by Pulse Pressure, PP, or $PP \propto SV/C$. Mean pressure is equal to Peripheral Resistance, R_p, times Cardiac Output: $P_{mean} = R_p \cdot CO$, and Cardiac Output equals Heart Rate times Stroke Volume, i.e., $P_{mean} = R_p \cdot SV/T$. Therefore $P_{mean}/PP \propto (R_p \cdot SV/T)/(SV/C) = R_p C/T$. With $R_p C/T$ being size-independent this implies that, with similar mean pressure, also Pulse Pressure, and systolic and diastolic pressure are the same in mammals. The ratio of Pulse Pressure and mean pressure, PP/P_{mean}, is called the fractional Pulse Pressure.

The finding that the heart period increases with body mass predicts, even in a single species, that heart period increases also with body length. This was indeed shown to be the case in the human (Fig. 32.2).

Since volumes are proportional to body mass, i.e., M^{+1}, so are cardiac volume and Stroke Volume [6]. With CO = HR·SV, it follows that CO is proportional to $M^{-0.25} \cdot M^1 = M^{1/4}$. Metabolic rate also relates to $M^{3/4}$ [7, 8].The result implies that the ratio of metabolic rate and CO is independent of mammal size. The importance of the relation between the cardiovascular system and metabolism form the basis of studies of the arterial system [11]. The size of the normal heart is proportional to body mass, about 0.58% of body weight [12], this size results in optimal external power production as shown in Chap. 18 [13].

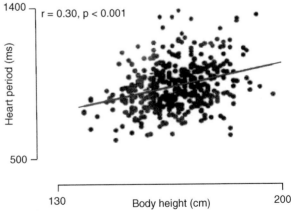

Fig. 32.2 Heart period relates to body height in humans. Slope is Length$^{0.9}$ or Mass$^{0.27}$, which is close to ¼ as found between mammals. (Adapted from Ref. [10], used by permission)

Other comparative data are scarce but if we assume similar material properties, and with volumes proportional to body mass [6], it follows that the slope of the diastolic and systolic pressure-volume relations, are proportional to M^{-1}, and also that total arterial compliance, C, is proportional to body mass. Thus, the coupling parameters CE_{min} and CE_{max} (see Chap. 31), are independent of body mass. For iso-volumic beats the ratio of E_{max} and E_{min} equals systolic over diastolic pressure and this ratio is similar in mammals, thus E_{max}/E_{min} is size independent. In the data published on the $E(t)$ curve, those of man and dog are not dissimilar in shape, when normalized with respect to time of peak and peak value [14]. Quantitative data on a whole range of mammals is not available yet.

When we plot the characteristic impedance and peripheral resistance as a function of body mass we find parallel lines again (Fig. 32.3). This implies that this ratio is similar in mammals. Therefore the aortic input impedance (Fig. 32.4) when scaled with respect to the characteristic impedance or peripheral resistance and plotted as a function of harmonic, i.e., as multiples of the Heart Rate (Appendix 1) is similar [9].

When a three-element Windkessel is assumed as acceptable model of the systemic arterial tree (Chap. 24), the normalized input impedance can be written as:

$$Z_{in}/Z_c = \left[1 + R_p/Z_c + i\cdot 2\pi\cdot n\cdot R_pC/T\right] / \left[1 + i\cdot 2\pi\cdot n\cdot R_pC/T\right]$$

where n is the harmonic number. With R_pC/T and R_p/Z_c independent of animal size, the normalized input impedance plotted as a function of harmonic number is basically similar for all mammals (Fig. 32.4, green line). Thus, the aortic pressure and flow wave shapes are related in a similar way in all mammals.

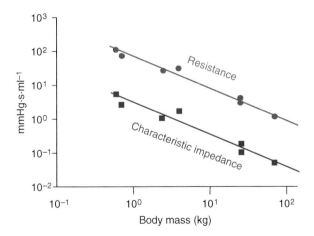

Fig. 32.3 Peripheral resistance and aortic characteristic impedance scale similarly with body mass. Therefore their ratio is independent of animal size. (Adapted from Ref. [9], used by permission)

Fig. 32.4 Normalized input impedance with respect to peripheral resistance, and plotted as a function of harmonic number is similar in mammals. This implies that pressure and flow wave shapes are the same. (see text)

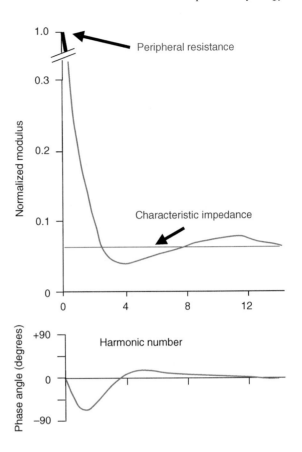

It has also been suggested that shear stress would be similar in mammals (Chaps. 29 and 30). Shear stress is proportional to Q/r_i^3, and since CO scales to $M^{3/4}$, and r_i to $M^{1/3}$, and the shear stress scales to $M^{3/4}/M = M^{-1/4}$. Shear stress is probably not very tightly controlled (Chaps. 29 and 30) and is not the same in different vessels and different in similar arteries between animals (Chap. 2).

The allometric relations of heart period and duration of diastole are given in Fig. 32.5. The slopes of the relations are not different, which means that diastole is a constant fraction of the heart period. Subendocardial perfusion mainly takes place in diastole, and thus depends on diastolic pressure and the duration of diastole. With similar diastolic pressures and similar coronary fractional perfusion time (Chap. 19) perfusion conditions are also similar in mammals [9].

32.1.2 Basal Whole Body and Cardiac Metabolism

As mentioned and explained above basal whole body metabolic rate and Cardiac Output are both proportional to body mass as $M^{3/4}$. Why CO is proportional to $M^{3/4}$

Fig. 32.5 Heart period and duration of diastole are plotted as a function of body mass. The parallel lines imply that diastole is a fixed fraction of the heart period. (Adapted from Ref. [9], used by permission)

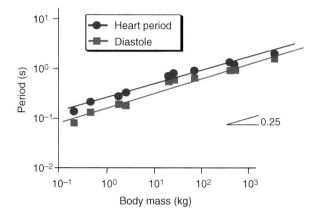

Fig. 32.6 Relative volumes of myofibrils and mitochondria of heart muscle. For smaller mammals the mitochondrial plus myofibrillar volume close to completely fills the muscle cells. (Compiled from Tables 1 and 4 of Ref. [16])

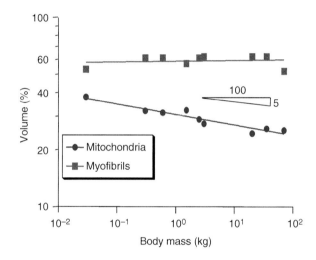

was explained above. Apparently metabolism is related to CO, but other suggestions have been given [15]. Basal metabolic rate and CO may be closely related because oxygen carrying capacity of the blood is similar in mammals.

Since cardiac metabolism also increases with body mass to the power ¾ and cardiac mass is proportional to body mass, and cardiac metabolism per gram heart tissue increases with body mass to the power –¼. This means that cardiac metabolism per gram is higher in small than in large animals.

Mitochondrial relative volume, as shown in Fig. 32.6, a measure of maximal energy expenditure per unit mass, decreases with body mass as $M^{-0.05}$ [16]. In other words, the difference between maximal metabolism and resting metabolism, i.e. the metabolic reserve is less in smaller than large mammals. Figure 32.6 shows also that the cardiac cells of the smallest mammals are almost entirely filled with (with somewhat more efficient, [17]) mitochondria and myofilaments suggesting a minimal size for mammals.

32.1.3 Pulse Wave Velocity and Reflections

Experimental data suggest that pulse wave velocity is independent of animal size. This can be seen from basic vascular data where the Youngs modulus of elasticity, E, and wall thickness over radius, h/r, are species independent and, as a consequence, wave speed (Moens-Korteweg equation), is independent of body size as well.

32.2 Physiological and Clinical Relevance

Comparative physiology has shown that the circulation is tightly linked with mammalian metabolism. Metabolism per gram in small animals is much larger than in large animals, as was also shown by experiments on cellular metabolism. This difference in metabolism should be kept in mind when using small animals as model of the human.

Comparative physiology of the cardiovascular system also shows that the heart and arterial system act to produce similar magnitude and wave shape of pressures and similar wave shapes of flow in mammals. This strongly suggests that pressure magnitude and wave shape are important. It has indeed been shown that high pressure, e.g., hypertension, is a strong indicator of cardiovascular pathology. Recent epidemiological data point to the strong relation between Pulse Pressure and cardiovascular morbidity and mortality [18, 19].

The magnitude of Pulse Pressure, together with the about 10^9 pulsations in a lifetime, may play a role in fatigue and fracture of components of the arterial wall. Martyn and Greenwald [20] argue that damage of elastance resulting from pulsations, is too rapid to keep up with repair of elastin. The decrease in elastin may be the reason that with age aortic diameter increases and the wall becomes stiffer, because vessel elasticity becomes gradually more determined by the collagen, which gradually replaces elastin.

The relation between lifespan at birth, Y, and body mass was shown to be $Y = M^{0.24} \approx M^{1/4}$ [21]. Indeed small animals with high Heart Rates live shorter than large animals [22]. It has been suggested that all mammals have the same number of heartbeats over their lifespan, a total of ~10^9. This suggests that lowering HR may prolong lifespan as has been tested in mice but the effect is smaller than expected [23].

Metabolism may also be a life limiting parameter. Small animals have a higher metabolic rate per gram tissue, lowering metabolism in small mammals has been shown to prolong lifespan. The relation between body height and heart period T in humans (Fig. 32.2) suggests that taller people might live longer, but this appears not to be the case [24]. However, taller subjects have reduced evidence of coronary artery disease [25].

References

1. Schmidt-Nielsen K. Scaling. Why is animal size so important? vol. 57. London/New York: Cambridge Univ Press; 1984.
2. Kleiber M. Body size and metabolic rate. Physiol Rev. 1947;27:511–41.
3. Dubois D, Dubois EF. A formula to estimate the approximate surface area if height and weight be known. Arch Int Med. 1961;17:867–71.
4. Takai S, Shimaguchi S. Are height and weight sufficient for the estimation of human body surface area? Hum Biol. 1986;58:625–38.
5. White CR, Seymour RS. The role of gravity in the evolution of mammalian blood pressure. Evolution. 2014;68:901–8.
6. White CR, Seymour RS. Mammalian basal metabolic rate is proportional to body mass2/3. Proc Natl Acad Sci U S A. 2003;100:4046–9.
7. Holt JP, Rhode EA, Kines H. Ventricular volumes and body weight in mammals. Am J Phys. 1968;215:704–14.
8. Altman PL, Dittmer DE (eds). Biological handbook. Bethesda, Fed Am Soc Exptl Biol. pp. 278, 320, 336–341; 1971.
9. Westerhof N, Elzinga G. Normalized input impedance and arterial decay time over heart period are independent of animal size. Am J Phys. 1991;261:R126–33.
10. Smulyan H, Marchais SJ, Pannier B, Guerin AP, Safar ME, London GM. Influence of body height on pulsatile hemodynamic data. J Am Coll Cardiol. 1998;31:1103–9.
11. Savage VM, Deeds EJ, Fontana W. Sizing up allometric scaling theory. PLoS Comput Biol. 2008;4(9):e1000171.
12. Kumar NT, Liestøl K, Løberg EM, Reims HM, Mæhlen J. Postmortem heart weight: relation to body size and effects of cardiovascular disease and cancer. Cardiovasc Pathol. 2014;23:5–11.
13. Elzinga G, Westerhof N. Matching between ventricle and arterial load. Circ Res. 1991;68:1495–500.
14. Senzaki H, Chen C-H, Kass DA. Single beat estimation of end-systolic pressure-volume relation in humans: a new method with the potential for noninvasive application. Circulation. 1996;94:2497–506.
15. West GB, Woodruff WH, Brown JH. Allometric scaling of metabolic rate from molecules and mitochondria to cells and mammals. PNAS. 2002;99:2473–8.
16. Barth E, Stämler G, Speiser B, Schaper J. Ultrastructural quantification of mitochondria and myofilaments in cardiac muscle from 10 different animal species including man. J Mol Cell Cardiol. 1992;24:669–81.
17. Dobson GP. On being the right size: heart design, mitochondrial efficiency and lifespan potential. Clin Exp Pharmacol Physiol. 2003;30:590–7.
18. Benetos A, Safar M, Rudnichi A, Smulyan H, Richard JL, Ducimetieere P, et al. Pulse pressure: a predictor of long-term cardiovascular mortality in a French male population. Hypertension. 1997;30:1410–5.
19. Mitchell GF, Moye LA, Braunwald E, Rouleau JL, Bernstein V, Geltman EM, et al. Sphygmomanometrically determined pulse pressure is a powerful independent predictor of recurrent events after myocardial infarction in patients with impaired left ventricular function. Circulation. 1997;96:4254–60.
20. Martyn CN, Greenwald SE. Impaired synthesis of elastin in walls of aorta and large conduit arteries during early development as an initiating event in pathogenesis of systemic hypertension. Lancet. 1997;3502:953–5.
21. Millar JS, Zammuto RM. Life histories of mammals: an analysis of life tables. Ecology. 1983;64:631–5.
22. Levine HJ. Rest heart rate and life expectancy. J Am Coll Cardiol. 1997;30:1104–6.

23. Gent S, Kleinbongard P, Dammann P, Neuhäuser M, Heusch G. Heart rate reduction and longevity in mice. Basic Res Cardiol. 2015;110:1–9.
24. Samaras TT, Elrick H, Storms LH. Is height related to longevity? Life Sci. 2003;72:1781–802. Review.
25. Reeve JC, Abhayaratna WP, Davies JE, Sharman JE. Central hemodynamics could explain the inverse association between height and cardiovascular mortality. Am J Hypertens. 2014;27:392–400.

Appendix 1. Times and Sines: Fourier Analysis

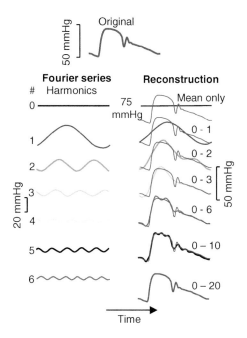

Fourier analysis is used to relate hemodynamic variables. When time signals, such as pressure and flow are related directly, i.e., in the 'time domain', the results are not meaningful (Chap. 6). One way to analyze a system is by relating sinusoidal signals (e.g., pressure and flow, or pressure and pressure). Fourier analysis allows for representation of hemodynamic variables as harmonics: their mean value (numbered zero) and a series of sine waves, numbered 1,2,3, etc.. The frequencies of the harmonics are multiples of Heart Rate. When Heart Rate is 72 bpm, or 1.2 Hz, the frequencies of the harmonics are 0 (mean), 1.2, 2.4, 3.6 Hz etc. Each harmonic, has an amplitude and a phase angle except the mean value which has an amplitude only.

© Springer International Publishing AG, part of Springer Nature 2019   283
N. Westerhof et al., *Snapshots of Hemodynamics*,
https://doi.org/10.1007/978-3-319-91932-4

Variables, e.g., pressure and flow, can now be related through their harmonics (of the same frequency) by dividing their amplitudes, and subtraction of their phase angles; zero harmonics have no phase angle and only the amplitude ratio is calculated, and for the pressure - flow relation resistance is obtained. For all harmonics the calculation is the same as applying Ohm's law, i.e., division of pressure and flow. Fourier analysis can only be performed when the signal is in the steady state of oscillation and thus the end-point and starting-point have the same value. Other limitations are not pertinent in biological signals (Dirichlet conditions). Relation of two signals is only meaningful when the signals are related through a linear system, i.e., a sine wave of one signal (pressure) produces a sine wave of the other signal (flow). Adapted from Ref. [1].

Description

Fourier analysis breaks a periodic signal up in a mean value and series of sine waves, called harmonics. Any repetitive physiological signal, such as pressure or flow in the steady state can be written as a Fourier series:

$$f(t) = \frac{a_0}{2} + \sum_{n=1}^{N}\left[a_n \cos \frac{2\pi}{T}t + b_n \sin \frac{2\pi}{T}t \right], \text{n harmonic number, and } N \geq 0$$

The Fourier coefficients a_n and b_n, can be straightforwardly calculated and are not obtained by curve fitting:

$$a_n = \frac{1}{T}\int_0^T f(t)\cos\left(n\frac{2\pi t}{T}\right)dt, \text{with n} \geq 0$$

$$b_n = \frac{1}{T}\int_0^T f(t)\sin\left(n\frac{2\pi t}{T}\right)dt, \text{with n} > 1$$

A practical way to write the Fourier series is in terms of modulus, M, and phase, φ.

$$M_n^2 = a_n^2 + b_n^2, \text{and} \tan \varphi_n = b_n / a_n.$$

Thus if, for example, the Fourier series of pressure and flow are expressed this way, the impedance modulus (Chap. 24) is obtained by division of the modulus of pressure and flow ($M_{n,p}/M_{n,q}$, harmonics with the same n), and the impedance phase angle is obtained by subtraction of the phase angles of pressure and flow harmonics ($\varphi_{n,p} - \varphi_{n,q}$) [1]. Similarly the transfer function can be obtained from two pressure signals at different locations (Chap. 27).

The software to perform Fourier analysis is now readily available and therefore Fourier analysis is easy to perform.

In the left part of the Figure in the Box the individual harmonics are given each having an amplitude and phase angle. The phase angle is best seen from the starting point of the sine wave. We see that for the higher harmonics the amplitudes are decreasing in amplitude. On the right hand side of the Figure in the Box, the reconstruction of pressure is presented, which is simply the addition of the sine waves at the same moments in time. Using 10 harmonics the signal is almost completely reconstructed, and with 20 harmonics the signal is completely described. This means that aortic pressure is described by approximately 15–20 harmonics. It turns out that the smoother the signal the fewer harmonics are required to describe it. Ventricular pressure can be described by about 10 harmonics. Thus, in general, the information in hemodynamic signals such as pressure, flow and diameter contains information up to 15 harmonics, i.e., 15 times the Heart Rate.

This knowledge is important with respect to measurement techniques. To describe a sine wave at least two time points are required (the Nyquist criterion [2]). Thus sampling should be done with at least twice the highest frequency, i.e. the highest harmonic, in the signal. In hemodynamics this means that the sampling rate should be at least twice as high as the frequency of the highest harmonic, thus ~2 × 15 = 30 times the Heart Rate. If dealing with human hemodynamics, with a Heart Rate of 60 bpm, the rate is 1 cycle per second (1 Hz) and sampling should be done with a rate higher than 30 samples per second. If we measure in the rat with a rate of 420 bpm, or 7 Hz, sampling rate should be at least 210 samples per second.

Along the same lines one can reason that equipment used in hemodynamics should be sufficiently fast so that 15 times the Heart Rate can be accurately measured. For instance, in the human at rest a pressure-manometer system should at least be accurate up to about 15 Hz, and when used during exercise with a Heart Rate of 180 bpm (3 Hz) at least up to 45 Hz.

In practice we use a large safety factor of about 3 or 4, and therefore a sampling rate of 100 Hz is generally be accepted as standard sample rate for the human at rest. In exercise the sampling rate should be increased by the same factor as the increase in Heart Rate.

Limitations

The following limitations apply to the use of Fourier analysis.

1. Fourier analysis may only be performed on periodic signals. In practice this means that the signal value at the start and end of the period to be analyzed should be the same. In other words only single heart beats or multiples of full beats, e.g., a respiratory cycle, where start values and end values of the signals are equal may be analyzed.

2. Fourier analysis can always be performed on signals in the steady state of oscillation. However, the calculation of *the relation* between two signals only leads to useful results when the system is linear, which means that sine wave input leads

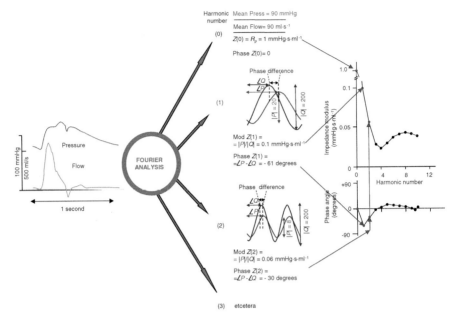

Fig. A1.1 Use of Fourier analysis in relating two time signals, here aortic pressure and flow. The analysis is used to calculate input impedance. For each harmonic the ratio of the moduli (amplitudes) and the difference their phase angles describes the pressure-flow relation for that harmonic. The mean terms, zero harmonic, have amplitudes only. Harmonics are multiples of Heart Rate

to sine wave output. The relations between pressure and diameter and pressure and flow etc., are in many situations not strictly linear, but the nonlinearity is limited and large errors do not result. However, the scatter in modulus and phase of the input impedance (Chap. 24) has been suggested to result at least to some extend from nonlinearity of the arterial system [3].

3. The system should also be time invariant. This means that over the period of sampling the system properties remain constant. The coronary arterial system is subject to cardiac contraction and varies over the heartbeat. Calculation of impedance is not giving useful information.

4. The amplitudes of the higher harmonics decrease in amplitude and are therefore more subject to noise than the lower harmonics. This, in part explains the scatter in the input impedance (Chap. 24).

5. Differentiation emphasizes the higher harmonics. Differentiation of $a_n \cdot \sin(n2\pi t/T)$ is equal to $a_n n2\pi/T \cdot \cos(n2\pi t/T)$, and the amplitude increase is a factor $n2\pi/T$. With $T = 0.8$ s this factor is ~7.5n; the first harmonic is multiplied by 7.5, the second by 15 etc. Thus differentiation leads to amplification of noise.

6. Fourier analysis gives data at multiples of the Heart Rate only. Thus the frequency resolution is limited. Pacing of the heart at different rates, including high Heart Rates, improves the frequency resolution and also produces more accurate high frequency information [4].

It is also advisable to analyze a number of beats (~10) in the steady state to reduce noise [5]. This can be done by analysis per beat, and averaging the derived harmonics of these beats. It is, in principle, equally accurate to analyze a series of beats. When the Heart Rate is 75 bpm, i.e., 1.25 Hz, and a series of 10 beats is analyzed, harmonics are obtained at multiples of 0.125 Hz. However, only the 10th, 20th, 30th, etc. harmonics, thus 1.25 Hz, 2.50 Hz, etc., then contain accurate information.

Physiological and Clinical Relevance

Fourier analysis teaches us that hemodynamic signals contain at most 10–20 harmonics. Higher harmonics disappear in the noise. Thus equipment should be able to measure frequencies up to 15–20 times the Heart Rate accurately. In the human pressure and flow measurement techniques to be used should thus have a flat frequency response up to 15 times the Heart Rate Hz. In the mouse, with a Heart Rate of 600 bpm the frequency response should be accurate up to at least 150 Hz. In practice a higher sample rate is advised as general accepted.

Fourier analysis and the subsequent calculation of the amplitude ratio and phase angle difference per harmonic of two hemodynamic signals may only be applied to linear and time invariant systems. An example is input impedance (Chap. 24). An important other example is the calculation of the pressure transfer function (Chap. 27).

Nonlinearity of the system e.g., cardiac valves, or a stenosis etc., cannot be studied based on Fourier analysis. For instance, systemic vascular resistance and impedance can be calculated from aortic pressure minus venous pressure and aortic flow but not from ventricular pressure minus venous pressure and flow.

The system under study is not allowed to change during the analysis period. The coronary arterial tree is affected by cardiac contraction and therefore time varying and cannot be studied with Fourier analysis.

The oscillatory flow theory is also based on sinusoidal relations between pressure drop over and flow through a segment of artery (Chap. 8).

Appendix 2. Basic Hemodynamic Elements

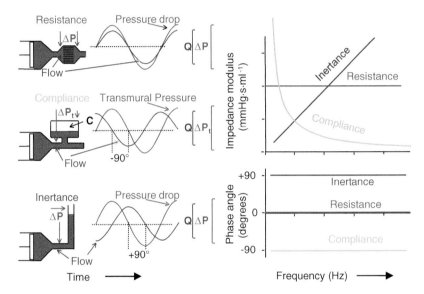

Left: The three basic hemodynamic elements are resistance, compliance and iner-tance. For steady flow only resistance has a meaning. Oscillatory flow theory demands the use of sine waves. Here the relations between sinusoidal pressure dif-ference (pressure drop, ΔP, or transmural pressure, ΔP_t), and flow are given for the three elements. The ratio of the amplitudes of pressure difference and flow gives the modulus of the impedance; the phase difference between them gives the phase angle. Right: For the resistance element pressure drop and flow are in phase, and the impedance is not frequency dependent. For the compliance the flow precedes the pressure difference by 90° for all frequencies and for an inertance flow lags by 90°. The amplitude ratio decreases for the compliance and increases for the inertance. These basic elements can, in combination, describe all oscillatory pressure-flow, and pressure-pressure relations of linear hemodynamic systems. The inertia and compliance are not defined at zero frequency. Adapted from Ref. [6].

© Springer International Publishing AG, part of Springer Nature 2019
N. Westerhof et al., *Snapshots of Hemodynamics*,
https://doi.org/10.1007/978-3-319-91932-4

Description

The impedance of the three basic hemodynamic elements (left) is shown in the right hand side of the Figure in the Box. For the resistance, the pressure drop and flow are in phase and their amplitude ratio gives the value of the resistance. For the compliance, the sine wave of flow precedes the pressure drop, and they are $-90°$ out of phase, i.e., a quarter of the whole sine wave for all frequencies. The modulus of the impedance, $|Z(\omega)|$ equals $1/\omega\,C$, with C compliance and ω the circular frequency, $\omega = 2\pi \cdot f$, with f the frequency in Hz (cycles per second). Increasing frequency implies decreasing impedance modulus. For the inertance the impedance modulus equals $|Z(\omega)| = \omega L = 2\pi \cdot f \cdot L$, the impedance increases with frequency, and the phase angle is $+90°$ for all frequencies.

Physiological and Clinical Relevance

All linear and time invariant hemodynamic systems, for instance the entire systemic arterial tree, the pulmonary vascular system (Chaps. 24 and 28), a pressure transfer function (Chap. 27), or the arterial transmural pressure-volume relation can be quantitatively described by (a combination) of these three basic elements. Linear means that when the input (e.g., pressure) is a sine wave, the output (e.g., flow) should also be a sine wave. Time invariant means that over the period of analysis the system does not change.

Limitations

The arterial system is not linear. For instance, the transmural pressure-volume relation of the arteries is not straight. Other aspects such as inlet length, curvature of vessels etc., result in nonlinear pressure-flow behavior. Nevertheless, in most practical applications the nonlinearity around a working point, 'piece-wise linearity', is sufficient and the results obtained correct. The 'piece-wise' linearity is sufficient: for a pressure range of 120/80 mmHg the system can be considered linear. Over a range 140–180 linearity may be assumed as well, but gives different system properties (Chap. 21). Over a large range of 160/80 mmHg linearity may not hold anymore. Thus, systemic vascular resistance and aortic input impedance can be calculated and this information is meaningful. However, the calculation of resistance from mean ventricular pressure and aortic flow rather than aortic pressure and flow does not contain useful information because of the strong nonlinearity of the aortic valves. Piece wise linearity accounts for changes in parameter between different working points. An example is the decrease in arterial compliance at higher mean blood pressure.

Appendix 3. Vessel Segment

Hydraulic representation **Electrical representation**

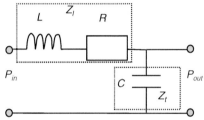

A segment of blood vessel is an important building block of arterial models. In principle, distributed models, single or two-tube models, and lumped models are based on these building blocks. The basic elements constituting the building block are inertance, $L = \rho l / \pi r_i^2$, resistance, $R = 8\eta l / \pi r_i^4$, and compliance, $C \approx 3\pi r_i^3 l / 2Eh$. When we express these parameters per unit length a prime is added, L', R', and $C' = C_A$, with C_A area compliance. The inertance and resistance describe the relation between pressure drop (ΔP) and flow (Q), and in combination are called the longitudinal impedance, $Z_l = i\omega L + R$. When one wants to account for oscillatory flow theory a combination of resistances and inertances are to be used, see Fig. A3.1. For large arteries resistance may be omitted, for very small arteries and arterioles only resistance remains. The compliance accounts for the change in diameter with transmural pressure (P_t). The diameter change implies storage of blood and relates to the difference of volumes into and out of the segment. The relation between the flow difference and transmural pressure is called transverse impedance, $Z_t = 1/i\omega C$. When accounting for viscoelastic wall properties a combination of resistances and compliances is required to describe C, see Fig. A3.2.

Description

The relation between the pressure drop and flow of a uniform segment of blood vessel is shown in the Figure in the Box. The relation consists of a longitudinal impedance, which is described by Womersley's oscillatory flow theory [7, 8]. The transverse impedance [9] describes the pressure-area (or volume) relation of the segment. The combination of longitudinal and transverse impedances gives characteristic impedance and wave propagation (Chap. 12).

The Longitudinal Impedance

The longitudinal impedance Z_l, is given in Fig. A3.1 and is described by Womersley's oscillatory flow theory (see Chap. 8) [7]. For small arteries, i.e., for small values of Womersley's α, the longitudinal impedance per length, Z_l', is described by Poiseuille's equation and $Z_l' \approx R' = 8\eta/\pi r_i^4$. For large values of α, i.e. for large arteries, the Z_l' reduces to an inertance only and equals $Z_l' \approx i\omega L' = i\omega(4/3)\rho/\pi r_i^2$ [8]. The Z_l' is often approximated by $i\omega\rho/\pi \cdot r_i^2$ when only L_1' is taken into account (Fig. A3.1).

The Transverse Impedance

The transmural pressure difference, i.e., the oscillatory pressure between lumen and external environment, is related to volume changes (see Chap. 11). Volume changes can be related to flow, and therefore we can use the term transverse impedance. The transverse impedance for a viscoelastic wall material is shown in Fig. A3.2 [9]. For large conduit arteries, where the wall is almost purely elastic, this can be simplified

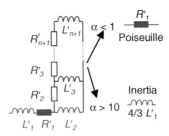

Fig. A3.1 The longitudinal impedance of a segment of artery is based on oscillatory flow theory with $Q(t) = \mathrm{Real}\left[\left(\pi r_i^2 \Delta P / i\omega\rho l\right) \times \left\{1 - 2\mathrm{J}_1\left(\alpha \cdot i^{3/2}\right) / \left(\alpha \cdot i^{3/2} \mathrm{J}_0\left(\alpha \cdot i^{3/2}\right)\right)\right\} e^{i\omega t}\right]$. In electrical terms this translates to a ladder network. For small arteries or low frequencies, low α, as in the periphery, resistance contributes only. For large arteries or high frequencies, large α, the inertia terms are only of importance and $Z_l' = (4\rho/3)/\pi r_i^2$. The $R''_n = 8\eta n/\pi r_i^4$ and $L'_n = \rho/(2n-1)\pi r_i^2$. (Adapted from Ref. [8], by permission)

Viscoelastic Purely Elastic

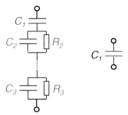

Fig. A3.2 The transverse impedance of a vessel segment with a viscoelastic wall can be described by $Zt'(\omega) = E_{inc} \cdot h \cdot (2r_i + h) / \left[i\omega \cdot 3\pi \cdot r_i^2 (r_i + h)^2 \right]$ with $E_{inc}(\omega) = \Sigma c_n(i\omega)^n / \Sigma d_n(i\omega)^n$, as shown by the electrical network below. Dashpot-spring representations are shown in Chap. 10. The ladder network (blue) results from the viscoelasticity. (From Ref. [9], by permission)

to a single compliance, C, and compliance per unit length is $C' = C_A = \Delta A / \Delta P$, with C_A area compliance (Chap. 11). The expression for compliance is:

$$C' = C / l = C_A = 3\pi \cdot r_i^2 (r_i + h)^2 / E \cdot h \cdot (2r_i + h),$$
$$\text{or when } h \ll r_i, \text{the } C' = C_A \approx 3\pi \cdot r_i^3 \cdot l / 2E \cdot h.$$

The transverse impedance per length is then $Z_t' = 1/i\omega \cdot C_A = 2E \cdot h/i\omega \cdot 3\pi \cdot r_i^3$

Large and Small Arteries

From the above formulas we see that inertance is proportional to r_i^{-2}, and resistance to r_i^{-4}. This implies that resistance increases most strongly towards the periphery and this is why it is the overriding element there. The area compliance is proportional to r_i^{-3}, and decreases towards the periphery, meaning that peripheral vessels contribute little to overall compliance. In other words compliance is mainly located in aorta and the conduit arteries. We should remember that all three basic hemodynamic elements are determined not only by the material properties but also by the geometry.

Physiological and Clinical Relevance

From the above we see that with smaller radius, as found towards the periphery, the importance of resistance becomes greater than inertance and compliance and in the very small arterioles only the resistance remains. Peripheral vessels smaller than 200 μm are often called 'Resistance Vessels'. In large conduit blood vessels, as the human aorta, the resistance term becomes negligible and inertance and compliance accurately describe the segment.

All models based on tubes. i.e., single tube, two-tube and distributed models, use the vessel segment as building block, and these building blocks are based on the description of longitudinal and transverse impedance.

Appendix 4. Basic Aspects

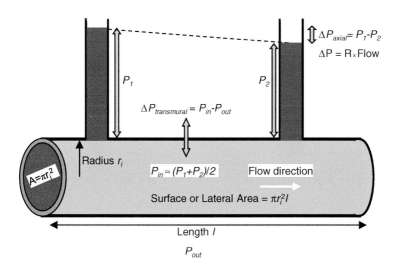

The pressure difference, $P_1 - P_2$, along the axis, inside the blood vessel, causes the flow. The axial pressure drop in large arteries is small. The pressure inside, which is about $P_{in} = (P1 + P2)/2$ *minus the pressure outside*, P_{out} is the transmural pressure. Changes in transmural pressure cause changes in diameter. Two areas are of importance: The cross-sectional area, $A = \pi r_i^2$, is where pressure acts to push blood forward (red), and the lateral area, which equals $A = 2\pi r l$, pertains to exchange with the environment (ochre).

© Springer International Publishing AG, part of Springer Nature 2019
N. Westerhof et al., *Snapshots of Hemodynamics*,
https://doi.org/10.1007/978-3-319-91932-4

Description

Pressure and Flow

Pressure is the force applied per unit area. In hemodynamics we always think of pressure in terms of a pressure difference. The pressure difference (drop) along the axis of a blood vessel, or pressure gradient, is the pressure that causes the flow of blood. The pressure difference between the inside and outside of a vessel or the heart, which is called transmural pressure, causes the wall distension and fluid transport over the wall (Starling equilibrium).

Flow (Q) is given in ml/s or in liters/minute (Cardiac Output), and variably called *flow*, *volume flow* or *flow rate*. The *velocity*, or *flow-velocity* of blood, v, is given in cm/s. The volume flow, and the flow velocity averaged over the cross-sectional area of a vessel are related through the cross-sectional area, A, equals $\int v(r) \cdot 2\pi r \, dr$, and can be approximated by $v \cdot A = Q$ (Chap. 2).

Pressure and flow result from the properties of the heart as a pump and the arterial system. However, the so generated pressure and flow, can be used to obtain the properties of the arterial system and the heart. For instance, aortic minus venous pressure divided by aortic flow gives total peripheral resistance. Stroke Volume over Pulse Pressure provides an estimate of total arterial compliance.

Pulsatile and Oscillatory Pressure and Flow

Pressure and flow vary during the cardiac cycle and are therefore called pulsatile pressure and flow. When pressure and flow are subjected to Fourier analysis and written as a series of sine waves (Appendix 1) we call them oscillatory pressure and flow. The zero term equals the mean value and the harmonics are the oscillatory terms. Womersley's oscillatory flow theory pertains to sinusoidal pressure-flow relations.

Areas

In the Figure in the Box the two areas of a blood vessel are shown. The area $A = \pi \cdot r_i^2$, the so-called cross-sectional area, is the area where the pressure acts to cause flow. The law of Poiseuille connects the pressure gradient to flow via this area to the second power, namely to r_i^4. The cross-sectional area of the human aorta is about 6 cm^2 and of an arteriole is about 30µm^2. The total cross-sectional area of all capillaries together is about 5000 cm^2 or 0.5 m^2.

The lateral area or exchange area is the area involved in the exchange of oxygen, substrates and metabolites between tissue and blood. This area is calculated as: $2\pi r \cdot l$, with l length. The total exchange area of all capillaries together is about 6000 m^2. The Starling equilibrium describes the water transport over the capillary

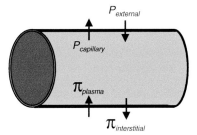

Fig. A4.1 The Starling equilibrium. The osmotic pressures of blood plasma and interstitial fluid, π, together with capillary blood pressure and interstitial pressure, i.e., transmural pressure, determine the transport of water over the capillary wall

wall Fig. A4.1). The P_{extern} (external or interstitial pressure) and the (blood) plasma colloid osmotic pressure move water inwards, while the capillary blood pressure and the interstitial fluid osmotic pressure move water outwardly. High capillary pressure, as in standing may cause edema in the legs.

Wave Speed Differs from Flow Velocity

Blood flow velocity is the speed with which the molecules and cells in the blood move from heart to periphery on the arterial side and back ('venous return') on the venous side. The, mean, velocity of blood in the aorta is about 15 cm/s, maximum velocity of blood in systole in the aorta is about 100 cm/s, and in the capillaries the average velocity is about 0.5 mm/s.

Wave speed or pulse wave velocity is the velocity with which the pressure wave, the diameter variation and the flow wave travel. The wave speed pertains to pulsatile phenomena, and depends on vessel size and vessel elasticity (Chap. 12). The values of wave speed are between 4 and 15 m/s, thus much higher than the blood flow velocity.

Wave speed and flow velocity are, in the context of this book, not related. Even without net blood flow-velocity, waves may be present.

The phase velocity (Moens-Korteweg; Frank; Newton-Young) is the wave speed in a reflection-less artery. When reflections are present the wave speed is called apparent phase velocity. The relation can be seen in Fig. 21.1

Volume, Flow, and Circulation Time

Volumes of compartments, flow and circulation time can be determined using an identifiable, nontoxic indicator that does not leave the compartment under study. Examples of indicators are dyes, radioactive tracers, or cold saline (thermodilution technique). For the last indicator a correction for disappearance from the circulation is made.

Blood volume can be determined by an intravenous injection of an amount, m_d, of a dye. The measurement of the concentration of the marker, $[C]$, in a blood sample, after complete mixing, allows for the calculation of the blood volume, V. When the concentration in the blood is $[C] = m_d/V$ it follows that $V = m_d/[C]$. The injection may be performed in any blood vessel and the sample may be taken from any vessel as well.

Blood flow can be determined from a rapid injection of an indicator, amount m_d, and measurement of the concentration-time curve of the indicator in the blood. This is called the indicator dilution technique to determine mean flow. The flow is calculated as m_d divided by the area under the time-concentration curve. In the indicator dilution technique, flow is determined at the location of injection, while the location of detection of the concentration-time curve is free. For instance, injection of a dye in the left atrium, guarantees good mixing, and allows for the estimation of Cardiac Output. The measurement of the concentration-time curve may take place in any artery and is thus rather free to choose.

In the indicator dilution technique cold saline is often used, and the method is then called the thermodilution technique. The most frequently used method is by flow guided catheter, injection of cold saline in the right atrium or right ventricle and measurement of the temperature in the pulmonary artery. The commercially available apparatuses correct for the heat loss.

Circulation time is obtained by rapidly injecting an indicator at one location, x_1, and measurement of the arrival time at another location, x_2. Circulation time alone is of limited use but in combination with flow it allows estimation of the vascular volume between the two points. The volume of vascular bed between x_1 and x_2 equals the circulation time between x_1 and x_2 times volume flow. The circulation time of the entire circulation is about 1 min.

The Navier-Stokes Equations

The Navier-Stokes equations form the basis of all fluid dynamics, including hemodynamics, and can be found in textbooks on fluid mechanics (Appendix 6). They are the equations of motion of the fluid due to the forces acting on it such as pressure and gravity, and the equations include the effect of fluid density and viscosity. It is a group of three sub-equations, each for one of the three spatial dimensions.

An exact mathematical solution of these general equations is not possible because of their nonlinear character, so that large computers are required to solve them for each situation. The software to solve the equations is available. One of the terms representing this method is Computational Flow Dynamics.

Under simplifying assumptions the Navier-Stokes equations can be solved. Poiseuille's law, Oscillatory Flow Theory and Bernoulli's equation, etc., are examples of simplified forms of the Navier-Stokes equations.

Appendix 5. Books for Reference

Aaronson PI, Ward JPT. The cardiovascular system at a glance. Indianapolis: Wiley; 2007.Bevan JA, Halpern W, Mulvany MJ. The resistance vasculature. New York/London: Springer Science & Business Media; 2012.

Bevan JA, Kaley G, Rubanyi GM. Flow-dependent regulation of vascuar function. New York/London: Springer; 1995.

Berne RM, Levy MN. Cardiovascular physiology. Edinburgh/London: Mosby; 2005.

Braunwald E, editor. Heart disease. 10th ed. Philadelphia/Sydney: WB Saunders; 2015.

Burton AC. Physiology and biophysics of the circulation. 2nd ed. Chicago: Year Book Medical Publ.; 1972.

Caro CG, Pedley TJ, Schroter RC, Seed WA. The mechanics of the circulation. Oxford/New York: Oxford Univ. Press; 1978.

Chien KR (Ed). Molecular basis of cardiovascular disease. Philadelphia/London: Saunders; 1999.

Cowen SC, Humphrey JD. Cardiovascular soft tissue mechanics. Dordrecht/Boston: Kluwer Acad. Publ.;2002.

Crawford MH, DiMarco JP, Paulus WJ. Cardiology. Edinburgh/London: Mosby; 2004.

Fung, YC. Biomechanics. Mechanical properties of living tissues. New York/Heidelberg: Springer; 1981.

Fung, YC. Biodynamics. Circulation. New York & Heidelberg: Springer; 1984.

Fung, YC. Biomechanics. New York/Heidelberg: Springer; 1990.

Fung, YC, Perrone N, Anliker M. Biomechanics. Englewood Cliffs: Prentice-Hall; 1972.

Glantz SA. Primer of biostatistics. New York: McGraw Hill; 2012.

Guccione JM, Kassab GS, Ratcliffe MB. Cardiovascular mechanics modeling and applications. New York/London: Springer; 2010.

Hall JE. Guyton and Hall textbook of medical physiology. 13th ed. Amsterdam/New York: Elsevier; 2015.

© Springer International Publishing AG, part of Springer Nature 2019
N. Westerhof et al., *Snapshots of Hemodynamics*,
https://doi.org/10.1007/978-3-319-91932-4

Hill AV. Trails and trials in physiology. Baltimore/London: Williams & Wilkins; 1965.

Hoppensteadt FC, Peskin CS. Modeling and simulation in medicine and the life sciences (texts in applied mathematics). 2nd ed. New York/London: Springer; 2002.

Hoskins PR, Lawford PV, Doyle BJ. Cardiovascular biomechanics. New York/London: Springer; 2017.

Humphrey JD. Cardiovascular solid mechanics. New York/London: Springer; 2013.

Hwang NHC, Normann NA. Cardiovascular flow dynamics and measurements. Baltimore: University Park Press; 1977.

Hwang NHC, Gross DR, Patel DJ. Quantitative cardiovascular studies. Baltimore: University Park Press; 1979.

Jaffrin MY, Caro CG. Biological flows. New York: Plenum Press; 1995.

Li J K-J. Dynamics of the vascular system. Singapore: World Scientific Publishing Co; 2004.

Milnor WR. Hemodynamics. 2nd ed. Baltimore/London: Williams & Wilkins; 1989.

Munson BR, Young DF, Okiishi TH. Fundamentals of fluid mechanics. 2nd ed. New York: Wiley; 1994.

Nichols WW, O'Rourke MF, Vlachopoulos C. McDonald's blood flow in arteries. 6th ed. Boca Raton: CRC Press Taylor & Francis; 2011.

Noble MIM. The cardiac cycle. Oxford/London: Blackwell Scientific Publications; 1979.

Noordergraaf A. Hemodynamics. In: Schwan HP, editor. Bio-engineering. New York: McGraw-Hill; 1969.

O'Rourke MF. Arterial function in health and disease. Edinburgh/London: Churchill Livingstone; 1982.

O'Rourke MF, Kelly RP, Avolio AP. The arterial pulse. Philadelphia: Lea & Febiger; 1992.

Ottesen JT, Olufsen MS, Larsen JK. Applied mathematical models in human physiology. Philadelphia: Society Industrial and Applied Mathematics (SIAM); 2004.

Safar ME, O'Rourke MF. Arterial stiffness in hypertension. Amsterdam: Elsevier; 2006.

Sagawa K, Maughan L, Suga H, Sunagawa K. Cardiac contraction and the pressure-volume relationship. New York/Oxford: Oxford University press; 1988.

Schmidt-Nielsen L. Scaling. New York: Cambridge Univ Press; 1984.

Spaan JAE. Coronary blood flow. Dordrecht/Boston: Kluwer Acad Publishers; 1991.

Strackee J, Westerhof N. The physics of heart and circulation. Bristol/Philadelphia: Inst of Physics Publishing; 1992.

Talbot SA, Gessner U. Systems physiology. New York/London: Wiley; 1973.

Weibel ER. Symmorphosis. Cambridge: Harvard Univ Press; 2000.

Westerhof N, Gross DR. Vascular dynamics. New York/London: Plenum Press; 1989.

Yin FCP. Ventricular/vascular coupling. New York.Heidelberg: Springer; 1986.

Appendix 6. Symbols

a	Acceleration
A	Area
A^*	Amplitude
AIx	Augmentation Index
BMr	Basal Metabolic rate
bpm	Heart Rate, HR
c	Pulse Wave Velocity or wave speed
$c_{f\text{-}f}$	Foot-to-foot wave velocity
c_{app}	Apparent wave velocity
C	Compliance $\Delta V/\Delta P$
C_A, C_D	Area, Diameter Compliance
CO	Cardiac Output
d	Derivative
∂	Partial derivative
d, D	Diameter
D	Distensibility
E	Elastance
E_d	End-Diastolic Elastance
E_{es}	End-Systolic Elastance
E_{inc}	Incremental modulus of elasticity
E_m	Murray energy term
E_{max}, E_{min}	Maximal, Minimal Elastance
E_p	Peterson modulus
EF	Ejection Fraction
ESPVR	End-Systolic Pressure-Volume Relation
$E(t)$	Time Varying Elastance
f	Frequency
F	Force
FFR	Fractional Flow Reserve

© Springer International Publishing AG, part of Springer Nature 2019
N. Westerhof et al., *Snapshots of Hemodynamics*,
https://doi.org/10.1007/978-3-319-91932-4

FMD	Flow Mediated Dilation
g	Gravity
g_f	Geometry factor
G	Gain – Conductance
h	(Wall) thickness
Hct	Hematocrit
i	$\sqrt{-1}$
iFR	Instantaneous Wavefree Ratio
J_o, J_1	Bessel functions, order 0, 1
l	Length
L	Inertia
l_{inlet}	Inlet length
m	Mass
m_d	Amount of substance
M	Body mass
P	Pressure
P_{es}	End-Systolic Pressure
P_f, P_r	Forward, Reflected Pressure wave
P_m	Measured Pressure wave
P_s, P_d	Systolic, Diastolic Blood Pressure
P_v	Venous filling Pressure
P_{mean}	Mean Blood Pressure
P_{O2}	Partial oxygen Pressure
PP	Pulse Pressure
PVA	Pressure Volume Area
Q	(Volume) Flow
Q_f, Q_r	Forward, Reflected Flow wave
r, r_i, r_o	radius, inernal, external radius
R	Resistance
R_c	Characteristic Resistance
R_p	Peripheral Resistance
Re	Reynolds number
RPP	Rate Pressure Product
SV	Stroke Volume
St	Strouhal number
t	Time
T	Transfer function
T	Heart Period
TTI	Tension Time Index
T_{su}	Surface tension
v	Velocity
V	Volume
V_d	Intercept Volume
V_{ed}, V_{es}	End-Diastolic, End-systolic Volume
V_{O2}	Oxygen Consumption

W	Work, Energy
WSS	Wall Shear Stress
x, z	Location, height
Z	(Input) Impedance
Z_c	Characteristic Impedance
ZSS	Zero Stress State
α	Womersley's parameter
β	Stiffness parameter (β − stiffness)
ε	Strain $\Delta l/l$
ε_t	Transverse strain
ϕ	Phase angle
γ	Shear rate
η	(Absolute or dynamic) viscosity
λ	Wave length
π	3.1415…
ρ	(Blood or muscle) density
σ	Stress and hoop stress
τ	Shear stress (Pa) and decay time (s)
ω	Circular frequency
Δ	Difference, 'gradient'
Γ	Reflection coefficient
K	Distensibility
θ	Angle (degrees)

Appendix 7. Units and Conversion Factors

	SI-system (kg m s)	cgs-system (g cm s)	Medical units (mmHg ml s)
Area compliance, C_A	$1\ m^2\cdot Pa^{-1} = 1\ m^4\cdot N^{-1}$	$10^3\ cm^4\cdot dyn^{-1}$	$1.33\cdot 10^6\ cm^2\cdot mmHg^{-1}$
Compliance, C	$1\ m^3\cdot Pa^{-1} = 1\ m^5\cdot N^{-1}$	$10^5\ cm^5\cdot dyn^{-1}$	$1.33\cdot 10^8\ ml\cdot mmHg^{-1}$
Bulk Modulus	$1\ Pa = 1\ N\cdot m^{-2}$	$10\ dyn\cdot cm^{-2}$	$7.5\ 10^{-3}\ mmHg$
Diameter compliance, C_D	$1\ m\cdot Pa^{-1} = 1\ m^3\cdot N^{-1}$	$10\ cm^3\cdot dyn^{-1}$	$1.33\cdot 10^4\ cm\cdot mmHg^{-1}$
Distensibility	$1\ Pa^{-1} = 1\ m^2\cdot N^{-1}$	$0.1\ cm^2\cdot dyn^{-1}$	$133\ mmHg^{-1}$
Density, ρ	$1\ kg\cdot m^{-3}$	$10^{-3}\ g\cdot cm^{-3}$	
Elastance, E	$1\ Pa\cdot m^{-3} = 1\ N\cdot m^{-5}$	$10^{-5}\ dyn\cdot cm^{-5}$	$7.5\cdot 10^{-9}\ mmHg\cdot ml^{-1}$
Energy – Work, W	1 Joule $= 1\ N\cdot m = Pa\cdot m^3$	$10^7\ erg\ (dyn\cdot cm)$	$7.5\cdot 10^3\ mmHg\cdot ml$ [a]
Flow, Q	$1\ m^3\cdot s^{-1}$	$10^6\ cm^3\cdot s^{-1}$ $= 10^6\ ml\cdot s^{-1}$	$1\ liter\cdot min^{-1}$ $= 16.7\ ml\cdot s^{-1}$
dQ/dt	$1\ m^3\cdot s^{-2}$	$10^6\ ml\cdot s^{-2}$	
Force, F	$1\ N = 1\ kg\cdot m\cdot s^{-2}$	$10^5\ dyn = 1\ g\cdot cm\cdot s^{-2}$	
Frequency, f	$Hz = s^{-1}$	$Hz = s^{-1}$	min^{-1} (60 bpm = 1 Hz)
Frequency circular, $\omega = 2\pi f$	Hz	Hz	
Inertance, L	$1\ Pa\cdot s^2\cdot m^{-3} = N\cdot s^2\cdot m^{-5}$	$10^{-5}\ dyn\cdot s^2\cdot cm^{-5}$	$7.5\cdot 10^{-9}\ mmHg\cdot s^2\cdot ml^{-1}$
(Incremental) Youngs Mod.	$1\ Pa = 1\ N\cdot m^{-2}$	$10\ dyn\cdot cm^{-2}$	$7.5\ 10^{-3}\ mmHg$
Phase angle, degrees	$(360° = 2\pi\ radians)$		
Power, W	$1\ Watt = 1\ J\cdot s^{-1}$	$10^7\ erg\cdot s^{-1}$	$7.5\ 10^3\ mmHg\cdot ml\cdot s^{-1}$
Pressure, P & stress, σ	$1\ Pa = 1\ N\cdot m^{-2}$	$10\ dyn\cdot cm^{-2}$	$7.5\ 10^{-3}\ mmHg$
dP/dt	$1\ Pa\cdot s^{-1}$	$10\ dyn\cdot cm^{-2}\cdot s^{-1}$	$7.5\ 10^{-3}\ mmHg\cdot s^{-1}$
Resistance, R	$1\ Pa\cdot s\cdot m^{-3} = N\cdot s\cdot m^{-5}$	$10^{-5}\ dyn\cdot s\cdot cm^{-5}$ $= 10^{-5}\ g\cdot cm^{-4}\cdot s^{-1}$	$7.5\cdot 10^{-9}\ mmHg\cdot s\cdot ml^{-1}$

(continued)

© Springer International Publishing AG, part of Springer Nature 2019
N. Westerhof et al., *Snapshots of Hemodynamics*,
https://doi.org/10.1007/978-3-319-91932-4

(continued)

	SI-system (kg m s)	cgs-system (g cm s)	Medical units (mmHg ml s)
Shear rate, γ	s^{-1}	s^{-1}	s^{-1}
(Shear) stress, τ	$1\ Pa = 1\ N{\cdot}m^{-2}$	$10\ dyn{\cdot}cm^{-2}$	$7.5\ 10^{-3}$ mmHg
Velocity (wave-)	$m{\cdot}s^{-1}$	$10^2\ cm{\cdot}s^{-1}$	$m{\cdot}s^{-1}$
Viscosity, η	$1\ Pa{\cdot}s = 1\ N{\cdot}s{\cdot}m^{-2}$	$10\ dyn{\cdot}s{\cdot}cm^{-2}$ $= 10$ Poise	
Youngs modulus	$1\ Pa = 1\ N{\cdot}m^{-2}$	$10\ dyn{\cdot}cm^{-2}$	$7.5\ 10^{-3}$ mmHg
Decay time $(R{\cdot}C)$	s	s	s
$L{\cdot}C$ [b]	s^2	s^2	s^2
1 ml O_2 [c]	~ 20 J	$20{\cdot}10^7$ erg (dyn·cm)	150 mmHg·ml = 4.8 cal
1 ml O_2/min [c]	~ 0.33 Watt	$0.33{\cdot}10^7$ erg·s^{-1}	2.5 mmHg·ml·s^{-1}

[a]Energy – Work: 1 Joule = 0.24 calories
[b]when L and C are expressed per length: $1/\sqrt{L'C} = $ m/s (velocity)
[c]for fatty acids and glucose metabolism; not for protein metabolism
1 kPa =7.5 mmHg = 10 cm H_2O = mN/mm^2
Contractile efficiency the inverse slope of the relation between Pressure Volume Area and O_2 consumption per beat
Economy of contraction is defined as oxygen consumption used for isovolumic contractions
Efficiency is the ratio of external mechanical power and input power (or oxygen consumption per time)
Strain, Reynolds number, and Womersley's parameter, have no dimension, but one must work in a single system

References

Appendix 1. Times and Sines: Fourier Analysis

1. Westerhof N, Sipkema P, Elzinga G, Murgo JP, Giolma JP. Arterial impedance. In: NHC H, Gross DR, Patel DJ, editors. Quantitative cardiovascular studies. Baltimore: University Park Press; 1979.
2. Hamming RW. Digital filters. Englewood Cliffs: Prentice Hall; 1977.
3. Stergiopulos N, Meister J-J, Westerhof N. Scatter in the input impedance spectrum may result from the elastic nonlinearity of the arterial wall. Am J Physiol. 1995;269:H1490–5.
4. Taylor MG. Use of random excitation and spectral analysis in the study of frequency-dependent parameters of the cardiovascular system. Circ Res. 1966;18:585–95.
5. Murgo JP, Westerhof N, Giolma JP, Altobelli SA. Aortic input impedance in normal man: relationship to pressure wave forms. Circulation. 1980;62:105–16.

Appendix 2. Basic Hemodynamic Elements

6. Westerhof N, Sipkema P, Elzinga G, Murgo JP, Giolma JP. Arterial impedance. *In*: Hwang NHC, Gross DR, Patel DJ. Quantitative cardiovascular studies. 1979, Baltimore; University Park Press.

Appendix 3. Vessel Segment

7. Womersley JR. The mathematical analysis of the arterial circulation in a state of oscillatory motion. Wright Air Dev. Center, Tech Report WADC-TR-56-614; 1957.
8. Jager GN, Westerhof N, Noordergraaf A. Oscillatory flow impedance in electrical analog of arterial system. Circ Res. 1965;16:121–33.
9. Westerhof N, Noordergraaf A. Arterial viscoelasticity. A generalized model. J Biomech. 1970;3:357–79.

Index

© Springer International Publishing AG, part of Springer Nature 2019
N. Westerhof et al., *Snapshots of Hemodynamics*,
https://doi.org/10.1007/978-3-319-91932-4

Printed by Printforce, the Netherlands